M000160118

Biosecurity and Bioterrorism

THE BUTTERWORTH-HEINEMANN HOMELAND SECURITY SERIES

Other Titles in the Series:

Other Related Titles of Interest:

Visit **http://books.elsevier.com/security** for more information on these titles and other resources.

Biosecurity and Bioterrorism

Containing and Preventing Biological Threats

Jeffrey R. Ryan *and* Jan F. Glarum

ELSEVIER

AMSTERDAM • BOSTON • HEIDELBERG • LONDON
NEW YORK • OXFORD • PARIS • SAN DIEGO
SAN FRANCISCO • SINGAPORE • SYDNEY • TOKYO

Butterworth-Heinemann is an imprint of Elsevier

Acquisitions Editor: Pamela Chester
Marketing Manager: Marissa Hederson
Project Manager: Jeff Freeland
Cover Design: Joanne Blank
Compositor: SPi Technologies India Pvt. Ltd.
Cover Printer: Phoenix Color Corp.
Text Printer/Binder: Sheridan Books

Butterworth-Heinemann is an imprint of Elsevier
30 Corporate Drive, Suite 400, Burlington, MA 01803, USA
Linacre House, Jordan Hill, Oxford OX2 8DP, UK

Copyright © 2008, Elsevier Inc. All rights reserved.
Exception: Cover image copyright © iStockphoto.

No part of this publication may be reproduced, stored in a retrieval system, or transmitted in any form or
by any means, electronic, mechanical, photocopying, recording, or otherwise, without the prior written
permission of the publisher.

Permissions may be sought directly from Elsevier's Science & Technology Rights
Department in Oxford, UK: phone: (+44) 1865 843830, fax: (+44) 1865 853333,
E-mail: permissions@elsevier.com. You may also complete your request online
via the Elsevier homepage (http://elsevier.com), by selecting "Support & Contact"
then "Copyright and Permission" and then "Obtaining Permissions."

♾ Recognizing the importance of preserving what has been written, Elsevier prints its books on acid-free paper
whenever possible.

Library of Congress Cataloging-in-Publication Data
Application submitted.

British Library Cataloguing-in-Publication Data
A catalogue record for this book is available from the British Library.

ISBN: 978-0-7506-8489-7

For information on all Butterworth–Heinemann publications
visit our Web site at www.books.elsevier.com

Printed in the United States of America
08 09 10 11 12 9 8 7 6 5 4 3 2 1

Working together to grow
libraries in developing countries

www.elsevier.com | www.bookaid.org | www.sabre.org

ELSEVIER   BOOK AID
            International   Sabre Foundation

Table of Contents

Foreword

The future ain't what it used to be.

Twenty-five years ago, when Yogi Berra uttered his famous oxymoron, few of us could have realized how very prescient those words were. At the time, our major concerns for security were nuclear, and our biggest fears stemmed from state-sponsored full-scale nuclear warfare. Governments as well as private citizens scrambled to create security through construction of fallout shelters, nuclear drills, stockpiling of food, and wholesale investment in the Cold War. Infectious agents were not even on the radar screen, and terrorism was something that happened only in other countries.

Today, our approach to hazards protection is quite different, and we recognize a broad spectrum of threats, not only nuclear, but also chemical, explosive, radiologic, and biologic. We need comprehensive and flexible packages to cover all. This book is designed to address the significant and wide-ranging threats posed by the biological agents—understanding the diverse nature of the biological threats that exist and promoting effective responses appropriate to each incursion.

Regarding biological security, we are faced with twin threats: a devastating event due to biological terrorism and the development of a pandemic due to Mother Nature. Biosecurity and biodefense are critical in preparing us for protection for either an intentional *or* an incidental event.

Terrorism is a form of "asymmetric warfare," designed to undermine economic, social, environmental, or political values. Targets and delivery mechanisms are highly variable, so preventive measures as well as control plans need to be flexible and comprehensive. In the case of biologic terrorism, targets are living organisms: humans, animals, or plants. Bioterror is aimed at humans and, as such, is capable of causing, if not mass morbidity or mortality, then mass hysteria, thereby undermining the whole fabric of society. This could be through dissemination of a disease agent that passes from person to person, or it could be through contamination of the food supply, causing illness through consumption of tainted food. But asymmetric threats may also be directed at agricultural animals or plants, with the purpose being to create economic devastation of the animal or crop industries that would initiate a cascade of negative events through multiple sectors of the economy.

In addition, the steady parade of emerging diseases, such as SARS or bird flu, has shown undeniably that destabilization and economic havoc can be wreaked by an emerging disease as well. These emerging diseases are spawned by globalization and the ever-expanding human population, allowing for possibilities for agents to move from comfortable domains into new unexplored niches. There have been tremendous increases in international trade and trafficking of people, animals, and animal products, all with potential for bringing animal, human, or plant diseases to new locations. The increasingly complex international transportation network can neither be predicted nor paused, creating well-founded concerns about emergence and incursion of diseases and subsequent public health or economic consequences. As articulated in several recent publications, we are creating the microbial equivalent of "a perfect storm." A human pandemic that emerges would be rapidly spread all over the globe. An agricultural epidemic could also have very severe consequences: production of sufficient food to feed the growing human population makes it imperative that we protect agriculture from emerging threats.

The key rule in limiting the damage caused by a biological event—whether it is bioterror, agroterror, or an emerging disease—is this: The amount of economic damage or human illness depends directly on how quickly the disease or contaminated food is detected and contained. If the first instance is recognized and adequate control measures implemented immediately, we will likely circumvent severe economic consequences and human illness. However, if the problem is not initially recognized and is allowed to spread to any extent, we will face dire consequences in our public or agricultural health. Our best defense against this serious damage is to increase awareness to a point where such an emergence or incursion is detected as early as possible and that effective local, state, and federal response capabilities are developed so that deleterious spread can be efficiently intercepted through rapid and appropriate actions.

In summary, these twin forces of terrorism and emerging diseases have made the possibilities of adverse biological events not just possibilities but probabilities. The threats are multifaceted and so preparedness and response plans must be also. There is not a "one size fits all" for biosecurity and biodefense. Generalized knowledge of biosecurity and biodefense are essential, and for each vulnerability that we recognize, there is an additional customized solution that can be applied. The same is true for emergency response plans. There is a general strategy, then for each potential scenario there are advanced solutions to optimal reaction.

This book is very timely and applicable, addressing the range and variety of threats and scenarios. The truth is that we do not know exactly what the future will bring in terms of threats, so we need the comprehensive and flexible understanding that is presented within these pages. In the words of Yogi Berra, once again, "You've got to be careful if you don't know where you're going because you might not get there." This book takes us as close as we can get, in an efficient and straightforward manner, preparing us for the panoply of possibilities.

Dr. Corrie Brown
Professor of Veterinary Medicine
University of Georgia, College of Veterinary Medicine

About the Authors

Dr. Jeff Ryan is a retired Army Lieutenant Colonel with an extensive background in preventive medicine, epidemiology, clinical trials, and diagnostics development. Dr. Ryan also served in the private sector, working for a biotech company, Cepheid, where he was a senior business developer and manager for its biothreat government business program. Dr. Ryan wrote more than 40 scientific, peer-reviewed journal articles and is the lead instructor and codeveloper of the Pandemic Influenza Planning and Preparedness course, taught at the Center for Domestic Preparedness (Department of Homeland Security) in Anniston, Alabama. Currently, Dr. Ryan serves as an Assistant Professor at the Institute for Emergency Preparedness, Jacksonville State University. His specialty areas include biosecurity, biodefense, medical aspects of emergency management, homeland security planning and preparedness, and terrorism studies.

Jan Glarum retired after 27 years in the emergency response field. He has an extensive background in emergency medical services, fire, and police special weapons and tactics operations. He served as the Medical Preparedness Officer for the state of Oregon Health Division and Executive Director of Development for the Portland Metropolitan Medical Response System. Mr. Glarum wrote the *Homeland Security Field Guide* and is codeveloper of the Pandemic Influenza Planning and Preparedness course, taught at the Center for Domestic Preparedness (Department of Homeland Security) in Anniston, Alabama. Currently, he works as a consultant for the Department of Homeland Security and the Department of Defense, both domestically and internationally.

Preface

This book is the result of much research, writing and thoughtful discussion with students, first responders, scholars, and thought leaders in the fields of biosecurity and biodefense. It comes at a time when emergency managers, public health professionals, clinicians, animal health professionals, and government officials are preparing themselves for acts of terrorism and the potential that weapons of mass destruction may be used against our citizens.

At the dawning of the 21st century, we moved very quickly from the Information Age to the Age of Terrorism. Certainly, historians will recall how the dark specter of terrorism raised its ugly head in the fall of 2001 as we witnessed the fall of the Twin Towers at the World Trade Center in New York and a direct attack on the Pentagon in Washington, D.C. Less than a month later, citizens of the United States were faced with the threat of a deadly and rare disease, anthrax, which was spread by a few letters introduced into the U.S. Postal System. Now, looking back, this period seems almost surreal to us. Even though these human-made disasters affected all of us in different ways, many Americans have already forgotten their personal feelings at the time. The global war on terrorism has been raging for several years now. Some would argue that taking the battle to the enemy on another front in a distant land has given us some modicum of protection. That may be true, but to this day we still do not know who perpetrated the anthrax attacks that killed five people and shocked a nation. Nonetheless, we are as vulnerable to the biological threat today as we were seven years ago.

In the wake of the terrorist attacks and anthrax assaults of fall 2001, U.S. policymakers developed the nucleus of a new regulatory framework to address the suddenly evident threat of bioterrorism (Dr. Julie E. Fischer, February 2006).

Accordingly, *Biosecurity and Bioterrorism: Containing and Preventing Biological Threats* introduces readers to global concerns for biosecurity including the history of biological warfare, bioterrorism, concerns for agroterrorism, and current initiatives in biodefense. Included is a thorough review of specific agents, the diseases they cause, detection methods, and consequence management considerations. Readers are introduced to international initiatives and federal legislation that address biosecurity and biodefense.

A comprehensive treatment of the subject is needed to promote understanding of the problem and the complex network of federal, state, and local assets for dealing with the threat. The book is intended to be used as a textbook or reference for security managers in the food industry, public health professionals, and emergency managers.

The primary goal of *Biosecurity and Bioterrorism: Containing and Preventing Biological Threats* is to give readers an understanding of the threat that biological agents pose to society. Accordingly, the book details the myriad threats posed to society by the

Department of Health and Human Services (HHS) Category A, B, and C agents. Readers are presented with a number of case studies that illustrate the impact of certain biological agents on society. Readers will be able to discuss federal programs and initiatives that encompass the government's vision of *Biodefense for the 21st Century*.

Terminal Learning Objectives

At the end of the course, students should be able to

- Discuss the history of bioweapons development and how those programs relate to the current threat of bioterrorism.
- Discuss what biological agents are and how they can cause illness and death.
- Understand that the scale of bioterrorist and natural events makes a tremendous difference in our ability to respond to them.
- Understand what criteria are important in placing the most serious pathogens and toxins into HHS Categories A, B, and C.
- Know the different biological agents in HHS Categories A, B, and C, what diseases they cause, and signs and symptoms of the associated disease. In addition, students will understand the natural history of each of these agents, their use in warfare and bioterrorism, and public health issues.
- Discuss specific case studies that examine bioterrorism and natural disease outbreaks.
- Demonstrate familiarity with sampling and detection methods.
- List the laws and presidential directives that apply to biodefense and biosecurity.
- Discuss many federal initiatives and programs designed to enhance biodefense and biosecurity in the United States.
- Understand the difference between quarantine and isolation and the challenges both present.
- Understand programs that are implemented by public health agencies to enhance preparedness for acts of bioterrorism and where this fits into emergency preparedness programs.

The Pedagogical Features of This Book

- **Objectives** and **Key Terms** at the beginning of all chapters guide the reader on chapter content and the topics to understand.
- **Scenarios** are placed at the beginning of some chapters to offer the reader a dose of reality and to increase interest in the chapter content.
- **Examples, illustrations,** and **figures** help explain concepts and relate theory to practice.
- **Boxed topics** are contained in each chapter to extend the depth of the information and to offer additional perspective on the issues.

- **Critical Thinking boxes** throughout the book help the reader to formulate alternative perspectives on issues and seek creative and improved solutions to problems.
- **Discussion Questions** at the end of each chapter reinforce content and provide an opportunity for the reader to review, synthesize, and debate major concepts and issues.
- **Web sites** at the end of each chapter provide direction for additional resources to enhance learning along topic lines and supplemental resources for student learning.
- An **interdisciplinary research base** was developed from books, journals, newsletters, magazines, associations, government, training programs, and other professional sources.

The book is organized into four thematic sections: Part I provides a conceptual understanding of biowarfare, bioterrorism, and the reasons why biosecurity and bio-defense are so important to modern day society. Part II investigates HHS Category A, B, and C agents; case studies; and recognition of the threat. Part III focuses on agricultural terrorism and food security. Finally, Part IV outlines and details federal and local initiatives for biodefense and biosecurity; included here are considerations for government officials, emergency management practitioners, public health professionals, and first responders. Each thematic section includes a short preface that draws together the key points and learning objectives of the chapters within them.

Acknowledgments

We both thank our families for taking the time to listen to our ideas and for pardoning us for our extended absences, idiosyncrasies, and preoccupation as we worked on researching and writing this book. We also give special thanks to Dr. Pam Ryan for critically reviewing each chapter, while balancing the rigors of a busy companion animal practice and a precocious three-year-old daughter. Finally, we thank the men and women in uniform, both military and civilian. They are the guardians standing on the front lines everywhere, protecting each other's families. Our hope is that they will find this compilation useful as they face the threat of asymmetric warfare.

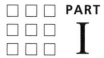
Biosecurity, Biodefense, and the Reason for Them

The first part of this book introduces the reader to the many foundational elements necessary to understand why biosecurity and biodefense have become so important. Both terms are described and differentiated. To get an appreciation for biosecurity and biodefense, one must first understand the importance of the biological threat as an element of terrorism.

To most Americans, these concepts and programs are transparent. The reality is that biosecurity and biodefense programs are very costly and slow to develop. Conversely, the threat of biological weapons is underlined by the unlimited potential for harm that they possess. The use of biological weapons by an aggressor could kill millions, disrupt societies, undermine economies, and alter life as we know it.

While the effects of a bioweapon attack could be horrible, the actual risk that such an attack would happen is, in the opinion of some experts, very low. Other experts believe with equal conviction that the risk is real and complacency will produce awful consequences when the impossible happens.

Much of our concern about bioweapons comes from a belief that some terrorist groups, like al Qaeda, wish to use bioweapons and are attempting to develop a capability. Why terrorists would want to develop bioweapons is a complicated question that defies simple answers. The decision to develop bioweapons likely involves perceptions that such weapons offer some political or military utility. Some would argue that technological barriers to the development and use of bioweapons are sufficiently low for terrorists to use them. Regardless, a key aspect of the perceived risk from bioweapons is that communities are extremely vulnerable to biological attacks. There is a dearth of recent articles in the scientific literature and popular media discussing how unprepared Western societies are for biological terrorism. The abundance of these works might seem to reinforce the utility of bioweapons in the eyes of terrorists, thus exacerbating the problem. Regardless, perceived terrorist motivations, increasing technological feasibility, and stated societal vulnerability have now merged to catalyze fears about bioweapon proliferation and use.

Chapter 1 is an introduction to the history of biowarfare and state-sponsored bioweapons programs. In addition, the reality versus the potential of bioterrorism is discussed and the reasons why biosecurity and biodefense have become so formidable in the United States. Chapter 2 provides a scientific foundation for all readers, no matter their professional discipline or background. As such, the different types of biological agents and some of their common characteristics are detailed. From here, the reader is introduced to terminology related to the clinical presentation of infectious disease and diagnostic processes. The information and understanding gained from these two chapters is essential to fully understanding the threat that will be explored in subsequent sections.

Seeds of Destruction

Destroy the seed of evil, or it will grow up to your ruin.
—Aesop

Objectives

The study of this chapter will enable you to

1. Understand the importance of the biological threat in its context of terrorism and weapons of mass destruction.
2. Discuss the terms *biosecurity* and *biodefense* and relate them to homeland security and defense, respectively.
3. Discuss the reality versus the potential of bioterrorism.
4. Discuss the history of biowarfare and the major events that are important in helping us understand the issues related to using biological substances against an adversary.
5. Understand why many of these threats have been used on a small scale and that going beyond that requires a high degree of technical sophistication and extensive resources.

Key Terms

biosecurity, biodefense, biowarfare, bioterror, bioterrorism, biothreat, pathogen, weaponization, zoonotic disease.

Introduction

The dawning of the 21st century will be characterized as the Age of Terrorism. Terrorism has affected most of us in one way or another. The shocking images of the September 11, 2001, attacks remind us of just how dramatic and devastating terrorism can be. In most developed countries, the concept of bioterrorism and many of the words associated with it are widely recognized. In the United States, *bioterrorism* became a household word in October 2001, when *Bacillus anthracis* (the causative agent of anthrax) spores were introduced into the U.S. Postal Service system by several letters dropped into a mailbox in Trenton, New Jersey (see Figure 1-1). These letters resulted in five deaths from

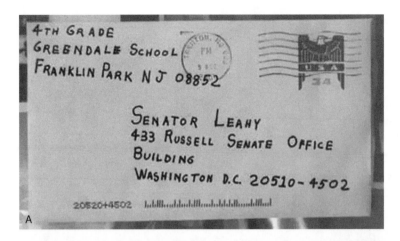

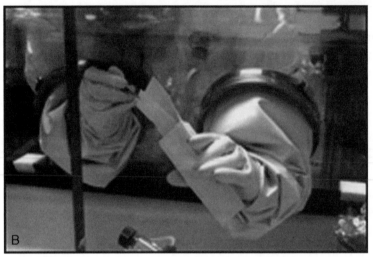

FIGURE 1-1 (A) This letter, postmarked October 5, 2001, was dropped into a mailbox near Princeton University in Trenton, New Jersey. It was addressed to Senator Patrick Leahy with a return address indicating a fourth grade class from Greendale School in Franklin Park, New Jersey. There is no such school, and the perpetrator of this crime has not been apprehended. (B) The infamous Leahy letter is opened by a scientist at the U.S. Army Medical Institute of Infectious Diseases, Fort Detrick, Maryland. (Photos are FBI file photos.)

pulmonary anthrax and 17 other cases of inhalation and cutaneous anthrax (Thompson, 2003). In the weeks and months that followed, first responders were called to the scene of thousands of "white powder" incidents that came as a result of numerous hoaxes, mysterious powdery substances, and just plain paranoia (Beecher, 2006). Public health laboratories all over the United States were inundated with samples collected from the scene of these incidents. Testing of postal facilities, U.S. Senate office buildings, and news-gathering organizations' offices occurred. Between October and December 2001, the Centers for Disease Control and Prevention (CDC) laboratories successfully and accurately tested more than 125,000 samples, which amounted to more than one million separate bio-analytical tests (CDC web site, www.bt.cdc.gov, 2007). Henceforth, there has been a national sense of urgency in preparedness and response activities for a potential act of bioterrorism.

Humankind has been faced with biological threats since we first learned to walk upright. In his thought-provoking book, *Guns, Germs and Steel*, Dr. Jared Diamond points out the epidemiological transitions we have faced since we were hunters and gatherers. More than 10,000 years ago, the human experience with biological peril was mostly parasitic diseases that affected individuals only. Following that, human societies began to herd and domesticate animals. The development of agriculture allowed for population growth and a shift from small tribal bands to concentration of people into villages. Larger groups of people could stand up to smaller elements, thereby enabling them to successfully compete for resources and better defend the ground that they held. Agriculture also brought some *deadly gifts*: animal diseases that also affected man (**zoonotic diseases**), outbreaks of disease due to massing of people and lack of innate immunity, and a growing reliance on animal protein (Diamond, 1999).

For ages, human societies and cultures have been looking for a competitive advantage over their adversaries. Advances in weapons of all types and explosives allowed military forces to defeat their enemies overtly on the battlefield and covertly behind the lines. Technologies leading to nuclear, biological, and chemical weapons have been exploited, as well. Indeed, each has been used legitimately and illegitimately on different scales to bring about a change in the tactics, the military situation, or the political will to face an enemy in battle. Biological agents are no exception to this rule. As such, **biowarfare** (biological warfare) has a historical aspect to it that must be considered here, for advances in the use of biological agents over the last century are one of the main reasons why bioterrorism exists today.

When President Richard M. Nixon said, in November 1969, that "Mankind already holds in its hands too many of the seeds of its own destruction," he was signing an Executive Order putting an end to the United States offensive capabilities for waging biowarfare. Arguably, this statement foretold the potential doom we might all face when then state-of-the-art technologies became commonplace techniques in laboratories all over the world today. Accordingly, this chapter derives its name from the preceding quote and should serve to remind the reader that the seeds we sowed so long ago have now sprouted. The question remains: How shall they be reaped?

The Reality versus the Potential

Bioterrorism is the intentional use of microorganisms or toxins derived from living organisms to cause death or disease in humans or the animals and plants on which we depend. Biosecurity and biodefense programs exist largely because of the potential devastation that could result from a large-scale act of bioterrorism. Civilian biodefense funding (CBF) reached an all time high following the anthrax attacks of 2001. Conversely, the reality of the situation is that these well-intended programs cost taxpayers billions of dollars annually. Rapid detection biothreat pathogen tools are available to assist responders with on-site identification of a suspicious substance. In addition, biosecurity and biodefense are "big business" in the private sector. Security measures to protect agriculture and certain vulnerable industries from acts of bioterrorism and natural biological threats are also in place.

Two detailed reports published in the journal *Biosecurity and Bioterrorism* (Schuler, 2005) show that U.S. government civilian biodefense funding between fiscal year (FY) 2002 and FY2006 amounted to more than $28 billion. Comparing FY2001 to

FY2005, there was an increase in CBF from $420 million to $7.6 billion. The Departments of Health and Human Services and Homeland Security, which together account for about 88% of the FY2006 request, have remained relatively constant in their funding. Other agencies, most notably the Department of Agriculture and the Environmental Protection Agency, have been more variable. These two agencies have seen increased budget requests in FY2006, focusing on programs that protect the nation's food and water supplies. Civilian biodefense spending, not including the BioShield bill, reached a consistent level of about $5 billion from FY2003 to FY2006. There was a decrease in government biodefense funding in FY2006 due to the end in programmed appropriations for the BioShield project (Schuler, 2005). Refer to Table 1-1 for a summary of CBF spending.

BioShield is a program that was designed to give the United States new medical interventions (e.g., vaccines, treatments) for diseases caused by a number of biothreat pathogens. When BioShield was conceived, it cost U.S. taxpayers a total of $5.6 billion and was programmed to be metered out to the Department of Health and Human Services over a 10-year period. Recently, reports have surfaced that suggest BioShield funds are being squandered and no useful products will be realized (Fonda, 2006).

The United States Postal Service spent more than $800 million developing and deploying its Biohazard Detection System (BDS). Currently, it spends more than $70 million annually to operate and maintain the system. The BDS is used only to provide early warning for the presence of a single biothreat pathogen, anthrax. Furthermore, the system screens letter mail that comes from sources like mailboxes and drops, which accounts for approximately 17% of all letter mail volume (Schmid, 2006). System upgrades are programmed to enable postal officials to screen large flats and provide detection for two other pathogens (plague and tularemia), which have been estimated to push the annual costs of the system and its disposable cartridges up to $120 million. The system was considered to be fully deployed in 2005. By the end of 2006, more than 3 million tests had been performed, screening 60 billion pieces of mail. It is interesting to note that, up to summer 2007, no positive test result was found in any of the billions of pieces of mail screened.

All this seems rather incredible when comparing the level of funding given to one of the greatest biological threats of our time, the human immunodeficiency virus (HIV), which causes acquired immunodeficiency syndrome (AIDS). An estimated 1 million people currently are living with HIV in the United States, with approximately 40,000 new infections occurring each year. Currently in the United States, approximately 75%

Table 1-1 Biodefense Funding (in Millions of Dollars) for Primary U.S. Government Agencies by Fiscal Year

Agency	2001	2002	2003	2004	2005	2006
Department of Health and Human Services	271	2,940	3,986	3,700	4,153	4,085
Department of Homeland Security*	—	—	418	1,704	2,946	554
United States Department of Agriculture	NA	NA	200	109	298	253
Environmental Protection Agency	20	187	133	119	97	129
Department of State	3.8	71	67	67	71	77
National Science Foundation	0	9	31	31	31	31
Total CBF	**295**	**3,207**	**4,836**	**5,730**	**7,592**	**5,123**

*The Department of Homeland Security was created in FY2003.
Source: Lam, Franco, and Schuler, 2006.

of the new infections in women are transmitted heterosexually. Half of all new infections in the United States occur in people 25 years of age or younger. Yet, the National Institutes of Health (NIH) budget for AIDS research is about $2.9 billion per year (NIH FY2004 budget document) compared to the $1.6 billion level funding it receives for biodefense.

The History of Biowarfare

Before delving into the subtleties of biosecurity and biodefense, one should explore the historical aspects of the use of biological agents in warfare and terrorism. The history presented here is not all inclusive. Rather, it is a fair assessment of key events and characterizations that can be examined in other more comprehensive documents.

Pathogens and biological toxins have been used as weapons throughout history. Some would argue that biological warfare began when medieval armies used festering corpses to contaminate water supplies. Over several centuries, this evolved into the development of sophisticated biological munitions for battlefield and covert use. These developments parallel advances in microbiology and include the identification of virulent pathogens suitable for aerosol delivery and large-scale fermentation processes to produce large quantities of pathogens and toxins.

However, the history of biological warfare is shrouded by a number of confounding factors. First, it is difficult to verify alleged or attempted biological attacks. These allegations might have been part of a propaganda campaign or due to rumor. Regardless, some of the examples we have been given cannot be supported by microbiological or epidemiologic data. In addition, the incidence of naturally occurring endemic or epidemic diseases during that time complicate the picture so that attribution is impossible (Christopher et al., 1997). More important, our awareness that infectious diseases are caused by microbes does not go back very far in human history. Germ theory, or the fact that infectious diseases are related to and caused by microorganisms, emerged after 1860 through the independent works of Pasteur, Lister, and Koch (Tortora, Funk, and Case, 1995). Therefore, how could the attacking or defending commander know that the festering corpses might cause disease, when people at that time thought that epidemics were related to "miasmas," the smell of decomposition, or heavenly "influences"? One need only consider the origin of certain disease names to appreciate this confusion. For instance, malaria gets its name from "malaria" or bad air—swamp gases (Desowitz, 1991). It was not until 1880 that we learned that the etiologic agents of malaria are protozoans in the genus *Plasmodium*. The name influenza refers to the ancient belief that the disease was caused by a misalignment of the stars because of some unknown supernatural or cosmic influence (Latin *influentia*). It was not until 1933 that we learned the flu was caused by the influenza virus (Potter, 2001).

Regardless of the lack of awareness of germs at the time, a few of the historic reports about the use of biological weapons in battle are worth noting here:

- In the sixth century BC, Assyrians poisoned enemy wells with rye ergot, a fungus.
- In fourth century BC, Scythian archers tipped their arrows with blood, manure, and tissues from decomposing bodies.
- In 1340 AD, attackers hurled dead horses and other animals by catapult at the castle of Thun L'Eveque in Hainault (northern France). Castle defenders reported that "the stink and the air were so abominable ... they could not long endure" and negotiated a truce.

- In 1422 AD at Karlstein in Bohemia, attacking forces launched the decaying cadavers of men killed in battle over the castle walls. They also stockpiled animal manure in the hope of spreading illness. Yet, the defense held fast, and the siege was abandoned after five months. Russian troops may have employed the same tactic using the corpses of plague victims against the Swedes in 1710.
- In 1495 AD, the Spanish contaminated French wine with the blood of lepers.
- In the mid-1600s, a Polish military general reportedly put saliva from rabid dogs into hollow artillery spheres for use against his enemies.
- Francisco Pizarro reportedly gave smallpox virus–contaminated clothing to South American natives in the 15th century.
- In a letter dated July 16, 1763, General Jeffrey Amherst, a British officer, approved the plan to spread smallpox to Delaware Indians (Robertson, 2001). Amherst suggested the deliberate use of smallpox to "reduce" Native American tribes hostile to the British (Parkman, 1901). An outbreak of smallpox at Fort Pitt resulted in the generation of smallpox contaminated materials and an opportunity to carry out Amherst's plan. On June 24, 1763, one of Amherst's subordinates gave blankets and a handkerchief from the smallpox hospital to the Native Americans and recorded in his journal, "I hope it will have the desired effect." (Sipe, 1929)
- The same tactic was employed during the Civil War by Dr. Luke Blackburn, the future governor of Kentucky. Dr. Blackburn infected clothing with smallpox and yellow fever virus, which he then sold to Union troops. One Union officer's obituary stated that he died of smallpox contracted from his infected clothing (Guillemin, 2006).

As previously mentioned, scientists discovered microorganisms and made advances toward understanding that a specific agent causes a specific disease, that some are food borne or waterborne, that an agent can cycle through more than one species, and, that insects and ticks are the vectors of disease. Furthermore, medical professionals established that wars, famines, and poverty opened populations to the risk of epidemics. Once these links were established, we learned that we could apply control and intervention methods. Scientific knowledge about disease transmission coupled with social stability and active public health campaigns aided human survival. Subsequently, it became possible for advanced populations to protect their citizens from the burden of some of the most insidious infectious diseases, such as plague, cholera, diphtheria, smallpox, influenza, and malaria. These epidemics swept across nations in previous centuries, hitting hardest in crowded urban centers and affecting mostly the poor (Guillemin, 2006).

At the opening of the Industrial Revolution, public health in cities had improved, water and food sources were monitored by the state, and vaccines and drug therapies were being invented as further protection. With many childhood diseases conquered, more people were living longer, and they were now dying of more "civilized" diseases like cancer, heart disease, and stroke (Diamond, 1999). In underdeveloped nations, public health did not develop; hence, epidemics were prevalent and continued to be devastating. The dichotomy between developed and developing nations remains marked by generally good health versus widespread, preventable epidemics (Guillemin, 2006).

As Western nations were taking advantage of innovations in public health and medicine to mitigate epidemics, their governments invented biological weapons as a means of achieving advantage in warfare (Diamond, 1999). The German military has the dubious honor of being the first example of using biological weapons following a state-sponsored program. However, during World War I, they used disease-causing organisms against animals, not people. The goal of their program was to interrupt the flow of supplies to the Allied frontlines. To do this, they targeted the packhorses and mules shipped from Norway, Spain, Romania, and the United States. In 1915, Dr. Anton Dilger, a German-American physician, developed a microbiology facility in Washington, D.C. Dilger produced large quantities of anthrax and glanders bacteria, using seed cultures provided by the imperial German government. At the loading docks, German agents inoculated more than 3,000 animals that were destined for the Allied Forces in Europe (Wheelis, 1999). From the German perspective, these attacks violated no international law. In addition, these activities were dwarfed by the atrocities of chemical warfare that was being waged on both sides of the line.

To counter the German threat and explore the potential of air warfare, the French sought to improve their integration of aerosols and bombs. At the same time as the French were signing the 1925 Geneva Protocol, they were developing a biological warfare program to complement the one they had established for chemical weapons during World War I (Rosebury and Kabat, 1947). Following World War I, the Japanese formed a "special weapons" section within their Army. The section was designated Unit 731. The unit's leaders set out to exploit chemical and biological agents. In 1936, they expanded their territory into Manchuria, which made available "an endless supply of human experiment materials" (prisoners of war) for Unit 731. Biological weapons experiments in Harbin, Manchuria, directed by Japanese General Shiro Ishii, continued until 1945. A post–World War II autopsy investigation of 1,000 victims revealed that most were exposed to aerosolized anthrax. More than 3,000 prisoners and Chinese nationals may have died in Unit 731 facilities. In 1939, the Japanese military poisoned Soviet water sources with intestinal typhoid bacteria at the former Mongolian border. During an infamous biowarfare attack in 1941, the Japanese military released millions of plague-infected fleas from airplanes over villages in China and Manchuria, resulting in several plague outbreaks in those villages. The Japanese program had stockpiled 400 kilograms of anthrax to be used in specially designed fragmentation bombs.

In 1942, shortly before the battle of Stalingrad, on the German-Soviet front, a large outbreak of tularemia occurred. Several thousand Soviets and Germans contracted the illness. Some estimate that more than 70% of the victims had inhalation tularemia, which is rare and considered to be evidence of an intentional release. It was determined later that the Soviets had developed a tularemia weapon the prior year (Alibek and Handelman, 2000).

During World War II, the Allies had great fear of German and Japanese biological weapons programs. Their fears were sparked by sketchy reports that the Japanese had an ongoing effort and British intelligence suggested that Germany might soon target Britain with a bomb packed with biological agents. Based on these fears, Great Britain began its own bioweapons program and urged officials in the United States to create a large-scale biological warfare program.

On December 9, 1942, the U.S. government convened a secret meeting at the National Academy of Sciences in Washington, D.C. The meeting was called to respond to Great Britain's request. Army officers had urgent questions for an elite group of scientists. Only a few months before, the president of the United States had grappled with the issue of biological weapons. President Franklin D. Roosevelt stated that "I have been loath to believe that any nation, even our present enemies, would be willing to loose upon mankind such terrible and inhumane weapons." Secretary of War, General Henry Stimson, thought differently. "Biological warfare is … dirty business," he wrote to Roosevelt, "but … I think we must be prepared."

President Roosevelt approved the launch of America's biological warfare program. For the first time, U.S. researchers would be trying to make weapons from the deadliest germs known to science. In spring 1943, the United States initiated its bioweapons program at Camp Detrick (now Fort Detrick), Maryland. The program focused primarily on the use of the agents that cause anthrax, botulism, plague, tularemia, Q fever, Venezuelan equine encephalitis, and brucellosis. Production of these agents occurred at Camp Detrick, Maryland, and other sites in Arkansas, Colorado, and Indiana. The British had made two primary requests of us: first, to mass produce anthrax spores so that they could be placed in bomblets and stored for later deployment against the Germans in retaliation for any future strike; secondly, the British supplied us with the recipe to make botulinum toxin and wanted to see if we could mass produce it. Naturally, the entire program was wrapped in a cloak of secrecy. Figure 1-2 is a collage of some important facilities built at Camp Detrick to produce and test bioweapons formulations.

The British program focused on the use of *Bacillus anthracis* (anthrax) spores and their viability and dissemination when delivered with a conventional bomb. Gruinard Island, off the coast of Scotland, was used as the testing site for formulations. At the time, British scientists believed that the testing site was far enough from the coast to cause any contamination of the mainland. However, in 1943, there was an outbreak of anthrax in sheep and cattle on the coast of Scotland that faced Gruinard. As a result, the British decided to stop the anthrax testing and close down the island site. Despite the cessation of experiments, the island remained contaminated for decades until a deliberate and extensive decontamination program rendered the island inhabitable again.

The U.S. bioweapons program continued to grow in scope and sophistication. Much of this was prompted by fear of a new enemy: the threat of communism, the Soviet Union, and its allies. Experiments to test bioweapons formulations were routinely carried out on a small scale with research animals. However, more comprehensive field and laboratory studies were carried out with human research volunteers exposed to actual live agents and some situational scenarios using surrogate nonpathogenic bacteria to simulate the release of actual pathogens inside buildings or aimed at cities.

In 1949, researchers from Detrick visited the Pentagon on a secret mission. Disguised as maintenance workers, they released noninfectious bacteria into the duct work of the building to assess the vulnerability of people inside large buildings to a bioweapons attack. The Pentagon trial was considered to be a success because it revealed that germs could be formulated and released effectively for a small-scale act of sabotage. However, there was considerable doubt that biological weapons could be effective against a target the size of a city. Accordingly, a number of tests were conducted on American cities (Miller, Engelberg, and Broad, 2001). In 1977, the U.S. Army admitted that there were 239 intentional releases of noninfectious bacteria in bioweapons experiments (Cole, 1988) . One such trial took place in San Francisco in September 1950, when a U.S. Navy ship sailed a course adjacent to the Golden Gate Bridge to release a plume of seemingly nonpathogenic bacteria (*Serratia marcescens*). This trial was intended to simulate the dispersion of anthrax spores on a large city. Based on results from monitoring equipment at 43 locations around the city, the Army determined that San Francisco had received enough of a dose for nearly all of the city's 800,000 residents to inhale at least 5,000 of the particles. Although the researchers believed that what they were releasing was harmless, one report shows that 11 people reported to area hospitals with severe infections due to the release of this agent, one of which was fatal (Cole, 1988).

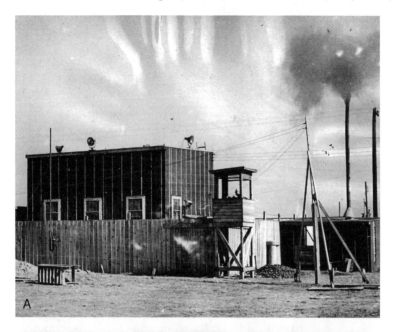

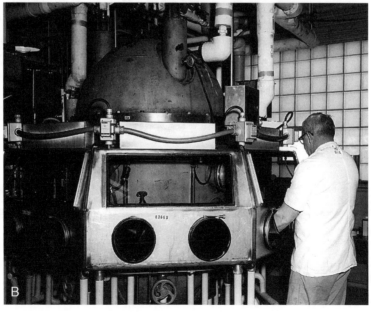

FIGURE 1-2 (A) The "Black Maria" was the first laboratory facility built at Camp Detrick to conduct top secret bioweapons research. The purpose of this tarpaper building was to produce Agent X (botulinum toxin) for the British. (B) A Camp Detrick researcher works with an aerobiology chamber to conduct a study with microbial aerosols, a biological weapons formulation.

(Continued)

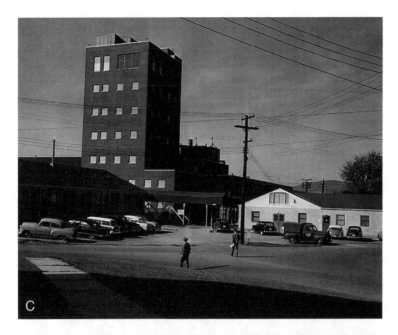

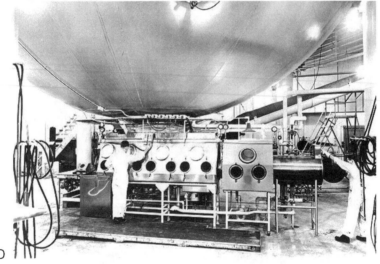

FIGURE 1-2—Cont'd (C) This is the old Pilot Plant (Building 470) at Fort Detrick. Here, experimental formulations of anthrax spores were made. The building had a reputation for mystery. Despite three decontamination procedures, it was never certified 100% clean. (D) Pictured here is a 1-million liter metal sphere workers called the *Eight Ball*. The largest aerobiology chamber ever constructed, it was used to test experimental bioweapons formulations at Fort Detrick. The last experiment in the Eight Ball was in 1969. (All images courtesy of the United States Army.)

Three years later, bioweapons experts took their secret exercises to St. Louis and Minneapolis, two cities that resembled potential Soviet targets, where sprayers hidden in cars dispersed invisible clouds of harmless *Bacillus* spores. In 1966, nonpathogenic *Bacillus globigii* spores were released into the New York subway system using a broken light bulb to demonstrate the ability of a specific formulation to make its way from a central point source to both ends of the system in less than an hour. Revelations of these experiments became known in 1977 when a Senate Subcommittee panel heard testimony from Pentagon officials (U.S. Department of the Army, DTIC B193427 L, 1977). Until that point, neither U.S. citizens nor their representatives in Washington knew almost nothing about the American germ program.

After nearly three decades of secret research aimed at producing the ultimate biological weapons and stockpiling them for use against our enemies, President Richard Nixon surprised the world by signing an executive order that stopped all offensive biological agent and toxin weapon research and ordered all stockpiles of biological agents and munitions from the U.S. program be destroyed. Accordingly, on November 25, 1969, he uttered these historic words in a speech to the nation on

> *...Biological warfare—which is commonly called "germ warfare." This has massive unpredictable and potentially uncontrollable consequences. It may produce global epidemics and profoundly affect the health of future generations. Therefore, I have decided that the United States of America will renounce the use of any form of deadly biological weapons that either kill or incapacitate. Mankind already carries in its own hands too many of the seeds of its own destruction.*

Subsequently, in 1972, the United States and many other countries were signatories to the Convention on the Prohibition of the Development, Production and Stockpiling of Bacteriological (Biological) and Toxin Weapons and on Their Destruction, commonly called the Biological Weapons Convention. This treaty prohibits the stockpiling of biological agents for offensive military purposes and forbids research into offensive use of biological agents.

Although the former Soviet Union was a signatory to the Biological Weapons Convention, its development of biological weapons intensified dramatically after the accord and continued well into the 1990s. In late April 1979, an outbreak of pulmonary anthrax occurred in Sverdlovsk (now Yekaterinburg) in the former Soviet Union. Soviet officials explained that the outbreak was due to ingestion of infected meat. However, it was later discovered that the cause was from an accidental release of anthrax in aerosol form from the Soviet Military Compound 19, a Soviet bioweapons facility. (This event is examined thoroughly in Chapter 7 as a case study to demonstrate the potential of weaponized anthrax.) The robust bioweapons program of the Soviet Union employed more than 60,000 people. Building 15 at Koltsovo was capable of manufacturing tons of smallpox virus annually. In Kirov, the Soviets maintained an arsenal of 20 tons of weaponized plague bacterium. By 1987, Soviet anthrax production capacity reached nearly 5,000 tons a year.

In the later part of the 1990s, the Russians disassembled their awesome bioweapons production capacity and reportedly destroyed their stocks. As the Soviet Union dissolved, it appeared that the threat of biowarfare would diminish. However, the Age of Bioterrorism emerged with the anthrax attacks of 2001. In addition, the U.S. Department of State published a report in 2004 that affirmed six countries had active bioweapons programs.

Table 1-2 summarizes some of these events.

Table 1-2 Seminal Moments in the History of Biowarfare and Bioterrorism

Date	Event	Significance
Sixth century, BC	Assyrians poisoned enemy wells with rye ergot	First known use of a biological toxin
1763	British soldiers give blankets infected with the smallpox virus to American Indians	Notable and documented use of virus against combatants
1915	Anton Dilger produces anthrax and glanders bacterium to infect horses intended for the war front	Notable and documented use of bacteria against animals
June 17, 1925	Delegates in Switzerland create a Geneva Protocol banning the use of chemical and bacteriological methods of warfare	First International effort to limit use of biologicals in warfare
1932	The Japanese Army gives General Ishii control of three biological research centers, including one in Manchuria	Most despicable character in bioweapons history gets his start
1934	Great Britain begins taking steps toward establishing its own biological weapons research project	Allies start to develop a program
July 15, 1942	Anthrax tested on Gruinard Island against sheep	Allies first field test of bioweapon
November 1942	British implore the United States to lead bioweapons production efforts; negotiations commence and President Roosevelt approves the program	Beginning of U.S. bioweapons program
Spring 1943	U.S. Bioweapons Program begins its activities at Camp Detrick, Maryland	Implementation of plans to begin U.S. Bioweapons program
May 1949	The U.S. Army Chemical Corps sets up a Special Operations Division at Camp Detrick to carry out field tests with bioweapons formulations	Tests conducted at the Pentagon show that biological weapons formulations are feasible for sabotage
1950	Navy warships spray the cities of Norfolk, Hampton, Newport News, and San Francisco	Tests show that large-scale deployment of a bioweapon from the sea is feasible
1953	Conduct of the St Jo Program stages mock anthrax attacks on St. Louis, Minneapolis, and Winnipeg using aerosol generators placed on top of cars	Tests show that large-scale deployment of a bioweapon from the land is feasible
1955	Operation Whitecoat uses human research volunteers to study the effects of biological agents on human volunteers	The operation will continue for the next 18 years and involve some 2,200 people
1957	Operation Large Area Concept kicks off to test the release of aerosols from airplanes; the first experiment involves a swath from South Dakota to Minnesota and further tests cover areas from Ohio to Texas and Michigan to Kansas	Tests show that large-scale deployment of a bioweapon from the air is feasible; some of the test particles travel 1,200 miles
November 25, 1969	Nixon announces that the United States will renounce the use of any form of deadly biological weapons that either kill or incapacitate	The end of an era in U.S. offensive biological weapons research, production. and storage
April 10, 1972	The Biological Weapons Convention, which bans all bioweapons, is completed and opened for signature	Seventy-nine nations signed the treaty, including the Soviet Union
March 26, 1975	The Biological Weapons Convention officially goes into force; the U.S. Senate also finally ratifies the 1925 Geneva Protocol	Political will to ban biological weapons on the international front

Table 1-2 Seminal Moments in the History of Biowarfare and Bioterrorism—Cont'd

Date	Event	Significance
April 1979	Nearly 70 people die from an accidental release of anthrax spores in the Soviet city of Sverdlovsk	The United States suspects that anthrax bacterial spores were accidentally released from a Soviet military biological facility
1984	The Rajneeshees contaminate food with *Salmonella* bacterium in a small town in Oregon to influence local elections	The first significant act of bioterrorism in the United States
1989	A Soviet defector from Biopreparat, Vladimir Pasechnik, reveals the existence of a continuing offensive biological weapons program in the U.S.S.R.	Evidence that the Soviet Union is violating the Biological Weapons Convention
April 1992	Russian President Boris Yeltsin admits the 1979 outbreak was caused by the Soviet military but gives few details	An admonition that the Soviet Union operated an offensive biological warfare program in violation of the Biological Weapons Convention
Fall 2001	Envelopes filled with anthrax spores are sent to various media and political figures in the United States; 22 people, from Florida to Connecticut, are infected; 5 die	A national movement begins to prepare a citizenry against the threat of bioterrorism, which has now become a household word

Modern-Day Bioterrorism

Biodefense programs and initiatives come out of a sense of vulnerability to biowarfare potentials. Bioterrorism is deeply founded in what has been gained from active biowarfare programs (Miller et al., 2001). In the early 1970s, the leftist terrorist group, the Weather Underground, reportedly attempted to blackmail an Army officer at Fort Detrick working in the Research Institute of Infectious Diseases (USAMRIID). The group's goal was to get him to supply organisms that would be used to contaminate municipal water supplies in the United States. The plot was discovered when the officer attempted to acquire several items that were "unrelated to his work." Several other attempts are worth mentioning here:

- In 1972, members of the right-wing group Order of the Rising Sun were found in possession of 30–40 kilograms of typhoid bacteria cultures that were allegedly to be used to contaminate the water supplies of several midwestern cities.
- In 1975, the Symbionese Liberation Army was found in possession of technical manuals on how to produce bioweapons.
- In 1980, a Red Army Faction safe house reportedly discovered in Paris included a laboratory containing quantities of botulinum toxin.
- In 1983, the FBI arrested two brothers in the northeastern United States for possession of an ounce of nearly pure ricin.
- In 1984, followers of the Bhagwan Shree Rajneesh contaminated salad bars with *Salmonella* bacteria in a small town in Oregon. It was the largest scale act of bioterrorism in U.S. history. More than 750 cases of salmonellosis resulted from the salad bar contamination. It was later discovered that the Rajneeshees wanted to influence the local county elections. Cult members obtained the *Salmonella* strain through the mail from the American Type Culture Collection (ATCC) and propagated the liquid cultures in their compound's medical clinic.

- In 1989, a home laboratory producing botulinum toxin was discovered in Paris. This laboratory was linked to a cell of the German-based Bäder Meinhof Gang.

- In Minnesota, four members of the Patriots Council, an antigovernment extremist group, were arrested in 1991 for plotting to kill a U.S. marshal with ricin. The group planned to mix the homemade ricin with a chemical that speeds absorption (DMSO) and then smear it on the door handles of the marshal's car. The plan was discovered and all four men were arrested and the first to be prosecuted under the U.S. Biological Weapons Anti-Terrorism Act of 1989.

- In 1995, Aum Shinrikyo, a Japanese doomsday cult, became infamous for an act of chemical terrorism when members released sarin gas into the Tokyo subway. What many people do not know about the group is that it developed and attempted to use biological agents (anthrax, Q fever, Ebola virus, and botulinum toxin) on at least 10 other occasions. Despite several releases, it was unsuccessful in its use of biologicals. This program is examined more thoroughly in Chapter 7.

□ □ □ ▬▬▬▬▬▬▬▬▬▬▬▬▬▬▬▬▬▬▬▬▬▬▬▬▬▬▬

The Public Health Security and Bioterrorism Response Act of 2002

On June 12, 2002 President George W. Bush uttered these remarks from the White House at the signing of H.R. 3448, the Public Health Security and Bioterrorism Response Act of 2002:

Bioterrorism is a real threat to our country. It's a threat to every nation that loves freedom. Terrorist groups seek biological weapons; we know some rogue states already have them ... It's important that we confront these real threats to our country and prepare for future emergencies.

Clearly, 9/11 and the anthrax attacks of 2001 sent the country to war and sparked a number of initiatives against all forms of terrorism.

▬▬▬▬▬▬▬▬▬▬▬▬▬▬▬▬▬▬▬▬▬▬▬▬▬▬▬ □ □ □

Weaponization

Biological agents have some unique characteristics that make weaponizing them attractive to the would-be terrorist. Most biological weapons are made up of living microorganisms, which means that they can replicate once disseminated. This possibility amplifies the problem and the effect of the weapon in several ways. First, some agents are capable of surviving in a variety of different hosts. The target might be humans, but the disease may manifest in other animal hosts, like companion animals (pets). In doing so, the problem may be more difficult to control. Second, when people become infected with a disease-causing organism, there is an incubation period before signs of illness are apparent. During this incubation period and the periods of illness and recovery, the pathogen may be shed from the victim causing the contagion to spread (a possibility only with diseases that are transmitted from person to person). There is no rule of thumb for how many people might be infected from a single patient. However, the nature of contagion clearly compounds the problem well beyond the initial release of the agent. In this instance, the initial victims from the intentional outbreak become more weapons for the perpetrator, spreading the problem with every step they take. As Grigg, Rosen, and Koop (2006) stated so precisely in their paper, "when the threat comes from the infected population, self defense becomes self-mutilation." Surely, the would-be terrorist could derive great pleasure from watching government officials and responders tread on the civil liberties of such victims as they attempt to limit the problem from spreading among the population.

Making an effective biological weapon is no easy undertaking. The process and complexity depends largely on the pathogen selected to be "weaponized." If the pathogen is a spore forming bacteria, like *Bacillus anthracis* (the causative agent of anthrax), there are five essential steps: germination, vegetation, sporulation, separation, and weaponization. The first three steps are designed to get small quantities of seed stock to propagate into a "starter culture," grow them to a significant stage of growth in the proper volume, and turn those active cells into spores. The goal of the last two steps is to separate the spores from the dead vegetative cells and spent media. All five steps have dozens of secondary steps. In addition, each of the five steps requires a fairly sophisticated and well-equipped laboratory if the goal is to develop a sizeable quantity of refined materials.

Weaponization is a term that applies to the processes necessary to purify, properly size, stabilize, and make biological agents ideally suited for dissemination. Stabilization and dissemination are important issues because of the susceptibility of the biological agents to environmental degradation, not only in storage but also in application. These issues are problems whether the end use is for biological weapons, pharmaceuticals, cosmetics, pesticides, or food-related purposes. Susceptibility of the organisms to inactivation by the environment varies with the agent. As an example, anthrax spores released into the environment may remain viable for decades, whereas plague bacterium may survive for only a few hours. Loss of viability or bioactivity is likely to result from exposure to physical and chemical stressors, such as exposure to UV radiation (sunlight), high surface area at air-water interfaces (frothing), extreme temperature or pressure, high salt concentration, dilution, or exposure to specific inactivating agents. This requirement of stabilization also extends to the methods of delivery, since the organisms are very susceptible to degradation in the environments associated with delivery systems.

The primary means of stabilization for storage or packaging are concentration; freeze drying (lyophilization); spray drying; formulation into a stabilizing solid, liquid, or gaseous solution; and deep freezing. Methods of concentration include vacuum filtration, ultrafiltration, precipitation, and centrifugation. Freeze drying is the preferred method for long-term storage of bacterial cultures because freeze-dried cultures can be easily dehydrated and cultured via conventional means. Freeze-dried cultures may remain viable for more than 30 years. Deep freezing of biological products is another long-term storage technique for species and materials not amenable to freeze drying. The method involves storage of the contained products in liquid nitrogen freezers ($-196°$ Celsius) or ultra-low-temperature mechanical freezers ($-70°$C).

Culturing viruses is a more costly and tenuous process because host cells are required for viral propagation. This means that cultures of host cells must be kept alive, often in an oxygen-deficient and temperature-stable atmosphere. In some cases, viruses may be more fragile when deployed as weapons, some becoming inactive on drying. Biological toxins can be quite difficult to produce and purify, each requiring its own special set of circumstances. Two specific examples are covered in subsequent chapters, when those agents are discussed in detail. However, past bioweapons programs have determined that these agents are most effective when prepared as a freeze-dried powder and encapsulated.

A Question of Scale

Apparently, biological attacks by a terrorist group are not easy to conduct or a practical option. If they were easy or practical, many terrorist groups and hostile states would have done so long ago and frequently. Our experience today with acts of biological terrorism has to do mainly with small-scale, limited attacks. However, if one were to acquire the means to produce the weapons, as described here or purchase viable, sophisticated materials on the black market, a small group of persons could bring about the infection of a large percentage of targeted persons. Clinical illness could develop within a day of dispersal and last for as long as two to three weeks. In a civil situation, major subway systems in a densely populated urban area could be targeted for a biological agent strike, resulting in massive political and social disorganization. It would take little weaponized material to bring about the desired effect. Looking at this potential comparatively on a weight-to-weight basis, about 10 grams of *Bacillus anthracis* (anthrax) spores could kill as many people as a ton of the nerve agent sarin.

With bioweapons in hand, small countries or terrorist groups might develop the capability to deliver small quantities of agents to a specific target. Under appropriate weather conditions and with an aerosol generator delivering 1–10 micron-particle-size droplets, a single aircraft could disperse 100 kg of anthrax over a 300 km^2 area and theoretically cause 3 million deaths in a population density of 10,000 people per km^2 (US DOD, ADA 330102, 1998).

Much has been made of the potential of aerosolized powders and respiratory droplets in factual and fictitious biothreat scenarios. The largest infectious disease outbreak in the history of the United States occurred in April 1993. The event was caused by an accidental waterborne contamination. The outbreak of cryptosporidiosis, which occurred in the greater Milwaukee area, was estimated to have caused more than 430,000 people to become ill with gastroenteritis among a population of 1.6 million (MacKenzie et al., 1994). About 4,400 people were hospitalized and about 100 people died as a result of the outbreak. The Milwaukee outbreak was attributed to failure of filtration processes at one of the two water treatment plants that served the city. A number of deficiencies were found at the plant, including problems relating to a change in the type of water treatment chemicals used for coagulation of contaminants prior to the filtration step. Weather conditions at the time were unusual, with a heavy spring snowmelt leading to high source water turbidity and wind patterns that may have changed normal flow patterns in Lake Michigan, the raw water source for the city.

The Genesis of Biosecurity and Biodefense

The secrecy of bioweapons programs of the previous century has been uncloaked. Some of the most insidious disease agents ever to afflict humans, animals, and plants have been mass produced and perfected for maximum effectiveness. Terrorist groups and rogue states may be seeking to develop bioweapons capabilities. These significant developments in bioweapons gave military leaders and politicians cause for great concern over the past few decades. The military necessity to protect the force and defend the homeland is the goal of a good biodefense program. Simply put, **biodefense** is the need for improved national defenses against biological attacks. These are national programs, mostly planned and carried out by military forces and other government agencies. Initially, biodefense programs require an intelligence-gathering capability that strives to determine what may be in the biological weapons arsenal of an aggressor. Intelligence is needed to guide biodefense research and development efforts aimed at producing and testing effective countermeasures (i.e., vaccines, therapeutic drugs, and detection methods). In addition, a real-time reporting system should be developed so that officials can be informed about an emerging threat before an agent has a chance to affect armed forces and millions of people in the homeland. The development of integrated systems for detecting and monitoring biological agents is instrumental to this goal. Although most biodefense initiatives rest with the military, civilian government agencies contribute greatly to the biodefense posture. This is quite evident by the increases in civilian biodefense funding over the past few years and will be discussed in great detail in Part IV of this book. **Biosecurity**, on the other hand, refers to the policies and measures taken for protecting a nation's food supply and agricultural resources from both accidental contamination and deliberate attacks of bioterrorism.

□ □ □ ▬▬▬▬▬▬▬▬▬▬▬▬▬▬▬▬▬▬▬▬▬▬▬▬▬▬▬▬▬

Critical Thinking
Describe the fundamental difference between biodefense and biosecurity.

▬▬▬▬▬▬▬▬▬▬▬▬▬▬▬▬▬▬▬▬▬▬▬▬▬▬▬▬▬ □ □ □

Essential Terminology

- **Biodefense.** The collective efforts of a nation aimed at improving defenses against biological attacks. Within these efforts are programs and agencies working toward increasing data collection, analysis, and intelligence gathering. The intelligence is applied to programs aimed at mitigating the effects of bioweapons by developing vaccines, therapeutics, and detection methods to increase the defensive posture. Ultimately, biodefense initiatives protect the military forces and the citizens from the effects of biological attack.
- **Biosecurity.** The policies and measures taken for protecting a nation's food supply and agricultural resources from both accidental contamination and deliberate attacks of bioterrorism.
- **Bioterrorism.** The intentional use of microorganisms or toxins derived from living organisms to cause death or disease in humans or the animals and plants on which we depend. Bioterrorism might include such deliberate acts as introducing pests intended to kill U.S. food crops, spreading a virulent disease among animal production facilities, and poisoning water, food, and blood supplies.

- **Biowarfare,** also known as *germ warfare.* The use of any organism (bacteria, virus, or other disease-causing organism) or toxin found in nature as a weapon of war. It is meant to incapacitate or kill an adversary.
- **Pathogen.** A specific causative agent of disease. Mostly thought of as being an infectious organism (e.g., bacteria, virus, rickettsia, protozoa).
- **Weaponization.** When applied to biologicals, the term implies a process of taking something natural and making it harmful through enhancing the negative characteristics of it. With biological agents, one might weaponize the agent by making more lethal, more stable, and more easily delivered or disseminated against an intended target. There is considerable debate about the use of this term.
- **Zoonotic disease.** An animal disease that may be transmitted to humans.

Discussion Questions

- How was the decision made to begin the U.S. biological weapons program?
- What are the significant events in the history of biowarfare? What makes them significant?
- When President Nixon said that "Mankind already holds in its hands too many of the seeds of its own destruction" in November 1969, what did he mean by that?
- Weaponizing a biological agent is easy to do, right?
- No one knows exactly who perpetrated the Anthrax attacks of 2001 and there has been no repeat of them since. Why do you think we have seen no repeat of the anthrax attacks since 2001.

Web Sites

The Center for Arms Control and Non-proliferation has an online course in Biosecurity. Type the URL that follows into your Internet browser and click on View Course and Select Unit 2: "The History of Biological Weapons." The six sections in this unit provide an excellent overview and reinforce the material presented in the subheading about the History of Biowarfare: www.armscontrolcenter.org/resources/biosecurity_course.

The CDC's Emergency and Preparedness web site offers a segmented video short lesson on the history of bioterrorism. The seven sections give a general overview on bioterrorism and separate vignettes on anthrax, plague, tularemia, viral hemorrhagic fevers, smallpox, and botulism: www.bt.cdc.gov/training/historyofbt.

References

Alibek, K., with S. Handelman. 2000. *Biohazard: The Chilling True Story of the Largest Covert Biological Weapons Program in the World—Told from the Inside by the Man Who Ran It.* New York: Random House.

Beecher, D. 2006. Forensic application of microbiological culture analysis to identify mail intentionally contaminated with Bacillus anthracis spores. *Applied and Environmental Microbiology* 72, no. 8:5304–5310.

Christopher, G. W., T. J. Cieslak, J. A. Pavlin, and E. M. Eitzen. 1997. Biological warfare: A historical perspective. *Journal of the American Medical Association* 278:412–417.

Cole, L. 1988. *Clouds of Secrecy. The Army's Germ Warfare Tests over Populated Areas.* Lanham, Maryland: Rowman and Littlefield Publishers.

Desowitz, R. S. 1991. *The Malaria Capers: More Tales of Parasites and People, Research, and Reality.* New York: W. W. Norton and Company.

Diamond, J. 1999. *Guns, Germs and Steel: The Fates of Human Societies.* New York: W. W. Norton and Company.

Eitzen, E., and E. Takafugi. 1997. A historical overview of biological warfare. Chapter 18 in *Medical Aspects of Chemical and Biological Warfare: A textbook in Military Medicine,* eds. F. R. Sidell, E. T. Takafugi, and D. R. Franz. Bethesda, MD: Office of the Surgeon General, Borden Institute, Walter Reed Army Institute of Reserach.

Fonda, D. 2006. Inside the spore wars. Controversial contracts, bureaucratic bungling—the Fed's biodefense drug program is a mess. How did it go so wrong? *Time* (January 3).

Grigg, E., J. Rosen, and C. E. Koop. 2006. The biological disaster challenge: Why we are least prepared for the most devastating threat and what we need to do about it. *Journal of Emergency Management* (January/February): 23–35.

Guillemin, J. 2006. Scientists and the history of biological weapons. A brief historical overview of the development of biological weapons in the twentieth century. *EMBO Reports* (July 7), Spec No: S45–49.

Lam, C., C. Franco, and A. Schuler. 2006. Billions for biodefense: Federal agency biodefense funding, FY2006–FY2007. *Biosecurity and Bioterrorism: Biodefense Strategy, Practice and Science* 4, no. 2: 113–127.

MacKenzie, W. R., N. Hoxie, M. Proctor, M. Gradus, K. Blair, D. Peterson, J. Kazmierczak, J. Addiss, K. Fox, J. Rose, and J. Davis. 1994. A massive outbreak in Milwaukee of Cryptosporidium infection transmitted through the public water supply. *New England Journal of Medicine* 331:161–167.

Miller, J., S. Engelberg, and W. Broad. 2001. *Germs: Biological Weapons and America's Secret War.* New York: Simon and Schuster.

Parkman, F. 1901. *The Conspiracy of Pontiac and the Indian War after the Conquest of Canada.* Boston: Little Brown and Company, p. 2.

Potter, C. W. 2001. A history of influenza. *Journal of Applied Microbiology* 91, no. 4:572–579.

Robertson, E. 2001. *Rotting Face: Smallpox and the American Indian.* Caldwell, ID: Caxton Press.

Rosebury, T., and E. A. Kabat. 1947. Bacterial warfare. *Journal of Immunology* 56:7–96.

Schmid, R. E. 2006. Postal testing increasing five years after anthrax deaths. Associated Press (October 3).

Schuler, A. 2005. Billions for biodefense: Federal agency biodefense budgeting, FY2005–FY2006. *Biosecurity and Bioterrorism: Biodefense Strategy, Practice and Science* 3, no. 2:94–101.

Sipe, C. H. 1929. *The Indian Wars of Pennsylvania.* Harrisburg, PA: Telegraph Press.

Thompson, M. K. 2003. *Killer Strain: Anthrax and a Government Exposed.* Collingdale, PA: DIANE Publishing Company.

Tortora, G. J., B. R. Funke, and C. L. Case. 1995. *Microbiology. An Introduction,* 5th ed., pp. 2–22. Redwood City, CA: Benjamin/Cummings Publishing, Company.

U.S. Department of the Army. 1977. *U.S. Army Activity in the U.S. Biological Warfare Programs,* vol. 2, Annexes. Washington, DC: U.S. Department of the Army Publication DTIC B193427 L, appendix IV to annex E.

U.S. Department of Defense, Office of the Under Secretary of Defense for Acquisition and Technology. 1998. *The Militarily Critical Technologies List Part II: Weapons of Mass Destruction Technologies*. Section III: "Biological Weapons Technology." ADA 330102.

U.S. Department of Health and Human Services. Centers for Disease Control and Prevention. 2007. *Examples of the Laboratory Response Network in Action*, available at www.bt.cdc.gov/lrn/examples.asp, downloaded August 15.

Wheelis, M. 1999. Biological sabotage in World War I. In *Biological and Toxin Weapons: Research, Development and Use from the Middle Ages to 1945*, eds. Erhard Geissler and John Ellis van Courtland Moon, pp. 35–62. New York: Oxford University Press.

Recognition of Biological Threat

Organisms are pretty complex machines.
—Dr. Joshua Lederberg, Nobel Laureate

Objectives

The study of this chapter will enable you to

1. Describe the general and common characteristics of most biological agents.
2. Define the terms *pathogen, toxin,* and *virulence.*
3. Discuss the physical attributes of bacterial, viral, and rickettsial pathogens.
4. Discuss the differences between bacterial, viral, and rickettsial pathogens.
5. Understand the difference between clinical presentation and diagnosis.
6. Describe the three tiers of diagnosis for infectious diseases and how differential diagnoses are used by clinicians.
7. Discuss the advantages and disadvantages of using biological agents as weapons.

Key Terms

bacteria, spores, rickettsia, virus, virion, prion, biological toxin, clinical presentation, signs, symptoms, differential diagnosis, tiered diagnostic system, virulence.

Introduction

Certain characteristics are common to most biological agents. First, all are obtained from nature, where they cause disease naturally. As such, they may be relatively easy to acquire—especially if you know where to find them and how to recover them. Second, biological agents are invisible to the human senses. They are too small to see with the naked eye, neither can you feel, taste, or smell them. Detection of the agents and diagnoses of the diseases they cause require sophisticated techniques and equipment, which will be covered in a later chapter.

Most biological agents are harmless and many are beneficial to humans, plants, and animals. Many microorganisms are essential to higher animals and plants. For instance, without some bacteria, animal digestive processes would not be efficient enough to fully break down food in the gut. Some plants rely on nitrogen-fixing bacteria to make nitrogen sources found in the soil available to the root system of the plant. Microorganisms play a key role in the overall breakdown of decaying organic matter, which is essential in returning key elements and nutrients to the soil.

Some biological agents are **pathogenic**, meaning that they have negative affects on the host, causing morbidity (illness) and mortality (death). Pathogenic microorganisms have a wide range of effects, from causing simple flulike illnesses and diarrhea all the way to seizures, coma, and death. **Virulence** is the degree of pathogenicity of a microorganism, as indicated by the severity of the disease produced and its ability to invade the tissues of a host. The severity of illness depends on a number of factors, such as the age and general health of the victim, the agent to which he or she is exposed, the dose received, and the way the agent gains entry into the body. Generally, bacteria and viruses do not produce immediate effects. Their populations need time to replicate within the host, which may or may not result in illness. The time frame from exposure to infection to illness is referred to as the **incubation period**.

Some biological agents are relatively easy to produce. If one can obtain a specimen of an organism and knows how to culture it (provide a suitable environment, provide nutrients, and allow it to reproduce), one can increase the quantity using basic procedures and commercially available equipment. Bioweapons programs built great capacities for mass production of specific agents. However, many advances in the mass production of microbes occurred long before the bioweapons programs of the 20th century. Beer fermentation, alcohol distilleries, pharmaceuticals, and cosmetics all rely on mass production of biologicals. Even though it may be "easy" to mass produce biological products, they are not generally easy to "weaponize" or put into a form that will be stable and viable for long periods.

Routes of Entry

Biological agents gain entry into the host through inhalation, ingestion, absorption, and injection.

Inhalation infection, or uptake of an infectious agent through the respiratory system, is of great concern when dealing with the release of biological agents. Terrorists have the potential to produce aerosols of biological agents. Release of aerosols would enable the agent to enter victims' lungs and initiate illness. Ideally, an aerosolized agent would be in a range of 1–10 microns (a micron is one millionth of a meter). This minute particle size is small enough to reach the deepest recesses of the lungs, but large enough not to be exhaled. Aerosols of this nature could be odorless, colorless, and invisible. Inhalation was the route of entry that caused the five deaths during the fall 2001 anthrax mail attacks.

Ingestion, or consumption through the digestive tract, of contaminated food or water is a simple method that can be used by a terrorist with minimal expertise and funding, because it is much easier to accomplish and requires little or no disseminating equipment. Biological agents can range from simple cultures grown in a refining broth to purified agents dried and concentrated; either preparation could be used to effectively contaminate a food source. Ingestion was used by members of the Rajneeshees to introduce *Salmonella* bacteria into residents of a community in Oregon.

Absorption occurs when a substance passes directly through the skin. Unlike some chemical agents, biological agents do not enter intact skin, because the skin provides a

Team Organization & Assignment

- Key Organizations (players) in Biological Attack Scenario

- Key Organizations (players) in Critical Infrastructure Attack Scenario

- Location maps, profiles, communications needed to conduct the scenarios
  - Biological attack
  - CI attack

very good biological defense. Tricothecene (T2) mycotoxins (e.g., yellow rain) would be a rare exception, as they can be absorbed directly through the skin. These fast-acting toxins produced by fungi reportedly were exploited by the Soviets and can produce effects similar to blister agents.

Injection occurs when something physically penetrates the skin and deposits a substance or agent. With respect to vector-borne diseases, this takes place when an infected insect (mosquito, deer fly, etc.) or tick bites someone and delivers the pathogen. Could the aggressor produce hoards of infected mosquitoes or ticks then release them to infect the targeted population? Producing infected insects is possible but very laborious, expensive, and time consuming. However, the Japanese demonstrated, in the early 1940s, that they could mass produce millions of fleas infected with the plague bacterium, pack them into clay bomblets, and drop them on villages. This insidious act introduced plague into Manchuria and probably resulted in the death of thousands of innocent people (Alibek and Handelman, 2000).

Injection as a means of delivering biological agents may also take place through the use of a syringe or other mechanical device. A primary example of this occurred in September 1978, when a Bulgarian dissident, Georgi Markov, received a lethal dose of ricin from the tip of an umbrella (Alibek and Handelman, 2000). This small-scale incident is more an example of international espionage and intrigue than bioterrorism. Although the targets have to be executed one victim at a time, it points out the feasibility and covert nature of using injection as a method of delivery for biological agents.

□ □ □ ▬▬▬▬▬▬▬▬▬▬▬▬▬▬▬▬▬▬▬▬▬▬▬▬▬▬▬▬▬▬▬▬

Critical Thinking

Biological agents are part of the natural world. So, what makes it wrong to use them in warfare?

▬▬▬▬▬▬▬▬▬▬▬▬▬▬▬▬▬▬▬▬▬▬▬▬▬▬▬▬▬▬▬▬ □ □ □

Bacterial Pathogens

Bacteria are single-celled organisms capable of causing a variety of diseases in animals, plants, and humans. Bacteria are living cells that carry out many complex metabolic functions. They may also produce extremely potent *toxins* inside the human body. In a laboratory setting, these single-celled organisms may be cultured in nutrient media and will grow in rather distinct colonies given a solid surface. They vary in shape and size from spherical cells (cocci) to long rod-shaped organisms (bacilli). The shape of the bacterial cell is determined by the rigid cell wall. Although they do not have a distinct nucleus, the interior of the cell contains the nuclear material (DNA), cytoplasm, and cell membrane necessary for the life of the bacterium. Going back far into the history of microbiology, bacteria have been divided into two major subdivisions: gram positive and gram negative. The basis for this classification lies with microscopic examination of the sample after staining the cells with Gram's stain. This differentiation was a useful tool decades ago, but provides little taxonomic resolution in this age of sophisticated molecular diagnostics and bacterial systematics. Figure 2-1 depicts the history of microscopy in characterizing bacterial pathogens.

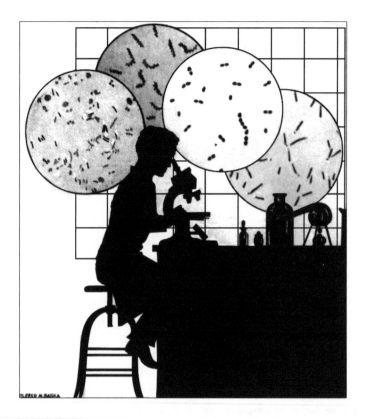

FIGURE 2-1 This historic illustration depicts a silhouette of a laboratory researcher sitting at a 1930s, lab bench and peering through a microscope. Within the circles in the background are artist's representations of different morphological forms of microbial pathogens. (Image courtesy of the CDC Public Health Image Library, No. 8583, originally provided by the Minnesota Department of Health, R. N. Barr Library.)

Under special circumstances some bacteria can transform into spores. *Spores* are a dormant form of the bacterium; like the seeds of plants, they can germinate when conditions are favorable. Formation of the spore is the cell's natural reaction given certain environmental stresses like extreme heat and drying. The spore of the bacterial cell is more resistant to cold, heat, drying, chemicals, and radiation than the vegetative bacterium itself. Bacteria generally cause disease in human beings and animals by one of two mechanisms: by invading host tissues or by producing poisons (toxins). Many pathogenic bacteria utilize both mechanisms. Figure 2-2 shows rod-shaped anthrax bacterium, *Bacillus anthracis*; vegetative cells and spores are obvious in this photomicrograph.

In general, bacteria that can enter and survive within eukaryotic cells are shielded from antibodies and can be eliminated only by a cellular immune response. However, these bacteria must possess specialized mechanisms to protect them from the harsh effects of digestive (lysosomal) enzymes encountered within the cell. Some bacteria (e.g., *Rickettsia*, *Coxiella*, and *Chlamydia*) grow only inside host cells; others (e.g., *Salmonella*, *Shigella*, and *Yersinia*) are facultative intracellular pathogens, invading cells when it gives them a selective advantage in the host. Regardless of the mechanisms for invasion and evasion, bacterial populations living within an infected individual compete for valuable nutrients, provoke an inflammatory response from the host, and cause host cells to die.

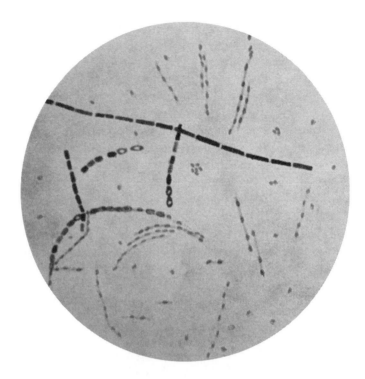

FIGURE 2-2 The anthrax bacteria, *Bacillus anthracis*, taken from an agar culture. Note the larger rod-shaped vegetative cells and smaller spores that show up well with a fuchsin–methylene blue spore stain.

Most bacterial infections can be effectively treated with antibiotic drugs, such as penicillin, ciprofloxacin, or tetracycline.

Rickettsial Pathogens

Rickettsiae are small, gram-negative bacteria that require a host cell. On infection, they reside in the cytoplasm or nucleus of the cell they invade. Many of the pathogenic rickettsial pathogens take up residence in red and white blood cells. Rickettsial pathogens frequently have a close relationship with arthropod vectors (e.g., ticks and fleas) that can transmit the organism to mammalian hosts. Normally, rickettsiae are inoculated into the dermis of the skin by a tick bite or through damaged skin from the feces of lice or fleas. The bacteria spread through the bloodstream and infect the linings of the vascular system. Rickettsial diseases vary in clinical severity according to the virulence of the *Rickettsia* and host factors, such as age, male gender, alcoholism, and other underlying diseases. The most serious rickettsial diseases are epidemic and scrub typhus, which kill a significant portion of infected persons. These diseases can be treated sufficiently early in the course of infection with an effective antimicrobial agent, usually doxycycline.

Viral Pathogens

Viruses are microorganisms much smaller than bacteria (approximately 2- to 60-fold smaller than a bacterium). Viruses were established as agents that cause human disease at the beginning of the 20th century. Like some bacteria, *all* viruses are obligate intracellular parasites. Meaning, they require living cells in order to multiply. Viruses are some of the simplest microorganisms. They are made up of an external protein coat (nucleocapsid) containing genetic material, either ribonucleic acid (RNA) or deoxyribonucleic acid (DNA). In some cases, an outer lipid (fat) layer also surrounds the viral particle. A virus particle is referred to as a **virion**. Viruses are totally dependent on the host cell for reproduction. Lacking a system for their own metabolism, viruses do not consume nutrients. These ubiquitous biological agents are found to infect virtually all living things; therefore, they have the potential to influence the entire biota of the planet. The host cells can be from humans, animals, plants, or bacteria. A virus typically brings about changes in the host cell that eventually leads to cellular death. The best way to control viral infections in a susceptible population is to prevent them from occurring through the use of a good vaccine. Vaccines have reduced the incidence of the viral diseases measles, mumps, and rubella by >99.7% in the United States and completely eliminated natural transmission of smallpox and poliovirus. Figure 2-3 is an electron micrograph of the Marburg virus, one of the hemorrhagic fever viruses.

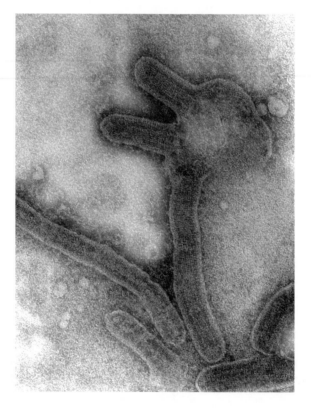

FIGURE 2-3 This negative stained transmission electron micrograph shows a number of Marburg virus particles (virions), which were in tissue culture cells. Marburg hemorrhagic fever is a rare, severe type of hemorrhagic fever that affects both humans and nonhuman primates. Caused by a genetically unique zoonotic (that is, animal-borne) RNA virus of the filovirus family, its recognition led to the creation of this virus family. The four species of Ebola virus are the only other known members of the filovirus family. (CDC Public Health Image Library, No. 7218, captured by F. A. Murphy in 1968.)

Prions

The conventional virus just described is not the simplest molecular pathogen. Protein-only pathogens called **prions** (pronounced PREE-ons) are the most basic pathogens known to exist. Presumably, prions replicate without a nucleic acid genome because they actually induce a structural or conformational change in other normal proteins. Prions are smaller than the smallest known virus and have not yet been completely characterized. They were discovered in 1982 by Stanley Prusiner, who at the time was studying what he thought to be slowly developing viral diseases. The name *prion* is supposed to be short for proteinaceous infectious particles. Given that design, their name should have really been *proin*, but Prusiner thought that *prion* was more catchy (Taubes, 1986). Much remains unknown about prions; however, the most widely accepted theory is that prions are mutated proteins. Prions cause degenerative neurological diseases called *spongiform encephalopathy* (sponge-like abnormalities of nervous tissues) in humans and other animals. These fatal neuron-degenerative disorders have attracted a great deal of attention because of their unique biological features and potential impact on public health (DeArmond and Prusiner, 1995).

This group of diseases includes kuru, Creutzfeldt-Jakob disease (CJD), Gerstmann-Straussler syndrome (GSS), and fatal familial insomnia (FFI) in human beings, as well as scrapie in sheep and goats and bovine spongiform encephalopathy (BSE or Mad Cow disease) in cattle. The primary symptom of the human prion-associated disorders is dementia, usually accompanied by manifestations of motor dysfunction. The symptoms appear insidiously in middle to late adult life and last from months to years prior to death. The abnormal protein is insoluble in all but the strongest solvents and highly resistant to digestion by proteases. It survives in tissues postmortem and is not destroyed by various rendering processes. The abnormal form of the protein is extremely resistant to heat, normal sterilization processes, and sunlight. It is also very resistant to most disinfectants and stable at a wide range of pH. The abnormal protein further does not evoke a detectable immune or inflammatory response in its host, so the body does not react to it as an invader.

Fungal Pathogens

When compared to bacteria and viruses, **fungi** are fairly complex microorganisms. Many of them are referred to as *molds* or *yeasts*. They are single-celled microbes that reproduce by a simple process known as budding. Normally, they play a very important role in the natural world by breaking down dead organic material, which ultimately adds to the cycle of nutrients through ecosystems. In addition, most plants could not grow without the symbiotic fungi, or mycorrhizae, that coexist with their roots to supply essential nutrients. Some fungi provide lifesaving drugs (e.g., penicillin) and foods (e.g., mushrooms, truffles, and morels).

Fungi cause many plant and animal diseases. In humans, they commonly cause ringworm and athlete's foot. More important, some fungal pathogens are highly pathogenic and capable of establishing an infection in all exposed individuals (e.g., *Histoplasma* and *Coccidioides*). Individuals that have a compromised immune system may develop infections from opportunist fungal pathogens (e.g., *Candida* and *Aspergillus*). In fact, these opportunistic fungi have become a major complication leading to the demise of many AIDS patients, since their immune systems are incapable of fighting off infection. Fungi are more physiologically similar to humans and other higher animals than other microbes; therefore, it can be fairly difficult to treat them. Some very serious plant diseases are caused by fungi. These include smuts, rusts, and leaf, root, and stem rots. Some early developments and efforts in the U.S. bioweapons programs centered on the use of fungal pathogens against crops.

Biological Toxins

Toxins are potent poisons produced by a variety of living organisms, including bacteria, plants, and animals. Some biological toxins are the most toxic substances known. Features that distinguish them from chemical agents, such as VX, cyanide, or mustard, include being not human made, nonvolatile (no vapor hazard), usually not dermally active (mycotoxins are the exception), and generally much more toxic per weight than chemical agents. Their lack of volatility is very important and makes them unlikely to produce either secondary or person-to-person exposures or a persistent environmental hazard.

Biological toxins are very large, complex molecules. A nerve agent, like sarin, has a molecular weight of approximately 140. Ricin, a potent toxin derived from the castor bean, has a molecular weight of about 66,000. Botulinum toxin is a very large molecule with a complex structure. Its molecular weight is approximately 150,000. The complex molecular structure of botulinum toxin is depicted in Figure 2-4.

Disease

Disease is defined by the Cambridge dictionary as "an illness of people, animals, plants, etc., caused by infection or a failure of health rather than by an accident." Here, it is appropriate to mention that we need to make a distinction between the agents and the disease or syndrome that a particular agent causes. *Infectious diseases are caused by an agent, typically referred to as an etiologic agent.* Are diseases transmitted or are their agents? To be exact, agents are transmitted. For example, the etiologic agent of anthrax is *Bacillus anthracis*. From the 2001 Amerithrax incident we often hear that "anthrax was sent through the mail." People cannot send diseases through the mail. Instead, we should say that *Bacillus anthracis* spores were sent through the mail. However, it is now so common to state it the other way around that it has become acceptable language.

A person who has a disease presents himself or herself to a medical authority for diagnosis. How that person presents him- or herself is referred to as clinical presentation. Here, the doctor describes the condition of the patient in a systematic fashion. Furthermore, a disease can have many different **clinical manifestations**. For instance, plague has many forms or manifestations. This is dependent on how the patient acquired the infection and how advanced the disease is. So, with plague, we could be talking about bubonic plague, septicemic plague, primary pneumonic plague, or secondary pneumonic plague. This becomes more apparent when we look at the specific diseases and their etiologies. **Etiology** is defined as the scientific study of the cause of diseases.

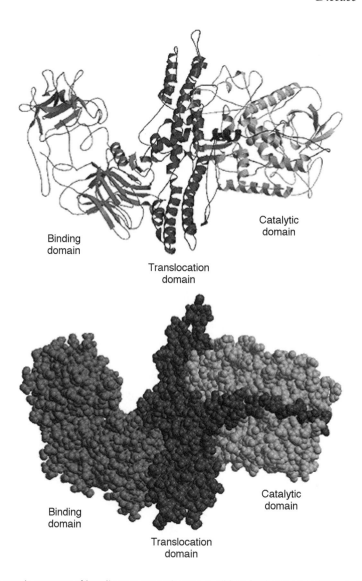

Binding
domain

Catalytic
domain

Translocation
domain

Binding
domain

Catalytic
domain

Translocation
domain

FIGURE 2-4 The atomic structure of botulinum neurotoxin type A. Ribbon (top) and space filling (bottom) models of the X-ray crystal structure of botulinum neurotoxin type A. The toxin consists of a binding domain, translocation domain, and catalytic domain. (Taken with kind permission from "Microbial Forensics," Chapter 7 in *Forensic Aspects of Biologic Toxins* by Dr. James D. Marks, Department of Anesthesia and Pharmaceutical Chemistry, University of California, San Francisco General Hospital, copyright © 2005 by Elsevier Inc.)

□ □ □

Critical Thinking

How will we recognize that a biological attack has occurred? What members of the community will be most at risk?

□ □ □

Tiered Diagnosis

Any small or large outbreak of reportable, unusual, or rare diseases should be evaluated as a potential bioterrorist attack (Pavlin, 1999). This initial investigation or inquiry should be sparked by a clinician's healthy suspicion. It need not be time consuming nor involve law enforcement. At first, clinicians should attempt to uncover the facts surrounding the outbreak to determine if anything seems unusual or indicative of bioterrorism. The disease outbreak might be due to a laboratory accident or it may be the result of a spontaneous outbreak of endemic disease, an outbreak of a new or reemerging disease, or an intentional release of a biological agent. Epidemiologists have many tools to determine the cause of the outbreak. However, health care providers stand on the front lines and must be the first to key public health officials that there is something out of the ordinary.

Disease goes hand in hand with diagnosis. Important patient management decisions depend on an accurate diagnosis. Reportable diseases and other diseases of public health significance often have a **case definition** to assist clinicians in their decision making. Typically, when a patient presents him- or herself to a clinician, there is a complaint. In the complaint, the patient will describe the way he or she feels, detailing to the clinician the abnormal condition. The complaint and its description constitute the **symptoms** of disease. The clinician examines the patient to observe any abnormal conditions. These observations constitute the **signs** of disease. The signs and symptoms of an infectious disease presented by the patient may be assembled by the clinician to classify them into a general syndrome (e.g., fever and rash, fever and cough). The clinician will order a number of diagnostic tests (or assays) to supplement the information already collected from the clinical presentation. Diagnostics may be performed locally at the medical treatment facility or sent off to a supporting or reference laboratory for more sophisticated technology (Snyder, 1999). Once the clinician has the test results, he or she will couple them with the clinical presentation to form an opinion as to what disease the patient may have.

In addition, the physician will often consider other probable or possible etiologies that present in the same manner. Here, a **differential diagnosis** approach is likely to be used to "rule in" or "rule out" the various possibilities. As more information is collected from the results of diagnostic tests and the development of other signs and symptoms, the physician will ultimately come to a conclusion. The diagnosis of many infectious diseases will be viewed in the context of a **tiered diagnostic system** (TDS), whereby the diagnosis will go from **suspected** to **probable** to **confirmed**. The three phases of the TDS are as follows:

- **Suspected.** This constitutes the first tier in the TDS. A suspected case is one that is compatible with the clinical description of the disease in the case definition and has an epidemiological link to a suspected disease origin. Consider Patient X who presents to a physician with fever, malaise, and a persistent, productive cough; and the patient had contact with a known tuberculosis patient several months ago. Given that scenario, the physician may consider Patient X to be a suspected case of TB.

- **Probable.** This constitutes the second tier in the TDS. Here, a probable case designation comes from a suspected case that also has a positive test result from an intermediary laboratory test. Given the preceding scenario, the clinician performed a tuberculin skin test on Patient X and the result came back positive. In addition, a chest X-ray shows a spot on the left lung of Patient X. Because of this, the doctor now considers the patient to have a probable case of TB.

- **Confirmed.** This constitutes the third tier in the TDS. Here, a suspected case or probable case is backed up by a definitive or confirmatory laboratory test. In the preceding scenario, a sputum sample from Patient X results in a positive culture, where the etiologic agent of TB, *Mycobacterium tuberculosis*, is grown in the laboratory. Further tests may be performed to determine the pathogen's sensitivity to specific antibiotics because antibiotic-resistant TB is a growing problem with serious consequences for the patient.

If the diagnosis turns out to be a reportable or rare disease, as in the scenario, the physician will contact the local public health agency. In addition, treatment may begin once a proper diagnosis has been formulated by the clinician. **Post-infection treatment** may begin at any point in the TDS as deemed prudent by the clinician. Typically, antibiotics are given to treat people infected with bacteria. However, antibiotics do nothing for viral infections. It may also be prudent for the clinician working in concert with public health officials to treat persons that have had contact with the infected patient. This type of treatment is referred to as **prophylactic treatment.** The goal of prophylactic treatment is to keep exposed individuals from becoming symptomatic and infectious to others, thereby reducing the chances that infection will spread among the population. Mass prophylaxis programs in the wake of a bioterrorist event can be very challenging, as large quantities of drugs or vaccines may need to be administered to the public in an orderly and efficient manner.

The medical expertise, laboratories, and communication networks needed to counter bioterrorism are the same resources that are needed to detect diseases in the community from any source, whether natural or deliberate. The Centers for Disease Control has developed diagnostic protocols that can be used to either "rule in" or "rule out" certain biological agents that represent a threat to the public. Nationally, the CDC has developed a network of laboratories, known as the Laboratory Response Network (LRN), that has a specified list of diagnostic tests and procedures to identify the bioterrorism agents. These tests can be performed on clinical and environmental samples. The LRN is fully explored in Chapter 12.

Probability of Use

All nations are vulnerable to the strategic, tactical, and terrorist use of biological weapons. This vulnerability comes from the fact that most agents in the arsenal come from rare diseases selected for their lethality and lack of innate or herd immunity of susceptible populations (Army, 1977). In that regard, we are universally vulnerable. We now know what types of biological agents constitute the threat.

However, many weapons of mass destruction are available to the would-be terrorist or state-sponsored aggressor. Commonly, explosives are used, as they are very effective in creating casualties and have an immediate and noticeable outcome whenever they are used effectively. So, why would an aggressor select a biological agent, and what factors are important in making that choice? To explore this, one might have to "think like a terrorist" and consider the advantages and disadvantages of using them.

One of the most ironic aspects of the United States' bioweapons program was that it probably created its own monster. Although it was designed to counter the threat to the United States, it in fact increased the threats on the same front. Today, there is an edict in military thinking about war and honor that puts the use of biological weaponry in a very negative context. Biological weapons are considered to be unfair, like something done covertly by an enemy who really lacks a sense of honor. Moreover, the threat of attack with biological agents creates psychological effects out of proportion to the threat. The fear factor is considerable, and in that regard, they are often considered to be weapons of mass "distraction" rather than mass destruction.

Depending on the desired outcome of a terrorist act, biological agents may offer considerable advantages to an aggressor who chooses to deploy them. However, the advantages must be weighed against some of the disadvantages. An attack using biological agents may be viewed as more sinister and insidious than an attack using conventional weapons because the effects are delayed and cryptic. By the time the index case is discovered, the agent will have already been consumed or inhaled by the masses. Because of this, more morbidity and mortality will result before medical and nonmedical interventions can mitigate the burden of disease. With minimal logistical requirements, biological weapons have the potential to inflict large numbers of casualties over a very wide area. In 1970, the World Health Organization published a document that discussed the threat of chemical and biological weapons and how they might be deployed against civilian populations. In this report, the WHO showed a table of casualty estimates produced by the release of approximately 110 pounds (50 kilograms) of various weaponized materials upwind of a population center of 500,000 people, given ideal weather conditions. Table 2-1 shows the mass casualty–producing potential highlights of these agents (WHO Report, 1970).

Some potential adversaries may overcome their conventional military inadequacies by choosing unconventional weapons that can be produced easily, cheaply, and with technology already available to them. It is considerably less expensive to produce biological weapons materials than chemical or nuclear agents. The cost advantage of biological weapons was demonstrated in a 1969 United Nations report that estimated the cost of operations against civilian populations at $1 per square kilometer for biological weapons versus $600 per square kilometer for chemical, $800 per square kilometer for nuclear, and $2,000 per square kilometer for conventional explosives.

Table 2-1 An Estimate of Mass Casualty Potential for Specific Biological Weapons

Disease/Agent	Downwind Reach (miles)	Human Casualties	
		Dead	Incapacitated
Rift Valley fever/RVF virus	>1	400	35,000
Tick-borne encephalitis/TBE virus	>1	9,500	35,000
Typhus/Rickettsia prowazeki	3	19,000	85,000
Brucellosis/Brucella species	6	500	100,000
Q fever/Coxiella burnetii	>12	150	125,000
Tularemia/Francisella tularensis	>12	30,000	125,000
Anthrax/Bacillus anthracis	>12	95,000	125,000

Note: Based on a hypothetical scenario estimating release of 50 kg (110 pounds) of the weaponized agent from a plane flying along a 2-km (1.2 miles) line upwind of a population center of 500,000 people in a developing country. (Adapted from WHO, 1970, p. 98.)

Aggressors might choose to covertly deploy biological weapons, since it is difficult for targeted communities to detect the presence of the agent and render some forms of treatment to the intended victims. Following an outbreak of disease, an aggressor may also be able to deny the use of such a weapon after casualties occur. This "plausible deniability" can be supported by claims or confusion that the outbreak is a natural occurrence. In addition, medical countermeasures needed to quell the outbreak in human populations may take a long time to field due to regulatory requirements imposing strict guidelines on the development and production of new vaccines and drugs for prophylaxis or treatment (NATO, 1992).

□ □ □ ▬▬▬▬▬▬▬▬▬▬▬▬▬▬▬▬▬▬▬▬▬▬▬▬

Advantages and Disadvantages of Using Biologicals

Advantages

- Low cost of producing many biological agents.
- Small quantities may have dramatic effects.
- Deadly or incapacitating effects on a susceptible population.
- Agent formulations may be easily disseminated.
- Difficulty in diagnosing index cases.
- Can result in fear, panic, and social disruption.
- Symptoms can mimic endemic, naturally occurring diseases.

Disadvantages

- Biological agents may affect the health of the aggressor.
- Agent desired may be difficult or impossible to acquire.
- Weather conditions directly effect dispersion.
- Weather conditions lessen the survivability of some organisms.
- May not generate immediate attention; incubation period to consider.
- Advanced technology needed to produce most formulations.

▬▬▬▬▬▬▬▬▬▬▬▬▬▬▬▬▬▬▬▬▬▬▬ □ □ □

To an aggressor, biological weapons may be a very attractive option from a variety of standpoints, which include low cost, natural availability, ease of dissemination, difficulty of detection, plausible deniability, and the ability to cause mass casualties, fear, panic, and social disruption. However, there are numerous disadvantages to using biological warfare agents, both to the target population and the aggressor forces. One major disadvantage is that they are classified as weapons of mass destruction. Their use by a sovereign state may bring about a retaliatory attack and immediate escalation of military conflict. As previously mentioned, we are universally vulnerable to the biological agents that have been the subject of past and present biological weapons programs. Therefore, the weapons themselves are dangerous to the aggressor as well as the intended victims. Historically, biological weapons have been difficult to control after release. Those that are communicable (person-to-person transmission) may spread from the intended target area to unintended targets. In Ken Alibek's book *Biohazard* (2000), he discusses an incident in the summer of 1942 where the Russians deployed *Francisella tularensis* (the etiologic agent of tularemia) in the Battle for Stalingrad. The intended target was thousands of German soldiers manning the front; however, thousands of Russian soldiers and tens of thousands of Russian civilians were also infected.

Many agents are not stable in the environment and their formulations have been greatly influenced by environmental conditions. The plague bacterium, *Yersinia pestis*, is a very fragile organism when it is not either inside the mammalian host or vectoring flea. Exposure to the sun, drying, and temperature extremes often kill bacteria and viruses after dissemination. Spore-forming bacteria are an exception to this. Areas where lethal spores have been deployed remained dangerous for decades (e.g., anthrax and Gruinard Island, Scotland).

Conclusion

Bacteria, rickettsia, viruses, fungi, and biological toxins are the agents that would most commonly be exploited for their use in a biological weapon. There are characteristics common to all of these agents. Most notably, they may be acquired naturally, especially if one knows where to look for them. All are invisible to the human senses and require incubation periods before disease conditions are noticeable; therefore, they might be deployed covertly and evidence of the event may not be apparent for days or weeks. The four routes of entry into the host are by inhalation, ingestion, absorption, and injection. Most biological weapons formulations have been adapted for entry by inhalation. Following infection, patients manifest signs and symptoms of disease. Clinical presentation results in a differential diagnosis, where many disease possibilities may be considered. Following that, a tiered diagnostic system may be employed so that as additional information is known about the patient the diagnosis may proceed from suspected to probable to confirmed. Clinicians must remain vigilant to the possibility that rare or unusual diseases may be due to an act of bioterrorism. The ever-present threat of biological weapons and emerging diseases has given rise to programs and initiatives in biodefense and biosecurity. Much has been done in the past five years, but we are all extremely vulnerable to their awesome potential.

Essential Terminology

- **Biological toxin.** A toxic substance originating from a living organism. Most biological toxins are used for defense; are very large, complex molecules; and are among the most toxic substances known to higher animals. Botulinum toxin is the most deadly substance known to humans.
- **Diagnosis.** The determination of the presence of a specific disease or infection, usually accomplished by evaluating clinical symptoms and laboratory tests.
- **Differential diagnosis.** Distinguishing among two or more diseases and conditions with similar clinical findings, including physical signs and symptoms, as well as the results of laboratory tests and other appropriate diagnostic procedures.
- **Incubation period.** Most biological agents require days to weeks before the effects are felt. Once the incubation period is completed, victims will begin to exhibit effects of

the exposure that occurred days or weeks before. The time required for a biological agent to gain access to the human body and cause harm is highly dependent on the dose a person receives and the pathogenicity of that agent. Periods may vary from a few hours with a toxin, to many days or weeks with a bacteria or virus.

- **Post-infection treatment.** Typically, antibiotics are given to treat people infected with bacteria. However, antibiotics do nothing for viral infections.
- **Prophylactic treatment.** General medical attention given to expected victims on discovery of possible exposure to biological events.
- **Signs.** Anything observed in a patient that indicates the presence of a disease.
- **Symptoms.** A change from normal function, sensation, or appearance, generally indicating disease or disorder. Typically, patients explain or describe their symptoms and health-care professionals note the signs.
- **Tiered diagnosis.** A systematic approach to reaching a definitive diagnosis after a patient presents with the signs and symptoms of illness. Within this approach, clinicians apply the signs and symptoms to a case definition to reach a *suspected* diagnosis. From here, some diagnostic tests can be applied to reach a *probable* diagnosis, if the tests turn out to be positive. Finally, definitive diagnostic tests coupled with patient presentation allow the physician to reach a *confirmed* diagnosis. When it comes to the agents most likely to be used in an act of bioterrorism, the Laboratory Response Network performs the definitive diagnostic test.
- **Virion.** A virus particle or unit.
- **Virulence.** The degree of pathogenicity of a microorganism, as indicated by the severity of the disease produced and its ability to invade the tissues of a host. It is measured experimentally by the median lethal dose (LD_{50}) or median infective dose (ID_{50}). By extension, the competence of any infectious agent to produce pathologic effects.

Discussion Questions

- In what ways can biological agents enter the body? Which ways might be practically exploited by bioweapons technology?
- What is the most common way to treat bacterial diseases?
- What is the best prevention for viral diseases?
- What is a tiered diagnostic system?
- What are the advantages and disadvantages of using biological agents as a weapon? In answering, think like a terrorist.

Web Sites

Centers for Disease Control and Prevention, home page for information about bioterrorism: www.bt.cdc.gov/bioterrorism.

The Microbiology Information Portal: www.microbes.info.

The Microbiology Network: www.microbiol.org.

BiodefenseEducation.org is a Biodefense Digital Library and Learning Collaboratory intended to serve as a source of continuing education on biodefense, bioterrorism, and biological warfare: www.biodefenseeducation.org.

National Biosecurity Resource Center: www.biosecuritycenter.org.

References

Alibek, K., with S. Handelman. 2000. *Biohazard: The Chilling True Story of the Largest Covert Biological Weapons Program in the World—Told from the Inside by the Man Who Ran It.* New York: Random House.

DeArmond, S. J., and S. B. Prusiner. 1995. Etiology and pathogenesis of prion diseases. *American Journal of Pathology* 146, no. 4:785–811.

Department of the Army. 1977. Special Report to Congress. *US Army Activities in the US Biological Defense Programs, 1942–1977*, vols. 1 and 2. Washington, DC: Department of the Army.

North Atlantic Treaty Organization. 1992. *NATO Handbook on the Medical Aspects of NBC Defensive Operations*, AMed-P6, part 2, Biological. Brussels, Belgium: NATO.

Pavlin, J. 1999. Epidemiology of bioterrorism. *Emerging Infectious Diseases* 5, no. 4:528–530.

Snyder, J. W. 1999. Responding to bioterrorism: The role of the microbiology laboratory. *American Society of Microbiology News* 65 (November 8):524–525.

Special Subcommittee on the National Science Foundation of the Committee on Labor and Public Welfare, U.S. Senate. 1969. *Chemical and Biological Weapons: Some Possible Approaches for Lessening the Threat and Danger.* Washington, DC: US Government Printing Office.

Taubes, G. 1986. The game of the name is fame. But is it science? Stanley Prusiner, "discoverer" of prions. *Discover.*

World Health Organization. 1970. *Health Aspects of Chemical and Biological Weapons: Report of a WHO Group of Consultants.* Geneva, Switzerland: WHO.

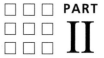

PART

II

The Threat to Human Health

Part II of this book provides essential, detailed information on the biological agents and diseases that pose the highest risk to national security. The Centers for Disease Control and Prevention published an updated list of what are considered some of the more critical biological agents we may face today.

The genesis of this listing began with a congressional initiative in 1999 aimed at upgrading national public health capabilities for response to acts of biological terrorism. Accordingly, the CDC was designated the lead agency for overall public health planning. In June 1999, nationally recognized infectious disease and public health experts, Department of Health and Human Services (HHS) agency representatives, military intelligence experts, and law enforcement officials met to review and comment on the threat potential of various agents to civilian populations. The expert panel considered factors such as agent-related morbidity and mortality, potential for distributing the agent based on its stability, ability to mass produce and distribute the agent, and the possibility for person-to-person transmission of the agent. The panel also considered the potential that the presence of the disease might result in public fear, panic, and possible civil disruption. In addition, special public health preparedness needs based on stockpile requirements, enhanced surveillance, or diagnostic needs were considered in developing the list of agents.

The resulting list of critical biological agents was divided into three categories (A, B, and C), based on the level of public health importance. High-priority agents include organisms that pose a risk to national security because they

- Can be easily disseminated or transmitted from person to person.
- Result in high mortality rates.
- Might cause public panic and social disruption.
- Require special action for public health preparedness.

The most serious threats have been placed in Category A. Category A agents and their diseases are both fascinating and vitally important to biodefense and biosecurity programs. These biological agents could be easily disseminated to many people in a given area, with the potential for a major public health impact.

Category B agents, although not as threatening as Category A, are serious threats to human and animal health. Many were considered to be "good candidates" for weapons of biowarfare due to their ease of dissemination and incapacitating effect. Realize that, if one were to use biowarfare as an option in battle, one may wish to make more soldiers sick than kill them. This would place a tremendous burden on the enemy.

Category C agents are often emerging or reemerging disease threats, something very much in the public eye. Think back to a time not so long ago when SARS raised its ugly head or West Nile fever appeared mysteriously in New York City in the summer of 1999. These agents may not be as promising a candidate for weaponization, but they may be exploited for the attention that they generate within the media.

You will find that many of these diseases are zoonoses, or animal diseases that also affect humans. As stated in Part I, there is a very good reason why many of these diseases and the pathogens that cause them have been so devastating to us. Whenever we consider this in biosecurity and biodefense programs, we should attempt to understand the inter-relatedness of the dynamics of disease, agent transmission, and the factors that make it all come together naturally. As such, we address these components whenever a zoonotic disease is detailed in this book. Consider the following for zoonotic disease pathogens.

An act of bioterrorism aimed at humans may have a secondary affect on the animals that live in close association with the victims. Animals secondarily infected in such a scenario may manifest the disease earlier than the human targets. In this way, the animals infected could be considered sentinels to alert us to the occurrence of an unusual or rare disease. In fact, once the pathogen gets into the animal population it may sustain or amplify the disease in the area for a longer duration.

Conversely, an act of agroterrorism aimed at animals may have a secondary affect on the humans that live nearby or work with the intended animal victims. As such, humans may manifest the disease earlier than the animal hosts and they could even sustain the disease in an area if attention to such a condition were overlooked or misdiagnosed. Although the correct use of terminology and the manner in which we view these situations may seem to be academic to many, it is important to remember that responders, health-care workers, public health officials, and animal health professionals must be prepared to face various biological agents, including those that are rarely encountered in the United States.

3

Category A Diseases and Agents

The single biggest threat to man's continued dominance on the planet is a virus.
—Joshua Lederberg, Ph.D., Nobel Laureate

Objectives

The study of this chapter will enable you to

1. List and explain the criteria used to define Category A agents.
2. Describe the signs and symptoms of anthrax, plague, tularemia, smallpox, viral hemorrhagic fever, and botulism.
3. Describe the clinical manifestations of anthrax, plague, tularemia, smallpox, viral hemorrhagic fever, and botulism.
4. Discuss prophylaxis and medical treatment strategies used to counter anthrax, plague, tularemia, smallpox, viral hemorrhagic fever, and botulism.
5. Understand the challenges that public health officials and emergency management practitioners face when an intentional release of a Category A agent occurs in their community.

Key Terms

Category A, anthrax, plague, tularemia, smallpox, viral hemorrhagic fever, contact, botulism, *Bacillus anthracis*, *Yersinia pestis*, *Francisella tularensis*, filovirus, arenavirus, flavivirus, bunyaviruses, *Clostridium botulinum*.

Introduction

Terrorism experts are most concerned with **Category A** agents because they have the greatest potential for harm if used in a bioterrorist attack. These agents can be easily disseminated or transmitted, cause high mortality, severely affect the public health, might cause public panic and social disruption, and require special action for public health preparedness (Rotz et al., 2002). Six diseases are caused by Category A agents (refer to Table 3-1 for a summary): anthrax, plague, tularemia, smallpox, viral hemorrhagic fever, and botulism. All six of these diseases and the agents that cause them are detailed here.

Table 3-1 Category A Diseases and Their Etiologic Agents: A Summary

Disease	Agent	Type of Agent	Zoonoses	Contagious Person to Person?
Anthrax	*Bacillus anthracis*	Bacteria	Yes	No
Plague	*Yersinia pestis*	Bacteria	Yes	Yes, in pneumonic form
Tularemia	*Francisella tularensis*	Bacteria	Yes	No
Smallpox	*Variola major*	Virus	No	Yes
Viral Hemorrhagic Fever	Several from Arenaviridae, Filoviridae, Bunyaviridae and Flaviviridae	Virus	Yes	Yes
Botulism	Botulinum toxin from *Clostridium botulinum*	Toxin	No	No

Anthrax

Anthrax, a disease of both humans and other mammals, is caused by the bacterium *Bacillus anthracis*. Anthrax was the first disease for which a microbial etiology was firmly established (in 1876) and the first bacterial disease for which immunization was available (in 1881). Although anthrax has been known since antiquity, it was not always clearly distinguished from other diseases with similar manifestations. Scholars have characterized the fifth and sixth biblical plagues as well as the "burning plague" described in Homer's Iliad as anthrax. However, it was Virgil (70–19 BC) who provided one of the earliest and most detailed descriptions of an anthrax epidemic in his Georgics. Virgil also noted that the disease could spread to humans (Sternbach, 2003).

Over the next 1,500 years, Europe witnessed sporadic outbreaks of anthrax, with the most acute outbreaks occurring in 14th-century Germany and 17th-century Russia and central Europe. Despite the threat these outbreaks posed to livestock, it was only in 1769 that Jean Fournier classified the disease as anthrax or *charbon malin*, a name undoubtedly derived from the black lesions characteristic of cutaneous anthrax. Anthrax has also been commonly referred to as woolsorter's disease, ragpicker's disease, malignant carbuncle, and malignant pustule. The bacterium and its associated disease get their name from the Greek word for coal, or anthracite, because of the characteristic coal-black sore that is the hallmark of the most common form of the disease (Sternbach, 2003). In fact, the Greek word *anthrakôsis* means "'malignant ulcer."

The Etiologic Agent of Anthrax

Bacillus anthracis is a gram-positive rod-shaped bacteria approximately 4 μm long by 1 μm wide. The anthrax bacterium is found nearly worldwide, with hundreds of different strains cataloged in numerous archives. The bacterium can take two forms: the vegetative bacilli and the spore. *Bacillus anthracis* is highly dependent on the spore form for survival. Within infected hosts, spores germinate to produce the vegetative forms, which release toxins and multiply, eventually killing the host. A proportion of these vegetative bacilli released by the dying or dead animal into the environment (usually the soil under the carcass) sporulate, ready to infect another animal. Vegetative forms of *B. anthracis* grow and multiply readily in normal laboratory nutrient agars or broths (e.g., sheep's blood agar, MacConkey's agar, trypticase soy broth).

When conditions are not conducive to growth and multiplication of the vegetative bacilli, *B. anthracis* forms spores. The process of sporulation occurs when vegetative cells encounter high temperature, low moisture, a nutrient-poor environment, or the presence of free oxygen. These spores are resistant to physical extremes of heat, cold, drying, pH, and even some of the chemicals used in disinfection or decontamination. Spores can survive for decades in soil, and it is through the uptake of spores that anthrax is contracted.

Humans appear to be relatively resistant to anthrax. Estimates as to how many anthrax spores must be inhaled to produce a fatal outcome in a human victim vary widely (2,500–55,000 spores) and can be quite controversial. Bear in mind that lethality estimates are based on primate studies conducted decades ago with specific *Bacillus anthracis* strains formulated by bioweapons specialists.

Anthrax: True Zoonoses

Anthrax is a disease that gravely affects humans and other animals. The disease most often occurs in herbivores (e.g., cattle, sheep, goats, camels, and antelope) but can also occur in humans and other warm-blooded animals. Carnivores (e.g., dogs, cats, and lions) and omnivores (e.g., swine) may become infected by eating uncooked meat from infected animals; however, many carnivores appear to have a natural resistance. Herbivores may become infected by ingesting spores while grazing in areas of high soil contamination (Dixon et al., 1999).

Anthrax is most common in temperate agricultural regions. Areas of high risk include South and Central America, southern and Eastern Europe, Africa, Asia, the Caribbean, and the Middle East. Natural incidence is extremely low in the United States, although outbreaks have been reported in California, Louisiana, Mississippi, Nebraska, North Dakota, Oklahoma, South Dakota, and Texas.

Human anthrax has three major clinical forms: **cutaneous, inhalation**, and **gastrointestinal**. If left untreated, all three forms can result in septicemia and death. Human exposures are usually occupational, resulting from handling infected livestock, infected wild animals, or contaminated animal tissues or products. The best documented evidence of this comes from studies in the 1960s in mills in which unvaccinated workers "chronically exposed" to anthrax had annual case rates of 0.6–1.4% (Dahlgren et al., 1960). In a study of two such mills, *B. anthracis* was recovered from the nose and pharynx of 14% of healthy workers; in another study, workers were inhaling 600–1,300 spores during the work day with no ill effect, although a well-documented outbreak of pulmonary anthrax occurred in one mill with a similar level of contamination (Albrink et al., 1960; Brachman, Kaufman and Dalldorf, 1966).

Cutaneous anthrax, rare in the United States, is common in parts of Asia and sub-Saharan Africa. Cutaneous anthrax results when *Bacillus anthracis* gains entry to the body through an abrasion or open lesion of the victim. A typical cutaneous anthrax lesion is depicted in Figure 3-1. Ingestion of undercooked meat from anthrax-infected animals results in gastrointestinal anthrax (AVMA, 2006a). Inhalation anthrax has been a hazard associated with slaughterhouse and textile workers; immunization has virtually eliminated this hazard in the Western nations. Anthrax as a weapon would most likely be delivered via an aerosol, resulting in inhalation anthrax.

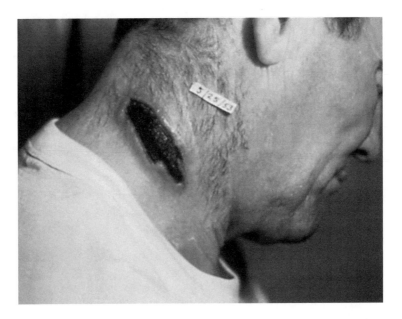

FIGURE 3-1 Photograph depicts cutaneous anthrax lesion on the neck of a patient. Note the "coallike" appearance of the lesion. Cutaneous anthrax is the most common clinical manifestation of anthrax, with most patients having some occupational exposure to infected animal product. (Image courtesy of CDC Public Health Image Library, No. 1934, photo taken in 1953.)

The incubation period for inhalational anthrax in humans is one to seven days. In the initial phase, it appears as a nonspecific illness characterized by mild fever, malaise, myalgia, nonproductive cough, and some chest or abdominal pain. The illness progresses within two to three days leading to fever, painful cough, cyanosis, wheezing, mediastinal widening, and subcutaneous edema of the chest and neck. The second stage of inhalation anthrax occurs within 24 to 36 hours and is characterized by high fever, difficulty breathing, cyanosis (a bluish discoloration of the skin and mucous membranes resulting from inadequate oxygenation of the blood), and shock (Swartz, 2001). Chest-wall edema and hemorrhagic meningitis may be seen late in the course of the disease.

☐ ☐ ☐ ▬▬▬▬▬▬▬▬▬▬▬▬▬▬▬▬▬▬▬▬▬▬▬▬▬▬▬▬▬

Anthrax Bacterium as a Terrorist Threat

The anthrax bacterium has several characteristics that make it a formidable bioterrorist threat. These characteristics include its stability in spore form, its ease of culture and production, its ability to be aerosolized, the seriousness of the disease it causes, and the lack of sufficient vaccine for widespread use (Eitzen, 1997).

▬▬▬▬▬▬▬▬▬▬▬▬▬▬▬▬▬▬▬▬▬▬▬▬▬▬▬▬▬ ☐ ☐ ☐

Early antibiotic treatment of cutaneous and gastrointestinal anthrax is usually curative; however, even with antibiotic therapy, inhalational anthrax is a potentially fatal disease. Although case-fatality estimates for inhalational anthrax are based on incomplete information, the historical rate is considered to be high (about 75%) for naturally occurring or accidental infections, even with appropriate antibiotics and all other available supportive care (Cieslak and Eitzen, 1999). During the entire 20th century, there were 18 diagnosed cases of inhalation anthrax, 16 of which were fatal (Sternbach, 2003). The best chance for survival is to receive antibiotics and medical care within the first 48 hours of the onset of signs. Interestingly, the survival rate after the recent intentional exposure to anthrax in the United States was 60% for the first 10 cases (Thompson, 2003).

Cutaneous anthrax cases in the United States early in the 20th century averaged 200 cases per year. During the second half of the century, this decreased to approximately six cases per year. Since the 2001 Amerithrax incident, there have been five cases of human cutaneous anthrax and one case of inhalation anthrax (CDC, Morbidity and Mortality Weekly Report [MMWR] summaries). All of these anthrax cases occurred in drum makers and were associated with the victims handling infected goat skins (MMWR 2006; ProMED Mail 2007).

Anthrax in Animals

Anthrax occurs in several forms in animals, defined mostly by the length of the clinical course of the disease. The incubation period of natural infection in animals is typically 3–7 days, with a range of 1–14 or more days. In cattle and sheep, the *peracute* course of the illness may last only one to two hours, during which one of the first clinical indications of disease may be the animal's sudden death. Clinical signs, such as fever up to 107°F, muscle tremors, respiratory distress, and convulsions, often go unnoticed. After death, there may be bloody discharges from the natural openings of the body, rapid bloating, and a lack of rigor mortis; blood may not clot (AVMA 2006a).

The acute form of anthrax in ruminants may run a course of 24–48 hours. Affected animals may exhibit a high fever, complete anorexia, diarrhea, severe depression, and listlessness. Pregnant cows may abort, milk production may drop severely, and what milk there is may be yellow or blood stained.

Outbreaks in the United States are most often associated with alkaline soil, and there are some areas where it is more endemic. Wet conditions followed by hot, dry weather in summer or fall are considered good conditions under which anthrax cases in livestock (cattle primarily) are likely to be seen.

Diagnosis of Anthrax

Anthrax is diagnosed by isolating *B. anthracis* from the blood, skin lesions, or respiratory secretions or by measuring specific antibodies in the blood of persons with suspected cases. An enzyme-linked immunosorbent assay (ELISA) was developed by the CDC for anthrax and was quickly qualified during the outbreak in the fall of 2001 (Quinn et al., 2002). It proved to be accurate, sensitive, reproducible, and quantitative. The nasal swab test was used as a screening tool during the 2001 Amerithrax outbreak to determine if anyone associated with the case patient might have been exposed. In this setting, the nasal swab method was used for a rapid assessment of exposure and as a tool for rapid environmental assessment. When the source of exposure is not known, nasal swabs can help investigators screen potential contacts. However, these tests are for screening purposes only and are not used for definitively diagnosing anthrax. Furthermore, they are not 100% effective in determining all who may have been exposed.

□ □ □

Acts of Biological Terrorism
Previous acts of biological terrorism have been small in scale.

The Potential
A 1993 report by U.S. Congressional Office of Technology Assessment estimated 130,000 to 3 million deaths following the aerosolized release of 100 kg of anthrax spores upwind of Washington, D.C.

The Reality
In the aftermath of the 2001 Amerithrax incident, the CDC conducted a telephone survey of 40 state and territorial health officials. According to the results of the survey, during the time period September 11 to October 17, 2001, more than 7,000 reports of suspicious powders had been received at the health departments. Approximately 4,800 of these reports required phone follow-up, and 1,050 reports led to testing of suspicious materials at a public health laboratory. In comparison, the number of anthrax threats reported to public health authorities from 1996 to 2000 did not exceed 180 reported threats per year.

The antibiotic ciprofloxacin was offered to many people in the aftermath of anthrax mailings in 2001. According to one report, 5,343 people were prescribed "cipro" for 60 days. Only 44% of those given the drugs adhered to the 60-day regimen. Amazingly, 57% of those taking the drug experienced side effects (diarrhea, abdominal pain, dizziness, nausea, and vomiting) from taking the drug.

□ □ □

Penicillin has been the drug of choice for anthrax for many decades, and only very rarely has penicillin resistance been found in naturally occurring isolates. Preliminary data from the Florida, New York, and Washington, D.C. isolates showed possible resistance to penicillin, so treatment with ciprofloxacin was recommended. Considerations for choosing an antimicrobial agent include effectiveness, resistance, side effects, and cost. No evidence demonstrates that ciprofloxacin is more or less effective than doxycycline for antimicrobial prophylaxis to B. anthracis. Widespread use of any antimicrobial will promote resistance. However, fluoroquinolone resistance is not yet common in these organisms. To preserve the effectiveness of fluoroquinolone against other infections, use of doxycycline for prevention of B. anthracis infection among populations at risk may be preferable.

In the United States, human anthrax vaccine is a cell-free filtrate, produced from an avirulent strain. The vaccine contains no whole bacteria, dead or alive. The vaccine was developed during the 1950s and 1960s for humans and was licensed by the FDA in 1970. Since 1970, it has been administered to at-risk wool mill workers, veterinarians, laboratory workers, livestock handlers, and military personnel. The vaccine is manufactured by BioPort Corporation. Vaccine side effects include injection site reactions. About 30% of men and 60% of women experience mild local reactions, which is a similar finding with other vaccinations. Approximately 1–5% of individuals experience moderate local reactions. Large local reactions occur at a rate of 1%. Beyond the injection site, from

5–35% of people will notice fever, muscle aches, joint aches, headaches, rash, chills, loss of appetite, malaise, and nausea. Serious events, such as those requiring hospitalization, are rare and happen about once per 200,000 doses. There have been no patterns of long-term side effects from the vaccine and neither persistent nor delayed side effects.

Plague

Plague is caused by the bacterium *Yersinia pestis*. Its potential as a biological weapon is based on an ability to produce and aerosolize large amounts of bacteria and its transmissibility from person to person in certain forms. An additional factor is the wide distribution of samples of the bacteria in research laboratories throughout the world. *Yersinia pestis* is easily destroyed by sunlight and drying. However, it can survive briefly in the soil and longer in frozen or soft tissues. Additionally, it is able to survive for up to one hour (depending on conditions) when released into air. This could increase its threat and aid in its dispersal as a potential bioterrorism weapon.

Plague has a very detailed past and long history. Throughout history, plague has caused several outbreaks (pandemics and epidemics) that led to large numbers of deaths (Riedel, 2005a). Justinian's Constantinople pandemic lasted from 540 AD to 590 AD and resulted in approximately 10,000 deaths per day at its height. It also contributed greatly to the fall of the Roman Empire. In the 14th century, plague was carried from outbreaks in India and China to Italy by merchants returning home. Soon after, plague spread to the rest of Europe (Slack, 1998). During this time, Venice instituted a 40-day period of detainment for docking ships, which gave us what is now known as the *quarantine*. Despite these efforts, plague quickly spread throughout all of Europe. Over one third of the European population died during the "Black Death pandemic." The decline in the population aided in the fall of the feudal system of government (Eckert, 2000). Another important plague epidemic occurred in 1665. Although limited to England, it killed approximately 100,000 (of the 500,000) inhabitants of London. During this outbreak, some of our modern public health practices were initiated (i.e., disease reporting, closing up of homes).

☐ ☐ ☐ ▬▬▬▬▬▬▬▬▬▬▬▬▬▬▬▬▬▬▬▬▬▬▬▬▬

The Great Plague
The Great Plague, also known as the Black Death, killed nearly one third of the population of Europe within a four year period (1347–1350).

▬▬▬▬▬▬▬▬▬▬▬▬▬▬▬▬▬▬▬▬▬▬▬▬▬ ☐ ☐ ☐

The United States has not been immune to the influence of plague. It entered the United States by way of Hawaii and San Francisco in 1899 (Link, 1955). Plague spread from infected rats aboard vessels in Californian ports to indigenous, sylvatic wild rodents throughout the western United States. Currently, it is well established in the Four Corners Region of the United States and parts of California. The last documented person-to-person transmission of plague occurred during the 1924 outbreak in Los Angeles.

Today, the World Health Organization categorizes plague as a Class 1 Quarantinable disease. This allows for detention and inspection of any vehicle or passenger originating from an area where a plague epidemic is in progress. Also personnel of the CDC Division of Quarantine and Global Migration are empowered to apprehend, detain, medically examine, or conditionally release a suspect having this illness. Plague in humans is a reportable disease, and in many states plague in animals is also reportable. The U.S. Public Health Service requires that all cases of suspected plague be reported immediately to local and state health departments and diagnosis be confirmed by the CDC. As required by the International Health Regulations, the CDC reports all plague cases to the World Health Organization.

Epidemiology—Natural Reservoirs

Humans acquire plague most often through the bite of an infected flea. The flea ingests a blood meal from an infected, bacteremic animal. The bacteria multiply and block the foregut of the flea. When the flea attempts to feed again, it regurgitates bacteria into a human or animal mammalian host. The flea *Oropsylla montana* is the primary vector for naturally occurring cases of plague. This flea is found mostly in rural rodent species, particularly the rock squirrel in New Mexico and Arizona (Orloski and Lathrop, 2003). Urban plague from rats has not occurred in the United States in over 70 years. This is due to good public health surveillance and control and improved sanitation measures. If an urban plague event (natural) were to occur, the flea *Xenopsylla cheopis*, or the "oriental rat flea" would be the most likely vector.

Urban (domestic) plague occurs when the infected fleas or rodents move into urban areas. Influx can also occur when there is significant development and expansion into wilderness areas (i.e., interface building that borders a city and outlying wilderness), as is seen in some parts of the Southwest. The epizootics may cause high mortality in commensal (domestic) rat populations, thereby forcing infected fleas to seek alternative hosts, including humans or domestic cats. Domestic cats in homes bordering wilderness areas pose a significant threat to humans because they may become infected with plague (i.e., hunting rodents) or transport rodent fleas into the home, thereby exposing their owners (AVMA, 2006b). Poverty, filth, and homelessness all contribute to urban plague transmission. The most common reservoirs for the bacteria are ground squirrels and wood rats.

Epidemiology—Transmission

Transmission occurs through the bite of an infected flea, respiratory droplets, or direct contact with a patient infected with pneumonic plague. Transmission by direct skin or mucous membrane contact with tissues and fluids of infected animals is less common. Infection via inhalation of infective respiratory droplets or aerosols is rare with naturally occurring plague in the United States, but is the most likely route of transmission in a bioterrorist event. Becoming infected naturally through the respiratory route requires direct and close (within 6 feet) contact with an ill person or animal and has not occurred in the United States for decades.

Incidence in the United States

Since 1900, plague has been endemic in the United States. Between 1970 and 2003, 2% of plague has been pneumonic, 83% has been bubonic, and 15% has been septicemic. Approximately 5–15 cases occur each year in the United States. The greatest concentration occurs in Arizona, Colorado, and New Mexico. But human cases have occurred in rural areas from the Pacific coastal region eastward to the Great Plains states. The last time person-to-person transmission occurred in the United States was during the epidemic of 1924–1925 in Los Angeles. During this outbreak, 32 pneumonic cases were reported with 31 resulting in death. Human cases of plague typically occur in April through November, when fleas and their hosts are most active and people are more likely to be outdoors. Ninety-three percent of human cases in the United States occurred during this period.

Plague exists in rodent populations on every inhabited continent except Australia. Approximately 1,500–3,000 cases of human plague are reported annually worldwide.

Worldwide, most cases of plague occur in Africa, with limited outbreaks in Asia and South America. In 2006, an outbreak of more than 600 suspected cases of pneumonic plague in the Democratic Republic of the Congo claimed the lives of 42 people (WHO, 2006).

Clinical Manifestations of Human Plague

Infection by inhalation of even small numbers of virulent aerosolized *Y. pestis* bacilli can lead to pneumonic plague, a highly lethal form of plague that can be spread from person to person. Natural epidemics of plague have been primarily bubonic plague, which is transmitted by fleas from infected rodents (Boyce and Butler, 1995). Plague usually presents as one of three principal clinical syndromes: bubonic, septicemic, or pneumonic.

Bubonic Plague

Bubonic plague is the most common form and accounts for roughly 80% of cases. The incubation period is 2–6 days. Signs and symptoms include fever, malaise, chills, headache, and very swollen, painful lymph nodes (called a *bubo*). Vomiting, abdominal pain, nausea, and petechiae may also occur. Without treatment 50–60% of bubonic cases are fatal. Infection is transmitted by the bite of an infected flea or exposure to infected material through a break in the skin. Bubonic plague *cannot* be transmitted from person to person. If bubonic plague is not treated, the bacteria can spread through the bloodstream and infect the lungs, causing a secondary infection of pneumonic or septicemic plague.

Septicemic Plague

Septicemic plague occurs when the bacteria enter the bloodstream and are dispersed throughout the body. This phase follows bubonic plague in most cases, but not all people will develop buboes. In addition to the preceding signs, prostration, circulatory collapse, septic shock, organ failure, hemorrhage, disseminated intravascular coagulation, and necrosis of extremities can be seen. This condition, often seen in the fingertips, tip of the nose, and toes, is the result of small blood clots blocking capillaries and the circulation to these areas (Figure 3-2). Without treatment 100% of septicemic cases are fatal.

Pneumonic Plague

Primary pneumonic plague occurs when *Y. pestis* is inhaled and the bacteria gain direct access to the lungs. Pneumonic is the least common form of plague, but the most fatal. Pneumonic plague patients must receive definitive medical treatment within 24 hours

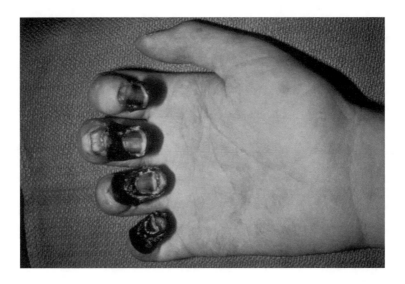

FIGURE 3-2 Hand of a plague patient displaying acral gangrene. Gangrene is one of the manifestations of plague and the origin of the term *Black Death* given to plague throughout the ages. (Image courtesy of the CDC Public Health Image Library, No. 1957.)

of becoming symptomatic. If not, pneumonic plague is considered to be universally fatal due to respiratory failure and shock. Pneumonic plague *can* be transmitted person to person through respiratory droplets with direct close contacts.

Primary pneumonic plague has a very rapid incubation period of 1–6 days. If septicemic plague is left untreated, it progresses to pneumonic plague (secondary pneumonic plague). A person with secondary pneumonic plague who coughs on another person can transmit plague in an aerosol and infect that person with a primary pneumonic infection. Symptoms include fever, chills, headache, septicemia, respiratory distress, and hemoptysis. Pneumonic plague is the only form of plague that can be transmitted person to person, but it usually requires direct or close contact with the ill person or animal.

Treatment of plague requires prompt antibiotic treatment and supportive therapy. Without treatment, most forms of plague are 100% fatal. Currently about 14% (1 in 7) of all plague cases in the United States are fatal. Fatalities in the United States are often linked to delay in seeking medical care or misdiagnosis. Penicillins and cephalosporins are not effective in treating plague. Prophylactic antibiotics should be administered to persons who have had close exposure (i.e., within 2 meters) to persons suspected of having pneumonic plague. Persons who have not had such exposure are unlikely to become infected, but should be monitored closely.

Critical Thinking

Consider a case of bubonic plague in the Emergency Room of a New York City hospital. Why would this be a "red flag" event for public health officials?

With any plague case, natural or bioterrorist, public health authorities need to conduct investigations to identify close contacts that need prophylaxis and to look for any additional cases, so that they may begin treatment as quickly as possible. By definition, a **contact** is anyone who has been within 2 meters of a coughing pneumonic plague patient in the previous seven days. If contacts are found to have fever or cough, they will be referred for evaluation. Those contacts that do not have fever or cough will be placed on antibiotics for seven days and monitored for the development of symptoms. Those that have contraindications to the antibiotics can be placed on a fever watch.

□ □ □ ▬▬▬▬▬▬▬▬▬▬▬▬▬▬▬▬▬▬▬▬▬▬▬▬▬▬▬▬

Short Case Study

On November 1, 2002, a 53-year old man and his 47-year old wife, traveled from Santa Fe County, New Mexico, to New York City (NYC). Both became ill and sought medical care in a NYC emergency room on November 5. The man reported two days of fever, fatigue, and a painful swelling in his groin area. His blood work showed that he had a serious infection. A blood culture grew *Yersinia pestis*. Plague was diagnosed. The man's treatment was initiated with several antibiotics (gentamicin, doxycycline, ciprofloxacin, and vancomycin). However, his condition deteriorated, he went into shock with septicemic plague and had to be admitted to the Intensive Care Unit (ICU). His wife presented with fever, fatigue, myalgia, and a painful swelling in her groin. Her blood work was normal, but she was presumed to have plague based on her husband's diagnosis. She was treated with antibiotics and recovered rapidly without complications. After six weeks in ICU, the man recovered and was discharged to a long-term-care rehabilitation facility.

The New Mexico Department of Public Health and the Centers for Disease Control and Prevention investigated the couple's New Mexico property. Trapped rodents and their fleas were tested for *Y. pestis* and found to be indistinguishable from the *Y. pestis* isolated from the male patient. Any time plague is suspected or diagnosed out of its endemic area (southwestern United States), suspicions should be raised about the source of the infection. In this case, the patients both had come from the endemic area. What if they had been from Boston?

This case also emphasizes the importance of early detection and diagnosis. This is important not only for patient care but also for implementation of any isolation or precautionary measures that may need to be implemented. (Case details were taken from CDC *Morbidity and Mortality Weekly Review* 52, no. 31 [2003]: 725–728).

▬▬▬▬▬▬▬▬▬▬▬▬▬▬▬▬▬▬▬▬▬▬▬▬▬▬▬▬ □ □ □

Tularemia

Tularemia is a potential bioterrorist agent because of its high level of infectivity and its ability to be aerosolized. Tularemia is caused by *Francisella tularensis*, which is a gram-negative, non-spore-forming intracellular bacterium that can survive at low temperatures for weeks. The disease is not transmitted from person to person; it spreads naturally from small mammals or contaminated food, soil, or water to humans. Natural infection may occur after inhalation of airborne particles (Dennis et al., 2001).

Tularemia is also known as *rabbit fever* and *deer fly fever*. The etiologic agent of tularemia is one of the most infectious bacterial agents known to man. Less than 10 cells inhaled into the lungs is sufficient to produce a lethal infection. The bacterium multiplies within white blood cells (macrophages) and the major target organs are the lymph nodes, lungs, spleen, liver, and kidney. The organism is relatively resistant in the environment, surviving 3–4 months in mud, water, or dead animals. Rabbit meat frozen at 5°F has remained infective for more than three years. Chlorination of water during water treatment will kill the organism. The organism is also easily destroyed by various disinfectants, including 1% hypochlorite (bleach), 70% ethanol, and formaldehyde. It can be inactivated by moist heat (121°C for at least 15 minutes) and dry heat (160–170°C for at least 1 hour). There are several subspecies (or biovars) of *Francisella tularensis*, which vary in virulence and distribution. Two of the four subspecies account for the majority of human illness: *Francisella tularensis* biovar *tularensis* (or Jellison type A) and *F. tularensis* biovar *palaearctica* (or Jellison type B). The other subspecies of *F. tularensis* are *mediasiatica* and *novicida*.

Tularemia was first described in humans in 1907. The disease was then discovered in the United States in 1911, in California ground squirrels suffering a plague-like illness. The organism was originally named *Bacterium tularense* named after Tulare County, California, where these first cases occurred. During the 1930–1940s, the Soviet Union and Europe experienced large waterborne outbreaks. In 1947, the organism was renamed *Francisella tularensis* in honor of Edward Francis, a U.S. Public Health Service surgeon who had dedicated his career (since 1914) to the study of all aspects of tularemia. In the 1950s and 1960s, the U.S. military was striving to develop bioweapons that aerosolized the organism.

The largest recorded airborne tularemia outbreak occurred in Sweden in 1966–1967. Over 600 patients were infected with the Type B strain. Most of those infected were exposed while doing farmwork that created contaminated aerosols, particularly when rodent-infested hay was being sorted and moved from field storage sites to barns. Most had the typical acute symptoms of fever, fatigue, chills, headache, and malaise. Although airborne exposure would be expected to principally manifest as pleuropneumonic infection, only 10% had symptoms of pneumonia, such as dyspnea and chest pains. Other "forms" of tularemia were noted in a variable proportion of patients: 32% has various skin exanthemas, 31% had pharyngitis, 26% had conjunctivitis, and 9% had oral ulcers. Patients responded well to treatment and no deaths were reported.

Tularemia is endemic on Martha's Vineyard, an island off the coast of Cape Cod, Massachusetts. In the 1930s, game clubs introduced cottontail rabbits from Arkansas and Missouri (endemic states) to Cape Cod and Martha's Vineyard. Shortly after this introduction, the first cases of tularemia were reported in Martha's Vineyard. The only two reported outbreaks of pneumonic tularemia in the United States occurred on Martha's Vineyard in 1978 and 2000. In 1978, the cluster of cases involved seven persons who lived together in a cottage. Epidemiological investigation attributed exposure to a wet dog, which aerosolized *F. tularensis* when it shook itself inside of the cottage. During the outbreak in 2000, 15 cases were identified; 11 of which had pneumonic tularemia, 2 had ulceroglandular form, and 2 experienced only fever and malaise with no localized signs. Epidemiologic investigation determined that the cases were primarily in persons occupationally associated with landscaping. Risk factors were increased for those that engaged in lawn mowing and bush cutting, which was thought to generate aerosols of the organism for dispersal. Investigation also proposed that *F. tularensis* was shed in animal (rodent) excrement and infected people after it was mechanically aerosolized and inhaled. One patient remembered cutting brush around a dead rabbit.

Incredibly, 14 species of ticks, 6 species of flies, several mosquito species, over 100 wild mammal species, and 25 species of birds serve as reservoirs for *F. tularensis*. A rodent-mosquito cycle has been described in Russia and Sweden. However, tularemia is commonly transmitted through the bite of an infected tick, including *Dermacentor andersonii*, *Dermacentor variabilis*, *Amblyomma americanum*, and less frequently the deer fly, *Chrysops discalis*. Transovarial transmission occurs in ticks. This means that the pathogen can be passed from an adult female tick to her progeny. Once infected, ticks can be infective for life. Flies are a less common source of transmission and are infective for only about 14 days. Tularemia has been rarely transmitted via bites and scratches from coyotes, squirrels, skunks, hogs, cats, and a dog whose mouth was contaminated by eating an infected animal (AVMA, 2006c). Transmission is possible through contaminated blood, tissue, or water coming in contact with eyes, mouth, or breaks in the skin. Transmission has also been documented through handling or ingesting undercooked meat (especially rabbits). Waterborne outbreaks can result from contaminated drinking water in rural areas. Person-to-person transmission has not been documented. Airborne outbreaks can occur from moving rodent-contaminated hay, threshing corn, or lab accidents.

Tularemia occurs in the temperate regions of the Northern Hemisphere (North America, Europe, Soviet Union, China, Japan, and Mexico). In the United States, tularemia occurs year-round and is a nationally notifiable disease. Typically, about 100 cases per year occcur in the United States. Most cases occur from June to September (corresponding to peak arthropod season) but a slight increase in winter has been associated with rabbit hunting. Tularemia has been reported in every state except Hawaii. Typically, more than half of all cases are reported from four states: Arkansas, Missouri, South Dakota, and Oklahoma. Tularemia is considered endemic in these states and ticks and rabbits are usually the sources of human infection. In Utah, Nevada, and California, biting flies are common vectors, while ticks are the primary vectors in states along the Rocky Mountains. Tularemia became a nationally notifiable disease in 2000.

In humans, the severity of infection and incubation period varies, depending on the subspecies, route of infection, and dose. The six clinical syndromes or manifestations of tularemia are based on the route of exposure to the agent. All forms initially present as flulike symptoms, including fever, chills, headache, and myalgia.

The ulceroglandular form is the most common presentation of tularemia. This usually occurs as a consequence of a bite from an arthropod vector which has previously fed on an infected animal. Some cases occur following the handling of infected meat, with infection occurring via cuts or abrasions. An ulcer develops at the site of infection, and the local lymph nodes are enlarged (Figure 3-3). The lymph nodes are painful, swollen and may rupture and ulcer. The ulcer may last from one week to several months. With a glandular presentation, there is no apparent primary ulcer, but there are one or more enlarged lymph nodes. Ulceroglandular and glandular presentations account for 75–85% of naturally occurring tularemia cases.

The oculoglandular form of tularemia is rare and occurs when the conjunctiva becomes infected. This may occur by either rubbing the eyes with contaminated fingers

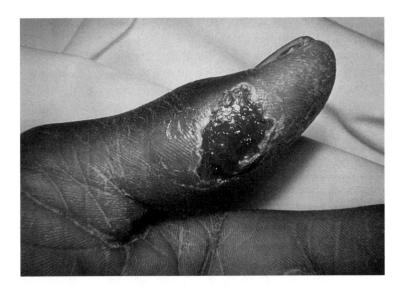

FIGURE 3-3 A characteristic lesion on the thumb of a patient with tularemia. (Image courtesy of the CDC Public Health Image Library, No. 1344, taken by Dr. Sellers of Emory University in 1964.)

or splashing contaminated materials in the eyes. Cleaning carcasses or rubbing the area of a tick bite then the eye can result in this form of tularemia. Clinical presentation involves initial flulike signs with conjunctivitis and painful swelling of the regional lymph nodes. In severe forms, the conjunctiva may be ulcerated and ocular discharge may be present.

The oropharyngeal presentation of tularemia occurs following ingestion of the organisms in either undercooked meat (especially rabbit) or contaminated water. Hand-to-mouth transfer can also occur. Infection may produce painful pharyngitis (with or without ulceration), abdominal pain, diarrhea, and vomiting. A pseudomembrane may cover tonsils and can be mistaken for diphtheria.

The most severe forms (and most fatalities) of tularemia are the typhoidal and pulmonary forms. The typhoidal form involves systemic infection and can develop from the oropharyngeal form of tularemia. Pulmonary tularemia is due to inhalation of infectious organisms or dissemination of organisms through the bloodstream. The pulmonary form of the disease results from 10–15% of the ulceroglandular and ~50% of the typhoidal cases. Organisms can become airborne as animals are skinned or eviscerated. Inhalation of infectious material may be followed by pneumonic disease or a primary septicemic (typhoidal type) syndrome with a 30–60% case-fatality rate if untreated. Although there have been descriptions of a triad of findings for tularemic pneumonia—ovoid opacities, pleural effusions, and hilar adenopathy—these radiologic manifestations are neither sensitive nor specific enough to render them diagnostically useful. Additionally, respiratory signs and symptoms may be minimal or absent and, when present, are often nonspecific.

Francisella tularensis is susceptible to a variety of antibiotics. Streptomycin is the antibiotic of choice, but gentamicin, doxycycline, and ciprofloxacin have also been used. The prognosis for tularemia varies with the form of disease that manifests and the subspecies of the organism. Type A (*F. tularensis tularensis*) organisms are more virulent, with an overall case-fatality rate of 5–15%. Typhoidal and pulmonary forms of disease account for most of these cases. Type B (*F. tularensis holarctica*) is less virulent and, even without treatment, produces few deaths. If untreated, general symptoms usually last one to four weeks but may continue for months. The mortality rate for all types of untreated tularemia is less than 8% and drops to less than 1% when treated. Treatment, however, is usually delayed due to misdiagnosis. Following recovery from infection, antibody titers can persist for years and subsequent infections may occur (Feldman, 2003).

Smallpox

Smallpox is considered one of the most dangerous potential biological weapons because it is easily transmitted from person to person, no effective therapy exists, and few people carry full immunity to the virus. The word *variola* (smallpox) comes from the Latin word *varius*, meaning "stained," or from *varus*, meaning "mark on the skin." It was also referred to by Native Americans as "rotting face." Although a worldwide immunization program eradicated smallpox disease in 1977, small quantities of smallpox virus still exist in two secure facilities in the United States and Russia. However, it is likely that unrecognized stores of smallpox virus exist elsewhere in the world. Today, any confirmed case of smallpox would constitute an international emergency and should be reported to public health authorities immediately (Barquet and Domingo, 1997).

The smallpox virus is a double stranded DNA virus in the genus Orthopoxvirus. Smallpox disease can be caused by *Variola major* or *Variola minor*. *Variola major* is the more common and severe form, causing an extensive rash and a higher fever. *Variola minor* is much less common and causes a less severe disease. Other orthopoxviruses include cowpox, vaccinia, monkeypox, and others. *Variola* is stable outside the host and retains its infectivity. Animals have never been found infected with or showing signs of smallpox; therefore, it is not a zoonotic disease.

Smallpox is believed to have appeared around 10,000 BC during the first agricultural settlements in northeastern Africa. The earliest evidence of skin lesions resembling those of smallpox is found on the faces of mummies (1570–1085 BC) and in the well-preserved mummy of Ramses V, who died as a young man in 1157 BC. While poxvirus was never isolated or identified in tissue samples from Ramses V, skin lesions were consistent with smallpox (Riedel, 2005b).

The devastating effects of smallpox gave rise to one of the first examples of biological warfare. In a letter written in 1763, Sir Jeffrey Amherst, commander-in-chief of British forces in North America, suggested grinding the scabs of smallpox pustules into blankets that were to be distributed among disaffected tribes of Indians. In the late 18th century in Europe, 400,000 people died of smallpox each year and one third of the survivors went blind. The case-fatality rate associated with smallpox varied between 20–60% and left most survivors with disfiguring scars. Many persons went blind as a result of corneal infection. The case-fatality rate in the infant population was even higher; among children younger than five years of age in the 18th century, 80% of those in London and 98% of those in Berlin who developed the disease died.

Physicians realized that smallpox survivors became immune to the disease. Thus, the method of variolation began, which involved taking samples (vesicles, pus, ground scabs) from benignly diseased patients and introduce the material into susceptible patients via the nose or skin. In China, powdered scabs of smallpox pustules were blown into the nostrils of healthy persons through a tube. Also in China, 100 years before Edward Jenner, healthy persons took pills made from the fleas of cows to prevent smallpox; this is the first recorded example of oral vaccination. In India, variolation took several forms, the most common of which was the application of scabs or pus from a person with smallpox to the intact or scarified skin of a healthy person. Children were exposed to organisms from persons with mild cases of smallpox, and various forms of material from persons with smallpox were administered to healthy adults in different ways. It was well known that milkmaids became immune to smallpox after developing cowpox. Variolation was practiced in England in the early 1700s. Variolation also spread to the New World, where in 1721, Boylston used the technique to stop the smallpox epidemic in Boston. By 1777, George Washington had all his soldiers variolated before beginning new military operations.

In Gloucestershire, England, on May 14, 1796, Jenner extracted fluid from a pustule on a milkmaid and used it to inoculate a healthy eight-year-old boy (James Phipps). Six weeks later, Jenner variolated the child but produced no reaction. Jenner, in combination with George Pearson and others, developed a vaccine using cowpox (see Figure 3-4). This prevented the vaccinee from developing smallpox if variolated or exposed to smallpox. Vaccination done by using pustule fluid spread rapidly. By 1800, it had reached most European countries and about 100,000 persons had been vaccinated worldwide. Cows were first used in the early 19th century for vaccine production. By 1801, over 100,000 persons in England had been vaccinated. In 1805, Napoleon himself insisted that all his troops who had not had smallpox should be vaccinated with the "Jennerian vaccine." He ordered the vaccination of French civilians one year later.

The World Health Organization began a smallpox eradication program in 1967 (Fenner et al., 1988). In that year, an estimated 10 million cases of smallpox caused 2 million deaths. However, the greatest triumph in public health history was realized in 1980, when smallpox was officially declared to be eradicated by the WHO. The total cost for this program was only about $400 million. By comparison, it cost $24 billion for the United States to put a man on the moon. The United States discontinued smallpox vaccinations in 1972 (World Health Organization, 1980).

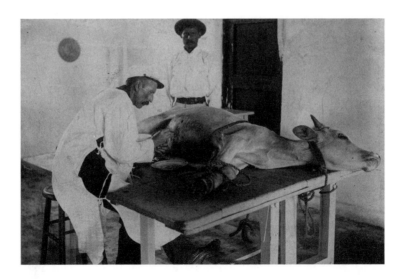

FIGURE 3-4 Edward Jenner discovered, in 1798, that people could be inoculated or vaccinated against smallpox by using the closely related cowpox. In this photograph from the early 1900s, cowpox fluid is being harvested from infected cows. (Image courtesy of the Armed Forces Institute of Pathology, National Museum of Health and Medicine, No. 2611.)

Eradication of smallpox was made possible for several reasons: a good, protective vaccine was available, there was no animal reservoir for smallpox, vaccinees were easily identifiable and could "vaccinate" friends and family through contact, and those who acquired smallpox were easily identifiable.

To sustain itself, the virus must pass from person to person in a continuing chain of infection and is spread by inhalation of respiratory droplets, typically within 2 meters or less. Generally, direct and fairly prolonged face-to-face contact is required to spread smallpox from one person to another. Smallpox also can be spread through direct contact with infected bodily fluids or contaminated objects, such as bedding or clothing. Rarely, smallpox has been spread by virus carried in the air in enclosed settings, such as buildings, buses, and trains. Smallpox spreads most readily during the cool, dry winter months but can be transmitted in any climate and in any part of the world. Smallpox is not transmitted by insects or animals.

A person with smallpox is sometimes contagious with onset of fever (prodromal phase), but the person becomes most contagious with the onset of rash (during the first 7–10 days). At this stage, the infected person is usually very sick and not able to move around in the community. The infected person is contagious until the last smallpox scab falls off. The incubation period for smallpox is 7–17 days but generally averages 12–14 days. Small red spots in the mouth and on the tongue are the initial signs of smallpox. Around the time the sores in the mouth break down, a rash appears on the skin, starting on the face. It then spreads to the arms and legs and then to the hands and feet. Usually the rash spreads to all parts of the body within 24 hours. As the rash appears, the fever usually falls and the person may start to feel better.

The two major forms of smallpox are *Variola major* and *Variola minor*. Variola major is the more common and severe form, causing an extensive rash and a higher fever (see the patient image in Figure 3-5). There are four forms of variola major: ordinary, modified, flat, and hemorrhagic. Variola minor is much less common and causes a less severe disease. In the ordinary (or discrete) form of variola major smallpox disease, the pustules remain separate and distinct from one another. This is the most frequent form of smallpox.

Hemorrhagic smallpox occurs in less than 3% of patients. There are two types of hemorrhagic smallpox, early and late, based on the time during the disease at which the hemorrhage appears. It causes the appearance of extensive petechiae, mucosal hemorrhage, and intense toxemia; death usually intervenes before the development of typical pox lesions can occur (McClain, 1997).

A patient with chickenpox has many pocks on his torso but very few on his arms or hands. A patient with smallpox manifests pocks more densely localized on the arms and legs than on the trunk. In smallpox, pocks are usually present on the palms of the hands and the soles of the feet. In chickenpox, there may be few or no lesions on the palms of the hands or the soles of the feet.

If a patient has been exposed to smallpox but is showing no signs of disease, vaccination within three days of exposure will prevent or significantly lessen the severity of symptoms in the vast majority of people and affords almost complete protection against death. Vaccination four to seven days after exposure likely offers some protection from disease or may modify the severity of disease. This person should also be quarantined and monitored for signs of disease. If the person is showing signs of smallpox, then isolation and supportive care are essential.

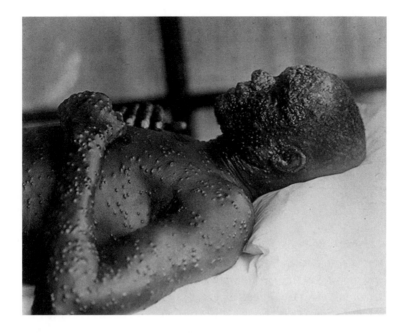

FIGURE 3-5 Man with characteristic smallpox lesions about the face, torso, and extremities. (Image courtesy of the Armed Forces Institute of Pathology, National Museum of Health and Medicine, No. 48135.)

Case fatality for smallpox caused by *Variola major* ranges between 20–40%. The flat and hemorrhagic forms are usually fatal. Fatality rates in vaccinated persons are around 3%. Blindness and limb deformities could also be sequelae from smallpox. *Variola minor* is a much less severe disease and had a case-fatality rate of 1%. Persons who recover from smallpox possess long-lasting immunity, although a second attack could occur in 1 in 1,000 persons after an intervening period of 15–20 years.

The only prevention for smallpox is vaccination. As described earlier, the practice of vaccination with vaccinia virus began in the early 20th century. The origins of vaccinia virus remain unknown, but this virus is distinct from both *variola* and cowpox. Some speculate the vaccinia virus is a hybrid between cowpox and *variola*. Vaccinia vaccine, derived from the calf lymph, was used in the United States until 1972. It is a lyophilized, live-virus preparation of infectious vaccinia virus. It contains no smallpox (variola) virus. The needle is dipped into the vaccine and then the vaccinee is jabbed 2 or 3 times on the upper arm (deltoid muscle) for the initial vaccine (15 times for a booster). Smallpox vaccination provides high level immunity for three to five years and decreasing immunity thereafter. If a person is vaccinated again later, immunity lasts even longer. Historically, the vaccine has been effective in preventing smallpox infection in 95% of those vaccinated. There is some evidence to indicate that some degree of immunity lasts much longer than three to five years.

If the vaccination is successful, a red, itchy bump develops at the vaccine site in three or four days. In the first week, the bump becomes a large blister, fills with pus, and begins to drain. During the second week, the blister begins to dry up and a scab forms. The scab falls off in the third week, leaving a small scar. People who are being vaccinated for the first time have a stronger reaction than those who are being revaccinated.

The ring vaccination strategy is the strategy that will be used if a case of smallpox were to break out in the United States. Contacts of the case will be found and vaccinated, as will contacts of those contacts. This appears to be the most effective way to contain an outbreak. There is currently enough vaccine available to vaccinate all Americans should the need arise.

Due to the events of September 11, 2001, the threat of a terrorist act on the United States was amplified. Government officials felt the threat of a smallpox attack on the United States was a real possibility. To protect its citizens, President Bush recommended, on December 13, 2002, that smallpox vaccination of health-care personnel and the military begin. In January 2003, the CDC began distributing smallpox vaccine and bifurcated needles to the states for voluntary vaccination of first responders in the health-care system.

Viral Hemorrhagic Fevers

Viral hemorrhagic fever (VHF) refers to a group of illnesses caused by several distinct families of viruses that effect humans and nonhuman primates. VHF is a severe multisystem syndrome characterized by diffuse vascular damage. Bleeding often occurs and, depending on the virus, may or may not be life threatening. Some VHFs cause mild disease, while others may cause severe symptoms and death. Viral hemorrhagic fevers encompass a group of similar diseases caused by four types of viruses:

- **Arenaviruses**, associated with Argentine, Bolivian, and Venezuelan hemorrhagic fevers, Lassa fever, and Sabia-associated hemorrhagic fever.
- **Bunyaviruses**, including Crimean-Congo hemorrhagic fever, Rift Valley fever, and hantavirus infection.
- **Filoviruses**, comprising Ebola and Marburg hemorrhagic fevers.
- Hemorrhagic **flaviviruses**, including yellow fever, dengue hemorrhagic fever, Kyasanur Forest disease, and Omsk hemorrhagic fever.

These viruses pose a risk from intentional exposure because, with very few exceptions, no vaccines or proven treatments exist and many of the diseases are highly fatal. Natural infections occur when people come in contact with rodents or insects that are infected or act as vectors. After human infection occurs, some VHFs can be transmitted from person to person through close contact or contaminated objects, such as syringes and needles.

Viral hemorrhagic fevers are caused by a long list of viral pathogens from a number of viral groups. We concentrate on those that are most likely candidates for bioterrorism or biowarfare.

VHF viruses are members of four distinct families: arenaviruses, bunyaviruses, filoviruses, and flaviviruses. All are RNA viruses enveloped in a lipid coating. The survival of these viruses is dependent on their natural reservoir, which in most cases is an animal or an insect host.

Arenaviruses

The first arenavirus was isolated in 1933 during an outbreak of St. Louis encephalitis virus. In 1958, the Junin virus was isolated in the plains of Argentina in agricultural workers. It was the first arenavirus found to cause hemorrhagic fever. Others soon followed, including Machupo virus in Bolivia in 1963 and Lassa virus in Nigeria in 1969. Since 1956, a new arenavirus has been discovered every one to three years, but not all cause hemorrhagic fever.

New and Old World rats and mice are chronically infected with arenaviruses. The virus is vertically transmitted from adult host to offspring with most viruses in this family. Transmission among adult rodents may also occur through bites and other wounds. Rodents shed the viruses into the environment through urine and fecal droppings. Humans can become infected when coming into contact with rodent excreta or contaminated materials such as contact through abraded skin or ingestion of contaminated food. Inhalation of rodent excreta may also result in disease. Person-to-person transmission has been documented in health-care settings through close contact with infected individuals and contact with infected blood and medical equipment.

Arenaviruses are found worldwide; however, the viruses responsible for causing hemorrhagic fever are restricted to two continents. Lassa virus is endemic to the region of West Africa, while Junin, Machupo, Guanarito, and Sabia viruses are all found in South America. The later are grouped together as the Latin American hemorrhagic fevers. Humans who have frequent contact with rodent excreta have an increased risk of developing an infection with an arenavirus. Agricultural and domestic exposures are the most common. Case fatality for arenaviruses ranges from 5–35%. Lassa and Machupo can cause explosive hospital-acquired outbreaks. The incubation period for arenaviruses is typically between 10–14 days. Disease onset begins with a fever and general malaise for two to four days. Most patients with Lassa fever recover following this stage; however, those infected with the Latin American hemorrhagic fever typically progress to more severe symptoms. The hemorrhagic stage of the disease quickly follows and leads to hemorrhaging, neurologic signs, leukopenia, and thrombocytopenia.

Bunyaviruses

Rift Valley fever (RVF) virus was first isolated in 1930 from an infected newborn lamb, as part of an investigation of a large epizootic of disease causing abortion and high mortality in sheep in Egypt. Crimean-Congo hemorrhagic fever (CCHF) virus was first recognized in the Crimean peninsula, located in southeastern Europe on the northern coast of the Black Sea, in the mid-1940s, when a large outbreak of severe hemorrhagic fever among agricultural workers was identified. The outbreak included more than 200 cases and a case fatality of about 10%. The discovery of hantaviruses traces back to 1951–1953, when United Nations troops were deployed during the border conflict between North and South Korea. More than 3,000 cases of acute febrile illness were seen among the troops, about one third of which exhibited hemorrhagic manifestations, and an overall mortality of 5–10% was seen. The family now consists of five genera, which contain 350 viruses that are significant human, animal, and plant pathogens.

Most bunyaviruses except for hantaviruses utilize an arthropod vector to transmit the virus from host to host. In some cases the virus may be transmitted from adult arthropods to their offspring. Humans are generally dead end hosts for the viruses and the cycle is maintained by wild or domestic animals. Crimean-Congo hemorrhagic fever virus is transmitted by ixodid ticks, and domestic and wild animals (such as hares, hedgehogs, and sheep) serve as amplifying and reservoir hosts. In contrast, Rift Valley fever virus is transmitted by *Aedes* mosquitoes resulting in large epizootics in livestock. Humans are incidentally infected when bitten by infected mosquitoes or when coming into contact with infected animal tissues. The virus is believed to be maintained by transovarial transmission between the mosquito and its offspring. Hantaviruses cycle in rodent hosts and humans become infected by coming into contact with rodent urine. Aerosolization of viruses and exposure to infected animal tissues are also two less common modes of transmission for some bunyaviruses.

Bunyaviruses are found worldwide, but each virus is usually isolated to a local region. RVF is found primarily in sub-Saharan Africa and was isolated in Saudi Arabia and Yemen in 2000. The case fatality rate in humans is generally around 1%. CCHF is found in most of sub-Saharan Africa, Eastern Europe, and Asia. The case fatality rate is 30% and nosicomial outbreaks have been documented through exposure to infected blood products. Hantaviruses are divided into two groups based on location: Old World viruses are found in Eastern Europe and eastern Asia while New World viruses are found in North and South America. Depending on the virus, case fatality rate can vary between 1–50%.

Most humans suffering from Rift Valley fever experience flulike symptoms and recover with no complications after an incubation period of 2–5 days. In 0.5% of cases, hemorrhagic fever develops following the initial febrile stage. Another 0.5% of cases develop retinitis or encephalitis 1–4 weeks following infection. Most human infections occur 1–2 weeks following the appearance of abortion or disease in livestock. In contrast to RVF, most humans infected with CCHF develop hemorrhagic fever. The incubation for the disease is 3–7 days and most patients will develop hemorrhagic fever 3–6 days following the onset of flulike symptoms. Hantaviruses generally cause one of two clinical presentations: hemorrhagic fever with renal syndrome, generally caused by Old World hantaviruses, or hantavirus pulmonary syndrome, generally caused by New World hantaviruses. Incubation period is 7–21 days followed by a clinical phase of 3–5 days. The severity of the illness depends on the virus.

Rift Valley fever causes severe disease in livestock animals. Abortion rates can reach 100%. Mortality rates in animals less than two weeks of age can be greater than 90%, with most animals succumbing to disease within 24–36 hours from the onset of fever. Older animals also suffer from a less severe febrile illness, with mortality rates ranging from 5–60%. In contrast, CCHF virus causes an unapparent or subclinical disease in most livestock species and is maintained in the herds through the bite of a tick. Rodents are persistently infected with hantaviruses but show no clinical signs. The virus is transmitted from rodent to rodent through biting, scratching, and possible aersolization of rodent urine.

Filoviruses

Marburg virus (see Figure 3-6) was first isolated in 1967 from several cases of hemorrhagic fever in European laboratory workers in Germany and the former Yugoslavia working with tissues and blood from African green monkeys imported from Uganda. Ebola virus was first reported simultaneously in Zaire and Sudan in 1976, when two distinct subtypes were isolated in two hemorrhagic fever epidemics. Both subtypes, later named *Zaire* and *Sudan*, caused severe disease and mortality rates greater than 50%. A third subtype of Ebola (Reston) was later found in macaques imported from the

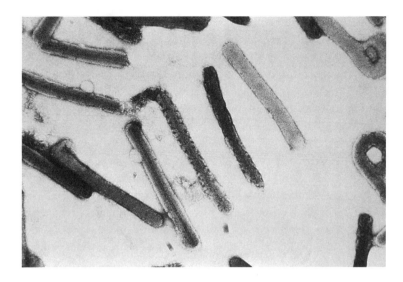

FIGURE 3-6 This electron micrograph depicts a number of Marburg virions responsible for causing Marburg hemorrhagic fever. Marburg hemorrhagic fever virus is caused by a genetically unique zoonotic, RNA virus of the filovirus family; its recognition led to the creation of this virus family. The Ebola viruses are the only other known members of this virus family. (Image courtesy of CDC Public Health Image Library, No. 5614, 1981.)

Philippines into the United States in 1989 and Italy in 1992. Four humans were asymptomatically infected and recovered with no signs of hemorrhagic fever. In 1994, a fourth subtype of Ebola was isolated from an animal worker in Côte d'Ivoire who had performed a necropsy on an infected chimpanzee. Scattered outbreaks have occurred periodically, with the latest being an outbreak of Ebola in the Republic of the Congo in 2003.

The reservoir for filoviruses is still unknown. Bats have been implicated for Marburg virus (Towner et al., 2007), but no evidence of Ebola viruses has been found in over 3,000 species of animals tested in the areas of human outbreaks. Intimate person-to-person contact is the main means of transmission of filoviruses for humans. Nosicomial transmission has been a major problem in outbreaks in Africa through the reuse of needles and syringes and exposure to infected tissues, fluids, and hospital materials. Aerosol transmission has been observed in primates but does not seem to be a major means in humans.

Marburg and Ebola subtypes Sudan, Zaire, and Côte d'Ivoire appear to be found only in Africa, and all three Ebola subtypes have been isolated from human cases only in Africa. The case fatality rate for Marburg ranges from 23–33% and 53–88% for Ebola, with the highest rates found in Ebola Zaire. The presence of Ebola Reston in macaques from the Philippines marked the first time a filovirus was found in Asia. The pattern of disease of humans in nature is relatively unknown except for major epidemics.

Filoviruses cause the most severe hemorrhagic fever in humans. The incubation period for both Marburg and Ebola is generally 4–10 days followed by abrupt onset of fever, chills, malaise, and myalgia. The patient rapidly deteriorates and progresses to multisystem failure. Bleeding from mucosal membranes, venipucture sites, and the gastrointestinal organs occurs followed by disseminated intravascular coagulation. Death or clinical improvement usually occurs around day 7–11. Survivors of the hemorrhagic fever are often plagued with arthralgia, uveitis, psychosocial disturbances, and orchitis for weeks following the initial fever.

Filoviruses cause severe hemorrhagic fever in nonhuman primates. The signs and symptoms found are identical to humans. The only major difference is that Ebola Reston has a high mortality in primates (~82%), while it does not seem to be pathogenic to humans.

Flaviviruses

Flaviviruses can cause an array of clinical manifestations. However, we concentrate on those causing hemorrhagic fever. Yellow fever was first described in 1648 in the Yucatan. It later caused huge outbreaks in tropical Americas in 17th, 18th, 19th, and 20th centuries. The French failed to complete the Panama Canal because their workforce was decimated by yellow fever. Yellow fever virus was the first flavivirus isolated (1927) and the first virus proven to be transmitted by an arthropod vector. Dengue virus, which was also found to be transmitted by an arthropod, was isolated in 1943. Major outbreaks of dengue with hemorrhagic fever occurred in Australia in 1897, Greece in 1928, and Formosa in 1931. Since the cessation of the use of DDT to control mosquito vectors, dengue has now spread to most of the tropical regions of the world.

Omsk hemorrhagic fever virus was first isolated in 1947 from the blood of a patient with hemorrhagic fever during an epidemic in Omsk and Novosibirsk Oblasts of the former Soviet Union. Kyasanur Forest virus was isolated from a sick monkey in the Kyasanur Forest in India in 1957. Since its recognition, 400–500 cases a year have been reported.

Flaviruses utilize an arthropod vector to transmit disease. Yellow fever is a zoonotic disease that is maintained in nonhuman primates. The virus is passed from primate to primate through the bite of an infected mosquito. This is known as the *sylvatic cycle*. Humans contract the disease when bitten by an infected mosquito, usually *Aedes aegypti,* and the disease can then be epidemically spread from human to human by these mosquitoes. This cycle is known as the *urban cycle*. Dengue virus is maintained in the human population and is primarily transmitted from human to mosquito to human, thereby concentrating cases in an urban setting.

Kyasanur Forest virus is transmitted by an ixodid tick. The tick can pass the virus from adult to eggs and from one stage of development to another. The basic transmission cycle involves ixodid ticks and wild vertebrates, principally rodents and insect-eating animals. Humans become infected when bitten by an infected tick. The basic transmission cycle of the Omsk hemorrhagic fever virus is unknown.

The yellow-fever virus is found throughout sub-Saharan Africa and tropical South America, but activity is intermittent and localized. The annual incidence is believed to be about 200,000 cases per year globally. Case-fatality rates range, greatly depending on the epidemic, but may reach up to 50% in severe yellow-fever cases. Dengue virus is found throughout the tropical Americas, Africa, Australia, and Asia. Cases of dengue hemorrhagic fever (DHF) have been increasing as the distribution of *Aedes aegypti* increases following the collapse of mosquito control efforts. Case fatality rates for DHF is generally low (1–10%), depending on available treatment. Kyasanur Forest virus is confined to the Mysore state of India but is spreading. The case-fatality rate is 3–5%. Omsk hemorrhagic fever virus is still isolated to the Omsk and Novosibirsk regions of the former Soviet Union. The case fatality is 0.5–3%.

Yellow fever can cause a severe hemorrhagic fever. The incubation period in humans is 3–6 days. The clinical manifestations can range from mild to severe signs. Severe yellow fever begins abruptly with fever, chills, severe headache, lumbosacral pain, generalized myalgia, anorexia, nausea and vomiting, and minor gingival hemorrhages. A period of remission may occur for 24 hours followed by an increase in the severity of symptoms. Death usually occurs on day 7–10. Dengue virus causes a mild, flulike illness on first exposure. If the person is then infected by a different serotype, dengue hemorrhagic fever can occur. The disease begins like a normal infection of dengue virus, with an incubation period of 2–5 days, but quickly progresses to a hemorrhagic syndrome. Rapid shock ensues but can be reversed with appropriate treatment. Kyasanur Forest virus in humans is characterized by fever, headache, myalgia, cough, bradycardia, dehydration, hypotension, gastrointestinal symptoms, and hemorrhages. Recovery is generally uncomplicated with no lasting sequelae. Omsk hemorrhagic fever virus has a similar presentation to Kyasanur Forest virus; however, hearing loss, hair loss, and neuropsychiatric complaints are commonly reported following recovery.

Yellow fever is maintained in nonhuman primates. Depending on the species, yellow fever may be an unapparent infection or a severe hemorrhagic illness. Dengue has been isolated from several nonhuman primates in Africa but does not cause clinical signs. Livestock may develop a viremia with Kyasanur Forest disease virus but generally do not show clinical signs. Omsk hemorrhagic fever virus is maintained in rodents but does not cause clinical signs.

Clinical Disease in Humans

Specific signs and symptoms vary by the type of VHF, but initial signs and symptoms often include marked fever, fatigue, dizziness, muscle aches, loss of strength, and exhaustion. More severe clinical symptoms include bleeding under the skin causing petechia, ecchymoses, and conjunctivitis. Bleeding may also occur in internal organs and from orifices (like the eye, nose, or mouth). Despite widespread bleeding, blood loss is rarely the cause of the death.

Clinical microbiology and public health laboratories are not currently equipped to make a rapid diagnosis of any of these viruses, and clinical specimens in an outbreak need to be sent to the CDC or the U.S. Army Medical Research Institute of Infectious Diseases, located in Frederick, Maryland. These are the only two level D laboratories in the laboratory response network. These laboratories can conduct serology, polymerase chain reaction (PCR), immunohistochemistry, viral isolation, and electron microscopy of VHF viruses.

Viral hemorrhagic fever patients receive supportive therapy, with special attention paid to maintaining fluid and electrolyte balance, circulatory volume, blood pressure, and treatment for any complicating infections. There is no other established treatment. No antiviral drugs have been approved by the U.S. Federal Drug Administration (FDA) for the treatment of VHF. Treatment with convalescent-phase plasma has been used with success in some patients with Junin, Machupo, and Ebola. If infection with a VHF virus is suspected it should be reported to health authorities immediately. Strict isolation of a patient is required.

Prevention of VHFs is done by avoiding contact with the host species. Because many of the hosts that carry VHFs are rodents, prevention should involve rodent control methods. Steps for rodent prevention include the control of rodent populations, discouraging their entry into homes, and safe cleanup of nesting areas and droppings. For VHFs that are spread by arthropod vectors, prevention efforts should focus on community-wide insect and arthropod control. In addition, people are encouraged to use insect repellant, proper clothing, bed nets, window screens, and other insect barriers to avoid being bitten.

The only established and licensed vaccine is for yellow fever. This live vaccine is safe and effective and gives immunity lasting 10 or more years. An experimental vaccine is under study for Junin virus, which provides some cross protection to Machupo virus. Investigational vaccines are in the development phase for Rift Valley fever, hantavirus, and dengue. For VHFs that can be transmitted person to person, including the Arenaviridae, the Bunyaviridae (excluding Rift Valley fever), and the Filoviridae, close physical contact with infected people and their body fluids should be avoided. One infection control technique is to isolate infected individuals to decrease person-to-person transmission.

Wearing protective clothing is also needed to reduce transmission between people. The WHO and CDC have developed practical, hospital-based guidelines, entitled *Infection Control for Viral Hemorrhagic Fevers in the African Health Care Setting*. The manual can help health-care facilities recognize cases and prevent further hospital-based disease transmission using locally available materials and few financial resources. Other infection control recommendations include proper use, disinfection, and disposal of instruments and equipment used in treating or caring for patients with VHF, such as needles and thermometers. Any disposable items, including linens, are placed in a double plastic bag and saturated with 0.5% sodium hypochlorite (1:10 dilution of bleach). Sharps are placed in the sharps container and saturated with the 0.5% solution, the containers are wiped with the 0.5% solution and sent to be incinerated.

Botulism

Botulinum toxin, which is produced by the spore-forming anaerobic bacterium *Clostridium botulinum*, is a highly toxic substance that presents a major threat from intentional exposure. The toxin is highly lethal and easily produced and released into the environment. Botulinum toxin is absorbed across mucosal surfaces and irreversibly binds to peripheral cholinergic nerve synapses. Seven antigenic types (A–G) of the toxin exist. All seven toxins cause similar clinical presentation and disease; botulinum toxins A, B, and E are responsible for the vast majority of food-borne illnesses in the United States.

□ □ □ ▬▬▬▬▬▬▬▬▬▬▬▬▬▬▬▬▬▬▬▬▬▬▬

Botulinum Toxin

Botulinum toxin is reported to be the *most toxic substance known*. Comparatively, it is 10–15,000 times more toxic than VX nerve agent.

▬▬▬▬▬▬▬▬▬▬▬▬▬▬▬▬▬▬▬▬▬▬▬ □ □ □

If evenly dispersed for inhalation, 1 gram of pure toxin is sufficient to kill 1 million people; however, such dispersion is technically impossible to achieve. The deadly toxin irreversibly blocks acetylcholine release from peripheral nerves, resulting in muscle paralysis. It has been developed as a biological weapon by many government research programs. As a biological weapon, it is a potent substance that is easy to produce and transport. A large population of victims requiring intensive care could easily overwhelm our health-care system (Horton et al., 2002).

Botulism is caused by poisoning from a toxin produced by the bacterium *Clostridium botulinum*. It is a gram-positive, spore-forming, obligate anaerobic bacillus. The clostridial spores are ubiquitous in soil and are very resistant to heat, light, drying, and radiation. Spores may survive boiling for several hours at 100°C; however, exposure to moist heat at 120°C for 30 minutes kills the spores. Specific conditions are required for the germination of spores. These include anaerobic conditions (such as rotting carcasses or canned food), warmth, and mild alkalinity (see Figure 3-7).

After germination, clostridial spores release neurotoxins. The seven antigenic types of neurotoxins are classified A–G. Typically, different neurotoxin types affect different species. Only a few nanograms of these toxins can cause severe illness. All cause flaccid paralysis in the species affected. Toxin is produced in improperly processed, canned, low-acid or alkaline foods, and in pasteurized and lightly cured foods held without refrigeration, especially in airtight packaging.

Botulism was first discovered by the German physician, Justinius Kerner in 1793. He called the substance *wurstgift*, since he found it in spoiled sausages. During this period of time, sausage was made by filling a pig's stomach with meat and blood, boiling it in water then storing it at room temperature. These were ideal conditions for clostridial spores to survive. Botulism gets it name from *botulus*, which is Latin for sausage. In 1895, Emile von Ermengem identified *Clostridium botulinum* as the actual source of a botulism outbreak in Belgium. Several outbreaks of botulism in the United States have led to federal regulations for food preservation. In 1919, an outbreak from canned olives (15 deaths) led to the use of high temperatures as industry standards for preserving foods. In 1973, an outbreak from canned soup led to further regulations for the safe processing of canned foods.

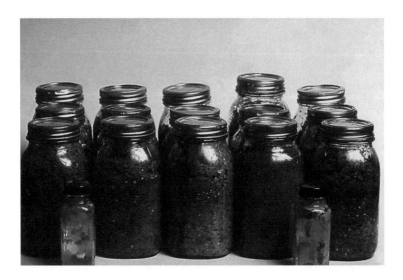

FIGURE 3-7 The jars of contaminated Jalapeño peppers involved in an outbreak of botulism in Pontiac, Michigan, April 1977. The bacterium *Clostridium botulinum* produces a nerve toxin that causes the rare but serious paralytic illness botulism. The seven types of botulism toxin are designated by the letters A through G; only types A, B, E, and F cause illness in humans. (Image courtesy of CDC Public Health Image Library, No. 3355, photo taken by Dr. Charles Hatheway, 1977.)

Botulism typically occurs through ingestion of the organism, neurotoxin, or spores. If the organism is ingested, it incubates in the stomach and produces spores, which then germinate to release neurotoxin. If spores are ingested, germination follows and neurotoxin is released. Finally, if spores have germinated within contaminated food, the neurotoxin itself is ingested, causing rapid progression of the disease. Other forms of transmission involve contamination of open wounds with clostridia spores. Additionally, inhalation of the neurotoxin is possible. This is the most likely bioterrorism method that would be used for this agent. No instance of secondary person-to-person transmission has been documented.

In the United States, on average, there are 110 cases of botulism per year. Typically, about 25% are food-related illnesses. Approximately 72% are the infant botulism form, and the remainder is wound related. To date, the largest botulism outbreak in the United States occurred in 1977 in Michigan. Fifty-nine people were affected after eating poorly preserved jalapeno peppers. Approximately 27% of U.S. food-borne botulism cases occur in Alaska. During 1950–2000, Alaska recorded 226 cases of food-borne botulism from 114 outbreaks. All were Alaska Natives and were associated with eating fermented foods, which is a part of their culture. Due to changes in the fermentation process (use of closed storage containers), an increase in botulism rates occurred in Alaska from 1970–1989.

Human botulism illness can occur in three forms: food-borne illness, infant botulism, and wound contamination. These forms vary by how the toxin is obtained. All forms of the disease can be fatal and should be considered a medical emergency. The incubation period can range from six hours to two weeks. However, signs typically occur 12–36 hours after toxin release. Humans can be affected by types A, B, E, and rarely F neurotoxins.

Food-borne botulism occurs when the preformed neurotoxin is ingested. The most common source of the preformed toxin is contaminated food, usually from improperly home-canned vegetables or fermented fish. Fifty percent of food-borne outbreaks in the United States are caused by type A toxins. The most commonly isolated neurotoxin is type A for canned foods and type E for improperly fermented fish products.

The most common form of human botulism occurs in infants. Annual incidence in the United States is two cases per 100,000 live births. Spores are ingested, germinate, then release their toxin and colonize the large intestine. It occurs predominantly in infants less than one year old (94% are less than six months old). The spores are obtained from various sources, such as honey, food, dust, and corn syrup.

Wound botulism is rare and occurs when the organism gets into an open wound and develops under anaerobic conditions. The organism typically comes from ground-in dirt or gravel. *Clostridium botulinum,* its spores, and neurotoxin cannot penetrate intact skin. This form has also been associated with addicts of black-tar heroin. It is thought to be contaminated with dirt or boot polish during its preparation process. There have been clusters of cases each year in these drug users, some resulting in fatalities.

In humans, the clinical signs of botulism are similar for all forms of the disease. Gastrointestinal signs (i.e., nausea, vomiting, and diarrhea) are usually the first to appear. They are followed acutely by neurological signs, such as bilateral cranial nerve deficits. The victim has double vision and difficulty seeing, speaking, and swallowing. This soon develops into a descending weakness to symmetrical flaccid paralysis. This paralysis can affect the respiratory muscles and lead to death.

Children less than one year of age with the following clinical signs should be suspected of infant botulism (sometimes referred to as *floppy baby syndrome*). These include lethargy, poor feeding, weak cry, bulbar palsies, failure to thrive, and progressive weakness. This can lead to impaired respiration and sometimes death if not treated promptly.

Clinical signs can provide a tentative diagnosis for botulism intoxication. The definitive diagnosis in humans involves identifying the toxin in serum, stool, gastric aspirate, or if available, the suspected food. Feces are usually the most reliable clinical sample in food-borne or infant botulism. Additionally, cultures of stool or gastric aspirate samples may produce the organism, but can take five to seven days. Electromyography can also be diagnostic. The most widely used and sensitive test for detecting botulism toxin is the mouse neutralization test. Serum or stool with the suspected botulism organism is injected into a mouse and observed for clinical signs of the disease. Results are available in 48 hours.

Airborne Botulinum Toxin

It is estimated that a point source aerosol release of botulinum toxin could incapacitate or kill 10% of persons within half a kilometer downwind of the point of release (*Journal of the American Veterinary Medical Association* 285 [2001]: 1059–1070). However, the CDC maintains a well-established surveillance system for reporting human botulism cases that would promptly detect such an event.

Most cases of botulism require immediate intensive care treatment. Due to respiratory paralysis, a mechanical ventilator is needed if respiratory failure occurs. An intravenous equine-derived botulinum antitoxin is available on a case-by-case basis from the CDC through state and local health departments. Botulism immune globulin was approved for use on October 23, 2003, for the treatment of infant botulism caused by types A and G.

Botulinum toxin has been used as an attempted bioweapon. Between 1990 and 1995, the Japanese cult Aum Shinrikyo used botulinum toxin aerosols at multiple sites in Tokyo. Fortunately, these attempts failed. As a potential bioterrorism agent, botulism toxin is extremely potent and lethal. It is easily produced and transported. Signs of a deliberate release of the toxin, either via aerosol or food, would be a large number of acute cases from no common source and occurring as a cluster. Additionally, uncommon toxin types, such as C, D, F, or G, may raise suspicion.

Critical Thinking

Discuss the reasons why each of the Category A agents discussed here is a threat to society. Apply the four Category A criteria to each of the agents and diseases.

Essential Terminology

- **Anthrax**. A serious zoonotic disease caused by *Bacillus anthracis*, a bacterium that forms spores. The three clinical manifestations of human anthrax are: cutaneous, inhalation, and gastrointestinal. Typically, the disease affects cattle and sheep in areas where it is endemic. The disease is not spread from human to human.
- **Botulism**. The result of poisoning from ingestion with botulinum toxin, which is produced by the bacterium *Clostridium botulinum*. Numerous cases occur in the United States every year due to adulterated food products.
- **Plague**. A serious zoonotic disease caused by *Yersinia pestis*, a bacterium. The three main clinical manifestations of human plague are bubonic, pneumonic, and septicemic. There are two lesser forms, plague meningitis and pharyngeal. Normally, the disease affects rodent species and is transmitted by the bite of an infected flea. The pneumonic form of plague is highly contagious from human to human.
- **Smallpox**. A serious, but eradicated, disease caused by smallpox virus. This pathogen is no longer found in nature, since a successful vaccination program eliminated it from human populations. It is not a zoonotic disease. A single case of smallpox today would prompt the World Health Organization to declare an international public health emergency.
- **Tularemia**. A serious zoonotic disease caused by *Francisella tularensis*, a bacterium. The six clinical manifestations of human tularemia are pneumonic, glandular, ulceroglandular, oculoglandular, oropharyngeal, and typhoidal. Normally, the disease affects rabbits and is transmitted by the bite of an infected flea. Tularemia is not spread by human-to-human contact.
- **Viral Hemorrhagic Fever (VHF)**. A group of illnesses caused by several distinct families of viruses that effect humans and nonhuman primates. VHF is a severe multisystem syndrome characterized by diffuse vascular damage. Bleeding often occurs and, depending on the virus, may or may not be life threatening. Some VHF viruses cause mild disease, while others may cause severe symptoms and death.

Discussion Questions

- What are the four criteria of HHS Category A?
- Why would a single case of smallpox be considered an incident of national significance, indeed an incident of international significance?
- In what ways could plague be used as a biological weapon?
- What is the most deadly biological toxin and how could it be practically employed to affect a large number of people?

Web Site

United States Department of Health and Human Services, Centers for Disease Control and Prevention, Emergency Preparedness and Response, Bioterrorism: A thorough listing of all agents covered in this chapter can be found at emergency.cdc.gov/bioterrorism.

References

Albrink, W., S. Brooks, R. Biron, and M. Kopel. 1960. Human inhalation anthrax: A report of three fatal cases. *American Journal of Pathology* 36:457–471.

American Veterinary Medical Association. 2006a. "Anthrax backgrounder." *Biosecurity Updates from the AVMA* (February 22), available at www.avma.org/reference/backgrounders/anthrax_bgnd.asp.>

American Veterinary Medical Association. 2006b. "Plague backgrounder." *Biosecurity Updates from the AVMA* (November 22), available at www.avma.org/reference/backgrounders/plague_bgnd.asp.

American Veterinary Medical Association. 2006c. "Tularemia backgrounder." *Biosecurity Updates from the AVMA* (November 27), available at www.avma.org/reference/backgrounders/tularemia_bgnd.asp.

Barquet, N., and P. Domingo. 1997. Smallpox: The triumph over the most terrible of the ministers of death. *Annals of Internal Medicine* 127:635–642.

Boyce, J., and T. Butler. 1995. *Yersinia* species (including plague). In: *Principles and Practice of Infectious Diseases* 4th ed., eds. G. L. Mandell and J. E. Bennett, pp. 2070–2078. New York: Churchill Livingstone.

Brachman, P., A. Kaufman, and F. Dalldorf. 1966. Industrial inhalation anthrax. *Bacteriology Reviews* 30:646–659.

Cieslak, Theodore J., and Edward M. Eitzen, Jr. 1999. Clinical and epidemiological principles of anthrax. *CDC: Emerging Infectious Diseases* (July 1).

Dahlgren, C., L. Buchanan, H. Decker, S. Freed, C. Phillips, and P. Brachman. 1960. *Bacillus anthracis* aerosols in goat hair processing mills. *American Journal of Hygiene* 72:24–31.

Dennis, D., T. Inglesby, D. A. Henderson, J. Bartlett, M. Ascher, E. Eitzen, A. Fine, A. Friedlander, J. Hauer, M. Layton, S. Lillibridge, J. McDade, M. Osterholm, T. O'Toole, G. Parker, T. Perl, P. Russell, and K. Tonat; Working Group on Civilian Biodefense. 2001. Tularemia as a biological weapon: medical and public health management. *Journal of the American Medical Association* 285:2763–2773.

Dixon, T., M. Meselson, J. Guillemin, and P. Hanna. 1999. Anthrax. *New England Journal of Medicine* 341:815–826.

Eckert, E. 2000. The retreat of plague from Central Europe, 1640–1720: A geomedical approach. *Bulletin of the History of Medicine* 74:1–28.

Eitzen, E. Use of biological weapons. Chapter 20 in *Medical Aspects of Chemical and Biological Warfare*. Washington, DC: Government Printing Office, 1997.

Feldman, K. 2003. Tularemia. *Journal of the American Veterinary Medical Association* 222:725–729.

Fenner, F., D. A. Henderson, I. Arita, et al. 1988. *Smallpox and Its Eradication*. Geneva, Switzerland: World Health Organization.

Horton, H., J. Misrahi, G. Matthews, and P. Kocher. 2002. Critical biological agents: Disease reporting as a tool for determining bioterrorism preparedness. *Journal of Law, Medicine and Ethics* 30:262–266.

Link, V. 1955. *A History of Plague in the United States of America*. Public Health Service Monograph No. 26. Washington, DC: Government Printing Office.

Morbidity and Mortality Weekly Report. 2006. Inhalation anthrax associated with dried animal hides—Pennsylvania and New York City, 2006. *Morbidity and Mortality Weekly Report 55* (March 17):280–282.

Orloski, K., and S. Lathrop. 2003. Plague: A veterinary perspective. *Journal of the American Veterinary Medical Association* 222:444–448.

ProMED Mail. 2007. Anthrax, animal skin. Connecticut, USA. Message No. 2930 (September 5).

Quinn, C., V. Semenova, C. Elie, S. Romero-Steiner, C. Greene, H. Li, et al. 2002. Specific, sensitive, and quantitative enzyme-linked immunosorbent assay for human immunoglobulin G antibodies to anthrax toxin protective antigen. *Emerging Infectious Diseases* [serial online], available at www.cdc.gov/ncidod/EID/vol8no10/02-0380.htm.

Riedel, S. 2005a. Plague: From natural disease to bioterrorism. *Baylor University Medical Center Proceedings* 18:116–124.

Riedel, S. 2005b. Edward Jenner and the history of smallpox and vaccination. *Baylor University Medical Center Proceedings* 18:21–25.

Rotz, L., A. Khan, S. Lillibridge, S. Ostroff, and J. Hughes. 2002. Public health assessment of potential biological terrorism agent. *Emerging Infectious Diseases* 8, no. 2:225–230.

McClain, D. 1997. Smallpox. Chapter 27 in *Medical Aspects of Chemical and Biological Warfare: A Textbook in Military Medicine,* eds. F. R. Sidell, E. T. Takafugi, and D. R. Franz, Bethesda, MD: Office of the Surgeon General, Borden Institute, Walter Reed Army Institute of Research.

Slack, P. 1998. The Black Death past and present. *Transactions of the Royal Society of Tropical Medicine and Hygiene* 83:461–463.

Sternbach, G. 2003. The history of anthrax. *Journal of Emergency Medicine* 24, no. 4:463–467.

Swartz, M. 2001. Recognition and management of anthrax—an update. *New England Journal of Medicine* 345:1621–1626.

Thompson, M. K. 2003. *Killer Strain: Anthrax and a Government Exposed.* 2003. Collingdale, PA: DIANE Publishing Company.

Towner, J., X. Pourrut, C. Albariňo, C. Nkogue, B. Bird, et al. 2007. *Marburg Virus Infection Detected in a Common African Bat.* PLoS ONE 2(8):e764. DOI:10.1371/journal.pone.0000764.

World Health Organization. 1980. Smallpot eradication. *Weekly Epidemiological Record*, no. 55: 33–40.

World Health Organization. 2006. Plague, Democratic Republic of the Congo. *Weekly Epidemiological Record* 81, no. 42:397–398, available at www.who.int/wer/2006/wer8142.pdf.

4

Category B Diseases and Agents

Infectious Disease is one of the few genuine adventures left in the world.
—Hans Zinsser (1878–1940)

Objectives

The study of this chapter will enable you to

1. List and explain the criteria used to define Category B agents.
2. Describe the signs and symptoms of brucellosis, glanders, melioidosis, Q fever, psittacosis, viral encephalitis, and ricin poisoning.
3. Describe the clinical manifestations of brucellosis, glanders, melioidosis, Q fever, psittacosis, viral encephalitis, and ricin poisoning.
4. Discuss prophylaxis and medical treatment strategies used to counter brucellosis, glanders, melioidosis, Q fever, psittacosis, viral encephalitis, and ricin poisoning.
5. Understand the challenges that public health officials and emergency management practitioners face when an intentional release of a Category B agent occurs in their community.

Key Terms

Category B, brucellosis, glanders, melioidosis, Q fever, viral encephalitis, Venezuelan equine encephalomyelitis, psittacosis, ricin, *Brucella* species, *Burkholderia mallei, Burkholderia pseudomallei, Coxiella burnetii, Ricinus communis, Chlamydophila psittaci.*

Introduction

This chapter provides the reader with detailed information on the biological agents and diseases that pose a moderate risk to national security. As discussed in the opening to Part II, the Department of Health and Human Services published a categorized list of what public health experts consider some of the more critical biological agents we face today. The most serious threats, detailed in Category A, were discussed completely in Chapter 3. Coverage of the threat continues with **Category B,** which consists of the second highest priority of agents, which are:

- Moderately easy to disseminate.
- Result in moderate morbidity rates and low mortality rates.
- Require specific enhancements for diagnostic capacity and disease surveillance.

A summary of all Category B diseases, agents, and some pertinent data is shown in Table 4-1. The discussion that follows this introduction will cover *most*, but not all, the diseases and agents found in Category B. Food-borne and waterborne disease pathogens and some of the toxins (SEB and *Clostridium perfringens* epsilon) were omitted so as not to overwhelm the reader.

Brucellosis

Brucellosis is a serious disease affecting humans and animals. In human medicine, brucellosis was previously known as *Malta fever* and is sometimes referred to today as *undulant fever*. In animal medicine, brucellosis was previously referred to as *Bang's disease* (Vella, 1964).

The causative organisms of brucellosis are small, aerobic, gram-negative coccoba-cilli in the genus **Brucella**. These bacteria can persist in the environment with varying degrees of success, depending on several environmental conditions (i.e., temperature, pH, and humidity). *Brucella* bacteria can persist indefinitely if frozen or protected in aborted fetuses or placentas. More important, most members of *Brucella* are facultative, intracellular pathogens, which require prolonged treatment with clinically effective anti-biotics whenever they cause infection.

Table 4-1 Category B Diseases and Their Etiologic Agents: A Summary

Disease	Agent	Type of Agent	Zoonoses	Contagious Person to Person?
Brucellosis	*Brucella* species	Bacteria	Yes	No
Glanders	*Burkholderia mallei*	Bacteria	Yes	No
Melioidosis	*Burkholderia pseudomallei*	Bacteria	Yes	No
Q fever	*Coxiella burnetii*	Rickettsia	Yes	No
Psittacosis	*Chlamydophila psittaci*	Bacteria	Yes	No
Food and water safety threats*	*Salmonella* species; *Shigella dysenteriae* Type 1; *Escherichia coli* O157:H7; *Vibrio cholerae; Typhi*	Bacteria	No	No
Viral encephalitis	Several arboviruses (e.g., VEE, WEE, EEE, SLE)	Virus	Yes	No
Epsilon toxin poisoning*	Clostridium perfringens epsilon toxin	Bacteria-derived toxin	No	No
SEB poisoning*	Staphylococcal Enterotoxin B (SEB)	Bacteria-derived toxin	No	No
Ricin poisoning	Ricin toxin from *Ricinus communis*	Plant-derived toxin	No	No

*Not covered in this chapter.

Table 4-2 Brucellosis: Brucella Species and Host Affected

Species	Biovar/Serovar	Natural Host	Human Pathogen
B. abortus	1–6, 9	Cattle	Yes
B. melitensis	1–3	Goats, sheep	Yes
B. suis	1, 3	Swine	Yes
	2	Hares	Yes
	4	Reindeer, caribou	Yes
	5	Rodents	Yes
B. canis	None	Dogs, other canids	Yes
B. ovis	None	Sheep	No
B. neotomae	None	Desert wood rat	No
B. maris		Marine mammals	?

Of the several species in the genus *Brucella* that cause disease, pathogenicity is relative to the host. Infection of nonprimary hosts may or may not result in disease. The relative pathogenicity in humans and primary hosts for each species and biovar of *Brucella* is summarized in Table 4-2. **Brucella melitensis** is considered to be the most pathogenic to humans, followed by **B. suis, B. abortus**, and finally, **B. canis**.

History

As a disease, brucellosis has a long history, which emanates from the Mediterranean region. Clinical conditions synonymous with brucellosis have been described since the time of Hippocrates. In approximately 400 BC, Hippocrates described a medical condition where people died after four months of intermittent, high fevers. Medical historians believe he was describing brucellosis (Vassalo, 1992). Two thousand years later, physicians described this intermittent, febrile condition as "undulant fever" for the paroxysms depicted on the victim's medical chart. These contagious fevers were documented on the island of Malta as early as 1530. In the Mediterranean region, there were many reports of undulant fevers in the 17th and 18th centuries. Local names, such as Rock fever of Gibraltar, Cyprus fever, Mediterranean fever, and Danube fever, were used. A British surgeon, J. A. Marston, wrote the first detailed account of Malta fever when he described his own illness (Vassalo, 1992). In 1887, another British Army physician, Sir David Bruce, discovered the microorganism responsible for Malta fever, which he called *Micrococcus melitensis*. His studies showed goats to be the primary reservoir for infection, which explained why soldiers that consumed goat's milk were much more likely to contract the disease. *Micrococcus* organisms responsible for brucellosis were later renamed *Brucella* in honor of Dr. Bruce (Ryan and Ray, 2004).

About the same time that physicians had noted brucellosis in humans, in 1897, Dr. Bernhard Bang discovered that an abortive disease affecting cattle in Denmark for more than a century was due to what he called *Bacterium* (a pseudonym for *Brucella*) *abortus*. Bang also determined that *Bacterium abortus* similarly affected sheep, goats, and horses. The disease became known as *Bang's disease*.

Brucellosis made its entry into the United States in 1905 from goats imported from Malta. In fact, an American bacteriologist, Alice Evans, is credited with establishing the link between human and animal infections. She noted similarities in the pathology of the disease and the morphological characteristics of Bang's *Bacterium abortus* and Bruce's *Micrococcus melitensis*.

Transmission

Brucella melitensis infection is primarily food-borne and most often results from consuming infected unpasteurized milk or dairy products (Nicoletti, 1992). It is one of the primary reasons why it is unlawful to sell or purchase raw milk. Human infections of *Brucella abortus* and *B. suis* are often due to contact with infected animal tissues, blood, urine, aborted fetuses, and placentas. *Brucella* can make entry into the body through breaks in the skin or the conjunctiva of the eye. It is also possible that infectious aerosols can lead to infection. These aerosols may be generated while cleaning out an infected animal pen or slaughter house. Person-to-person transmission is very rare but has been reported as a result of bone marrow transplants, breast-feeding, blood transfusion, and sexual contact between infected laboratory workers and their spouses. People that slaughter or process swine are at much higher risk for *B. suis* infections (Doganay and Aygen, 2003).

□ □ □ ▬▬▬▬▬▬▬▬▬▬▬▬▬▬▬▬▬▬▬▬▬▬▬▬▬▬▬▬▬▬▬

Critical Thinking

Brucellosis is a serious problem in many parts of the world. Pasteurization of dairy products greatly reduces the incidence of human brucellosis. Surveillance programs have managed to reduce the incidence of animal brucellosis. For more than 40 years, animal health professionals have been attempting to eradicate brucellosis from the United States (Cutler, Whatmore, and Commander, 2005). Why is it so elusive?

▬▬▬▬▬▬▬▬▬▬▬▬▬▬▬▬▬▬▬▬▬▬▬▬▬▬▬▬▬▬▬ □ □ □

Transmission of *Brucella* in animals appears to be due primarily to consumption of or contact with infected tissues or body fluids. Placenta and aborted fetuses are the most important sources of infection for other animals. Sexual transmission is known to occur with sheep, goats, and swine.

Incidence

Brucellosis is recognized worldwide as a reportable disease (Doganay and Aygen, 2003). Some countries have been able to eradicate it, while others have merely reduced its prevalence. In some areas, the incidence of infection may be significantly higher than the numbers reported because cases often go unrecognized. Currently, brucellosis in humans and animals appears to be on the rise in Eastern Europe, Latin America, Asia, and parts of Africa. In the Mediterranean and Middle East countries, annual incidences of more than 75 cases per 100,000 people have been reported (Pappas et al., 2006). In some areas of the Middle East with intensive dairy farm operations, infection with *B. melitensis* exceeds that of *B. abortus*. Infections due to *Brucella suis* are a major problem in most of the world where swine is produced.

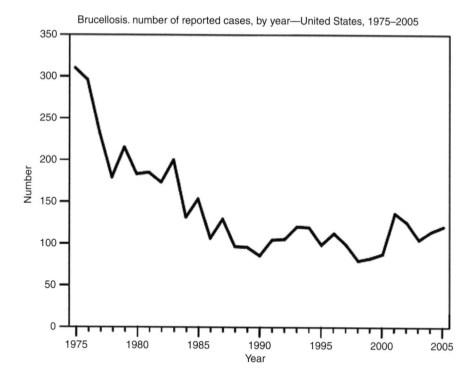

FIGURE 4-1 This graph shows the incidence of human brucellosis cases in the United States from 1975 to 2005. This reportable disease remains in the United States due to ongoing risk for infection with *Brucella suis* acquired from contact with feral swine and *B. melitensis* and *B. abortus* acquired through exposure to raw milk products. (Figure courtesy of the Centers for Disease Control and Prevention.)

The United Kingdom, Denmark, Holland, and Canada are free from brucellosis. Australia and the United States have reduced the prevalence to a very low level, but it remains a persistent problem. Due to the fact that *B. suis* infection is established in the feral swine population, animal health officials in both countries believe it unlikely that eradication efforts will be successful.

The Cooperative State Federal Brucellosis Eradication Program has nearly eliminated *B. abortus* infections among herds in the United States. Therefore, the risk of humans acquiring the infection from occupational exposure or food consumption is minimal. In fact, most cases in the United States are associated with the consumption of unpasteurized, imported milk products. There is an average of about 100 reported cases of brucellosis in the United States each year, with most cases coming from California, Florida, Texas, and Virginia. Figure 4-1 is a summary of the incidence of human brucellosis in the United States.

Clinical Presentation

Brucellosis can involve any organ or organ system. Infected persons present with varying clinical signs and symptoms. The incubation period of brucellosis in humans is 7–21 days but may be several months in some individuals. This latency of clinical signs can lead to difficulty in making a diagnosis. The one common sign in all patients is an intermittent and irregular fever of varying duration. In its acute form (<8 weeks from illness onset), nonspecific and flulike signs and symptoms like fever, sweats, malaise, anorexia, head-ache, myalgia, and back pain are reported. In chronic form (>1 year from onset), symptoms may include chronic fatigue and depressive episodes. Illness can be very protracted and painful resulting in an inability to work.

A frequent complication of brucellosis appears to be involvement of the bones and joints. Arthritis of hips, spine, knees, and ankles also occurs, with back pain and stiffness being the primary complaint. Additionally, the liver often becomes involved in most cases of brucellosis, resulting in hepatomegaly, or an enlarged and sometimes tender liver. When food-borne exposure occurs, the gastrointestinal complications are likely to include nausea, vomiting, anorexia, weight loss, and abdominal discomfort. In males, genitourinary complications can occur, with the testicles becoming inflamed and tender. While sexual transmission has not been proven in humans, *Brucella* bacteria have been detected in sperm bank specimens.

Neurological complications, such as depression and mental fatigue, are common complaints with brucellosis. Cardiovascular complications are rare; however, endocarditis is often the primary cause of death from this disease. In fact, the case-fatality rate in untreated cases is 2% or less, typically from endocarditis caused by *B. melitensis* infections.

Diagnosis and Treatment

Brucella bacteria may be isolated from the blood, bone marrow, and other tissues of infected hosts. Unfortunately, *Brucella* is very slow to grow in artificial media, so culture attempts must be kept for as much as eight weeks before declaring the culture negative. Antibodies for *Brucella*-specific antigens appear 7–14 days after infection. Identification of *B. abortus, B. melitensis*, and *B. suis* is often achieved through a serum agglutination test. *Brucella canis* infection determinations require a specific test. Polymerase chain reaction (PCR) tests for *Brucella* species have been developed by the CDC and USDA for use in their reference laboratories. These tests are fairly quick and definitive, with a high degree of accuracy (specificity and sensitivity). Currently, animal health professionals are using a rapid field test, referred to as a *card test*, for *Brucella* infection in production animals. It is a rapid, sensitive, and reliable procedure for diagnosing brucellosis infection. It is similar to the blood agglutination test but employs disposable materials contained in compact kits. *Brucella* antigen is added to the blood serum on a white card. Results of the test are read four minutes after the serum and antigen are mixed.

As previously stated, prolonged treatment with clinically effective antibiotics is necessary to defeat these intracellular pathogens. Combination therapy with doxycycline and streptomycin has shown the best efficacy for treatment in adults. In addition, doxycycline in combination with rifampin for six weeks has also been used with success. Patients that develop endocarditis require long-term treatment along with surgical replacement of damaged heart valves.

Given an accurate diagnosis and a good course of antibiotic therapy, the prognosis is good for most cases of brucellosis. However, disability from this disease can be quite severe and depends on the localization of infection and response to treatment. Approximately 5% of treated cases relapse weeks to months after therapy has ended. This is often due to the patient not completing the antibiotic regimen, or infection so severe that surgical intervention is required. Antibiotic-resistant strains of *Brucella* have been reported, but the clinical importance of this fact is not completely understood.

□ □ □

Brucellosis in Biowarfare

Laboratory-acquired infections emphasize the tremendous potential for use of the pathogen as an agent of biowarfare (Yagupsky and Baron, 2005). A bioterrorism scenario was evaluated using an aerosolized *Brucella melitensis* agent spread along a line with the prevailing winds and optimal meteorological conditions. It assumed the infectious dose to infect 50% (ID_{50}) of a human population would require inhalation of 1,000 vegetative cells. Once disseminated, the environmental decay of the organism is estimated at 2% per minute. Some assumptions were made in the construction of the scenario. First, persons close to the point of origin would inhale 1–10 times the ID_{50}. Second, half of the people affected would be hospitalized and remain so for 7 days. If not hospitalized, they would make 14 outpatient visits and receive parenteral gentamicin for 7 days followed by oral doxycycline for 42 days. Approximately 5% of case patients would relapse and require 14 outpatient visits in one year. Third, the case fatality rate would be 0.5%. In looking at the economic impact of such a threat, one must consider the cost of premature human death, and all the costs related to hospitalization and outpatient visits. The minimum cost of exposure would be around $477.7 million per 100,000 persons exposed.

Source: Kaufmann, Arnold F., Meltzer, Martin I., and Schmid, George P., "The Economic Impact of a Bioterrorist Attack: Are Prevention and Post-attack Intervention Programs Justifiable?" *Emerging Infectious Diseases* 3, no. 2 (April–June 1997): 85.

□ □ □

Glanders and Melioidosis

Glanders and melioidosis are two serious zoonoses that are caused by etiologic agents in the genus *Burkholderia*. *Burkholderia* bacteria are commonly found in the soil and in groundwater worldwide. Many species of *Burkholderia* are environmentally important because of their ability to break down toxic substances. However, some *Burkholderia* are animal and plant pathogens. In fact, the genus name comes from the researcher Walter Burkholder, who discovered a plant pathogen previously known only to cause onion bulbs to rot but mysteriously caused an outbreak in vegetable growers in New York state (Moore and Elborn, 2003).

Burkholderia are gram-negative bacilli, which may remain viable for several months in warm moist environments. They tend to form slender rods in culture media, appearing bipolar or safety-pin shaped after staining. *Burkholderia* can withstand drying for 2–3 weeks but are destroyed by sunlight and high temperature. Due to high infectivity and environmental stability, two species of *Burkholderia* have been exploited as biological weapons and are considered potential agents for biological terrorism.

Glanders

Glanders is an infectious disease caused by the bacterium ***Burkholderia mallei***. It primarily affects horses, but it can also affect mules, donkeys, goats, dogs, and cats. Glanders is commonly seen among domestic animals in Africa, Asia, the Middle East, and Central and South America. Glanders is transmitted to humans through direct contact with infected animals. The bacteria enter the body through the skin, eyes, and nose; the symptoms depend on the route of infection. Glanders may manifest in humans as localized, pulmonary, bloodstream, or chronic infections (CDC, "Glanders," pars. 1–12). There have been no human cases of glanders in the United States since 1954.

Melioidosis

Burkholderia pseudomallei is the causative agent of **melioidosis,** a serious disease affecting both humans and animals. Infection with *B. pseudomallei* can lead to septicemia and pneumonia in susceptible individuals (Godoy et al., 2003). Melioidosis is also referred to as *Whitmore's disease.* Melioidosis is clinically and pathologically similar to glanders, but the ecology and epidemiology of melioidosis are different from glanders. Melioidosis occurs in the tropics, especially in Southeast Asia, where it is endemic. *Burkholderia pseudomallei* bacteria are found in contaminated soil and water and spread to humans and animals through direct contact with the contaminated source.

History

During World War I, the Germans deliberately introduced glanders along the Eastern Front into Russian horse and mule herds. They did so to affect the Russian's ability to move supplies, troops, and artillery pieces throughout the war. Human cases of glanders also increased in Russia during and after World War I.

We also know that the Japanese deliberately infected horses, civilians, and prisoners of war with glanders during World War II. The U.S. biowarfare program considered *Burkholderia* as a possible bacteriological weapon in 1943 but did not weaponize it. Likewise, Biopreparat in the former Soviet Union was interested in glanders as a potential biological weapon agent after World War II.

Glanders was eradicated from the United States in the 1930s. However, six laboratory workers developed glanders in 1945 after working on a bioweapons project at Camp Detrick, Maryland. More recently, another laboratory-acquired case of glanders from Fort Detrick occurred in 2000. A diagnosis of glanders was not confirmed until two months after the onset of symptoms, though a tentative diagnosis was suspected due to the victim's work history. This delay in diagnosis gives credence to the third attribute of a Category B disease: They require specific enhancements for diagnostic capacity and disease surveillance.

□ □ □ ▬▬▬▬▬▬▬▬▬▬▬▬▬▬▬▬▬▬▬▬▬▬▬▬▬▬▬▬▬▬▬▬

Critical Thinking

Burkholderia pseudomallei and *B. mallei* are considered important bioterrorism agents due to their ready worldwide availability and their ability to be transmitted by aerosol. An intentional release of *Burkholderia* could affect hundreds or thousands of people, depending on the method of release and the setting. Would clinicians in the United States manage to recognize a case of glanders in a patient? What would be the burden to the health-care system?

▬▬▬▬▬▬▬▬▬▬▬▬▬▬▬▬▬▬▬▬▬▬▬▬▬▬▬▬▬▬▬▬ □ □ □

Transmission

Despite the efficiency of spread in a laboratory setting, glanders has been only an infrequent disease in humans. No epidemics of human disease have been reported. Glanders is transmitted to humans by direct contact with infected animal secretions and tissues. Normally, *Burkholderia* gain entry to the host through a break in the skin or mucosal linings of the eyes, nose, and mouth. The bacteria may be acquired through inhalation of infectious material. There are no known cases of human intestinal glanders, so infection through ingestion appears to be unimportant. Human-to-human transmission of glanders is possible and has been reported.

Glanders is mostly a disease of horses, donkeys, mules, and goats. Donkeys and mules have been regarded as most likely to experience the acute form of the disease, horses a more chronic form of the disease. Many carnivores are susceptible to glanders if they consume infected meat. Swine and cattle are resistant to infection from *Burkholderia mallei*.

In animals, glanders is introduced into horses by other diseased animals. The main route of entry is through ingestion. In fact, transmission appears to be facilitated by animals sharing feed and water sources. Experimental evidence suggests that inhalation of the organism is less likely to result in typical cases of the disease. Acquiring the disease through skin or mucous membranes is possible but regarded as of minor importance in the natural spread of the disease.

At one time, glanders was widespread throughout the world. However, the disease has been eliminated from many countries due to successful eradication efforts. Currently, glanders is found in parts of the Middle East, Africa, Asia, the Balkan states, and some of the former Soviet Republics. Sporadically, cases occur in South America and Mexico. Serological evidence for the prevalence of glanders is often confused by cross reactivity with specific antibodies for melioidosis (*Burkholderia pseudomallei*).

Clinical Presentation

Humans with occupational exposure to potentially infected animals are at the greatest risk for infection. This includes animal health professionals, ranchers, wranglers, and abattoir workers. The four distinct clinical manifestations of glanders in humans are a localized cutaneous form, a pulmonary form, a septicemic form, and, a chronic form. Generalized symptoms of glanders include muscle aches, chest pain, fever, muscle tightness, and headache. Occasionally, infected individuals complain about excessive tearing, sensitivity to light, and diarrhea. Untreated, 95% of glanders cases lead to death.

In the cutaneous form of glanders, a localized infection with inflammation and ulceration develops within 1–5 days at the site where the bacteria entered the body. This condition may lead to lymphadenopathy (swollen lymph nodes and nodules). Infections involving the mucous membranes result in increased mucus production from the affected sites. Infectious nodules, which appear along the course of the affected lymphatic pathway, form ulcers and leak a highly infectious exudate.

Pulmonary glanders may occur after inhalation of aerosolized *Burkholderia mallei* or invasion of the lungs following bacteremia. Here, the incubation period is 10–14 days. Pulmonary abscesses, pneumonia, and pleural effusions may occur.

The septic form of glanders occurs when *Burkholderia mallei* bacteria enter the bloodstream in large enough numbers to cause a generalized bacteremia. This form of glanders has an incubation period of 7–10 days. Septicemic glanders may occur independently or as a result of the pulmonary or cutaneous forms. Symptoms include high fever, chills, muscle pain, chest pain, and rash. Rapid heart beat, jaundice, sensitivity to light, and diarrhea can also occur. This is a very serious condition, where a 60% case fatality rate is seen, even with antibiotic treatment.

Chronic glanders is sometimes referred to as *farcy*. This form produces multiple abscesses with the muscles of the arms and legs. Chronic glanders may even lead to abscesses forming in the liver, spleen, and joints. This, too, is a serious medical condition with a treated case-fatality rate of 60%. Some of those with chronic glanders relapse long after treatment is complete and deemed to be successful.

□ □ □

Glanders in Biowarfare

Glanders has several characteristics that make it a potential agent for biological warfare and terrorism. Very few *Burkholderia mallei* organisms are required to cause disease and the organism is easily produced. In a single year in the 1980s, the Soviet Union produced more than 2,000 tons of formulated *B. mallei*. When the bacteria are inhaled as an aerosol, the disease has a very high mortality rate. Additionally, diagnosis and treatment of glanders is confounded by the lack of knowledge of this disease among health-care providers and diagnosticians. Patients who recover do not develop a protective immunity, therefore the agent could be reused.

□ □ □

Diagnosis and Treatment

Human glanders may be confused with a variety of other diseases, including typhoid fever, tuberculosis, syphilis, yaws, and melioidosis. Glanders is diagnosed in the laboratory by isolating *Burkholderia* from the blood, sputum, urine, or skin lesions of the host. As with *Brucella*, cultures are very slow to grow in artificial media, making them less useful than an accurate and more expedient test like PCR.

Limited information exists regarding antibiotic treatment of glanders since the disease had largely disappeared by the time antibiotics became available. Long-term treatment, up to 12 months, may be necessary for chronic and pulmonary forms of glanders. Currently, no proven pre- or postexposure prophylaxis is available. BioSafety Level (BSL) 3 containment practices are required for laboratory staff when working with *Burkholderia*. Glanders is reportable to state veterinary offices. A vaccine is not available for humans or animals.

Q Fever

Q fever is a very interesting disease and its use in biowarfare has an extensive past (Riedel, 2004). The agent that causes Q fever was a prime candidate in the U.S. bioweapons programs. Q fever is caused by **Coxiella burnetii**. It became a reportable disease in the

United States in 1999; however, reporting cases of Q fever is not required in other countries. The true incidence and prevalence of Q fever is unknown because public health officials believe this disease is underreported.

Coxiella burnetii is an obligate, intracellular, gram-negative, rickettsial pathogen. It replicates in some of the host's white blood cells (macrophage and monocytes). *Coxiella burnetii* has remarkable stability and can reach high concentrations in animal environments (Reimer, 1993). *Coxiella burnetii* forms unusual spore-like structures, making it highly resistant to environmental conditions and many disinfectants. *Coxiella burnetii* can survive up to 10 days on wool at room temperature, 1 month on fresh meat in cold storage, up to 4 months in dust, and more than 40 months in skim milk. Fortunately, the organism is killed by pasteurization (Reimer, 1993).

The primary reservoirs of *C. burnetii* are cattle, sheep, and goats. However, infection with *C. burnetii* has been reported in many other animals, including other production animals and domesticated pets (Maurin and Raoult, 1999). *Coxiella burnetii* spores are resistant to heat, drying, and many common disinfectants, enabling the bacteria to survive for long periods in the environment. Infection in humans usually occurs by inhalation of these organisms from air containing barnyard dust contaminated by dried placental material, birth fluids, and excretions of infected herd animals. Humans are very susceptible to the disease; very few organisms may be required to cause infection. Ingestion of contaminated milk is a less-common mode of transmission; other modes of transmission to humans, including tick bites and person to person, are rare (CDC, "Q Fever," pars. 1–12).

History

In 1935, Q fever, or "Query" fever, was first reported in Brisbane, Australia. This observation came after several outbreaks of febrile illness in abattoir workers in Queensland (Derrick, 1937). The organism was successfully isolated from the Queensland illnesses by Burnet. A similar organism was isolated by Davis and Cox from ticks in Montana and subsequently found to be the same organism as that in Queensland. In 1938, the organism was named *Coxiella burnetii* in honor of Cox and Burnet, who had identified the organism as a new rickettsial agent. In 1944, there were outbreaks among British and American troops stationed in Italy and the Persian Gulf region during World War II.

□ □ □ ▬▬▬▬▬▬▬▬▬▬▬▬▬▬▬▬▬▬▬▬▬▬▬▬▬▬▬▬▬▬

Critical Thinking

Low mortality and long-term morbidity was expected from an attack with Q fever. Formulation of *Coxiella burnetii* spores was perfected. As such, *C. burnetii* became a primary agent of the U.S. bioweapons program. Think of it this way: If we release a lethal agent in warfare, we might kill 1,000 soldiers. If we use Q fever, we might make 1,000 soldiers sick for several months and it will take 10,000 people to care for them!

▬▬▬▬▬▬▬▬▬▬▬▬▬▬▬▬▬▬▬▬▬▬▬▬▬▬▬▬▬▬▬▬▬▬ □ □ □

Transmission

Q fever is another example of an animal disease brought to humans through the domestication and production of animals. Ruminants are the most common source of *Coxiella burnetii*. It is transmitted to humans in many ways. Inhalation of the spore-like form of *C. burnetii* is the primary mode of transmission in humans. Since *Coxiella burnetii* is so persistent in the environment, dried infective material can contaminate dust or soil. In fact, *Coxiella burnetii* has been found in airborne particles contaminated by bodily fluids and infected tissues. This resulted in cases of patients with no evident contact with animals. Outbreaks have been reported in persons residing downwind from farms where infected animals were kept.

Normally, animals become infected with *Coxiella burnetii* when they are exposed to other infected animals, either through direct contact with contaminated material or aerosol exposure. *Coxiella burnetii* are shed into the environment when infected animals are giving birth. Transmission also occurs when infected animals are slaughtered. Organisms shed in the excreta of infected animals serve as a source of water, soil, or fomite contamination. Therefore, waterborne transmission is possible. *Coxiella burnetii* is also shed into the milk of infected mothers, but the pasteurization process renders the pathogen nonviable. A variety of arthropods can serve as a vector of *Coxiella burnetii*. The organism has been isolated from ticks, cockroaches, beetles, flies, fleas, lice, and mites. More than 40 tick species are naturally infected with *C. burnetii*.

Person-to-person transmission is extremely rare, with the exception of transplacental transmission. Transmission from blood transfusions and bone marrow transplants have been reported. Sexual transmission of *Coxiella burnetii* has been documented in rodents and suspected in a few human cases. Companion animals have been the source of some limited urban outbreaks.

Incidence

Q fever is a true zoonosis with a worldwide distribution, having been reported on all continents. Many animals can serve as a reservoir for *Coxiella burnetii*, including wild and domestic mammals, birds, and arthropods.

Naturally, Q fever is considered an occupational hazard in persons having contact with domestic animals, such as cattle, sheep, and goats. Persons at risk include farmers, animal health professionals, slaughterhouse workers, and laboratory personnel performing culture and diagnostics with *Coxiella burnetii*. Recently, there have been reports of cases of Q fever in people living in urban areas that have had limited contact with farm animals or contact with companion animals.

The map in Figure 4-2 details the geographic distribution of Q fever reported to the CDC in the year 2005. In the United States, Q fever became a nationally reportable disease in 1999; however, epidemiologic data is limited. Much of this is due to the sometimes benign nature of the disease in most individuals. Between the years 1948–1977, a total of 1,168 cases of Q fever were reported to the CDC (58.4 cases per year). More than 65% of these cases were reported from California.

Clinical Presentation

Most cases of Q fever are asymptomatic and without clinical consequence. Medical experts estimate that half of all the people infected with *Coxiella burnetii* show signs

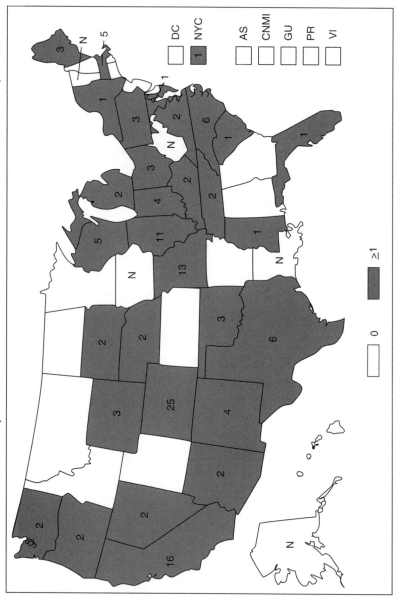

Q FEVER. Number of reported cases—United States and U.S. territories, 2005

Q fever became nationally notifiable in 1999. To capture as many cases of Q fever as possible, the Q fever case definition is intentionally broad. However, identification and reporting of Q fever remains incomplete, and the numbers of cases reported might not represent the overall distribution or regional incidence of disease.

FIGURE 4-2 The figure represents the incidences of human cases of Q fever by state in the United States in the year 2005. Q fever became a nationally notifiable disease in 1999; its case definition is intentionally broad to capture as many cases as possible. The CDC estimates that identification and reporting of Q fever is still incomplete, which makes the overall picture of distribution in the United States unreliable. N = Report of disease is not required in this state. (Figure courtesy of the Centers for Disease Control and Prevention.)

of clinical illness. Humans are considered dead-end hosts and therefore not important in the natural history of the disease. The incubation period in humans ranges from 2–40 days. Generally, there are two clinical forms of the disease: acute (less than six months, duration) and chronic (greater than six months, duration) Q fever.

Symptoms of acute Q fever vary in severity and duration. Normally, acute Q fever manifests as a self-limited febrile or flulike illness. Case patients experience high fever, chills, profuse sweating, fatigue, anorexia, malaise, myalgia, chest pain, and intense headaches around the eyes. Acute Q fever lasts from 1–3 weeks. Approximately half of the patients with symptomatic illness develop pneumonia. In severe cases, a nonproductive cough, hepatitis, and pleural effusion may develop. Only 2% of acute infections require hospitalization, and a similar percentage result in death.

Chronic Q fever, a condition where the infection lasts longer than six months, is relatively uncommon. Typically, chronic Q fever develops in persons with a preexisting cardiac condition. Pregnant women and individuals with a compromised immune system are also at greater risk for the chronic form of Q fever. Endocarditis is found in the majority of chronic Q fever cases. The infection can also affect the liver, resulting in hepatitis or cirrhosis. Involvement of skeletal and arterial systems has been reported in some patients. Incredibly, some acute Q fever patients developed the chronic form up to 20 years after their initial infection.

Diagnosis and Treatment

As always, the clinical presentation and patient history are important in the differential diagnostic process. A number of serological assays have been developed and are useful in making the differential diagnosis of Q fever. These tests include immunofluorescence assay (IFA), complement fixation (CF), and enzyme-linked immunosorbent assay. Indirect IFA is the most dependable and widely used method. However, a number of next-generation diagnostic assays are also useful in detecting *Coxiella burnetii* in patient samples. Specifically, immunohistochemistry (IHC) and polymerase chain reaction have been used with great sensitivity and specificity. Isolation of the organism is possible; however, *Coxiella burnetii* is a BSL 3 agent, making isolation problematic for most agencies.

Q fever case patients respond well to antibiotic therapy but more so when an early diagnosis is made. Doxycycline is the primary antibiotic used for the treatment of Q fever. Chronic Q fever patients may require antibiotic therapy for 2–3 years. Active chronic disease is usually fatal if untreated. Patients with chronic Q fever and a resultant endocarditis need valve replacement surgery. The case fatality rate for these patients may be as high as 65%.

□ □ □ ▬▬▬▬▬▬▬▬▬▬▬▬▬▬▬▬▬▬▬▬▬▬▬

Q Fever in Biowarfare

Because of its highly infectious nature, stability in the environment, and aerosol route of transmission, *C. burnetii* is considered a potential agent for acts of biowarfare and bioterrorism. Although the overall mortality associated with the disease is low, it is considered a debilitating agent. *Coxiella burnetii* was extensively researched in the U.S. bioweapons program. In fact, William Patrick, a prominent figure in that program, made great strides in formulating this agent. At one time, the United States had a project and plan aimed at releasing *C. burnetii*, along with other agents, in an attack against Cuba (Miller, Engelberg, and Broad, 2001). Fortunately, the plan was not implemented. The World Health Organization estimated that, if *C. burnetii* were aerosolized in a city of approximately 5 million people, there would be 125,000 ill and 150 deaths. The WHO estimate predicted that the agent would travel downwind more than 20 km.

Psittacosis

Psittacosis is the term used to describe human infection with **Chlamydophila psittaci**. When birds are infected with *Chlamydophila psittaci,* the term avian *chlamydiosis* is used. The disease in birds is also known as *parrot fever* and *ornithosis* (Avian chlamydiosis, 1996).

The etiologic agent of psittacosis is *Chlamydophila psittaci*. Psittacosis causes flu-like symptoms, which can lead to severe pneumonia and other health problems. With appropriate treatment, the disease is rarely fatal. Most human cases have been associated with exposure to pet birds, poultry, or free-ranging birds. Infection in humans occurs when a person inhales viable *Chlamydophila psittaci* aerosolized from the dried feces or respiratory tract secretions of infected birds (Smith et al., 2005).

Chlamydophila psittaci is an obligate intercellular organism, a small bacterium, undergoing several transformations during its life cycle. It exists as an elementary body (EB) in between hosts. The EB is not biologically active but is resistant to environmental stress, able to survive outside of the host. The EB is shed by an infected bird and inhaled into the lungs of a new host. Once in the lungs, the EB is taken into the endosome of host cells through the process of phagocytosis. Elementary bodies are then transformed into reticulate bodies (RB), which begin to replicate within the endosome. Reticulate bodies use host cell components to replicate. The RBs convert back to elementary bodies, are released back into the lung, and subsequently cause the death of the host cell. The new EBs released from the dead cells are able to infect new cells, either in the same host or another one. Thus, the life cycle of *C. psittaci* is an interesting dichotomy, including both a reticulate body, which can replicate but is unable to cause new infection, and an elementary body, which is able to infect new hosts but cannot replicate.

Chlamydophila psittaci is very resistant to drying. Elementary bodies have been shown to retain viability in canary feed for two months, in poultry litter for up to eight months, and in straw and on hard surfaces for 2–3 weeks (Johnston et al., 1999).

History

The first recognized outbreak of psittacosis occurred in 1879. Ritter described the disease in seven patients who had a history of recent contact with sick parrots. The largest epidemic occurred in 1929–1930, which resulted in approximately 750 sick people. The outbreak experienced in Europe and the United States was due to importation of infected exotic birds from Argentina. Approximately 20% of the patients associated with these outbreaks died from the disease. Since the 1930 epidemic, many countries have instituted an importation ban on psittacine birds. However, smuggling exotic birds out of tropical environments is common due to the price that some of these birds will bring.

Incidence

Between 1988 and 2002, the CDC received 923 reports of cases of psittacosis. However, CDC officials believe that this is likely an underrepresentation of the actual number of cases, because psittacosis is difficult to diagnose and cases often go unreported. Overall, pet store employees, owners of pet birds, and poultry processing plant workers account for the majority of the reported cases.

Figure 4-3 is a chart depicting the annual cases of psittacosis in the United States from 1972 to 2002. Case numbers vary dramatically from year to year due to periodic outbreaks. The increase in reported cases from the 1970s to the 1980s is probably due to increased use of diagnostic tests in respiratory patients following the onset of AIDS in the United States. The decrease in cases in the 1990s may be due to improved diagnostic tests and better disease control methods.

Transmission

Chlamydophila psittaci is found in the feces and nasal discharges of infected birds. The organism can remain infectious for several months if it remains moist and cool, such as

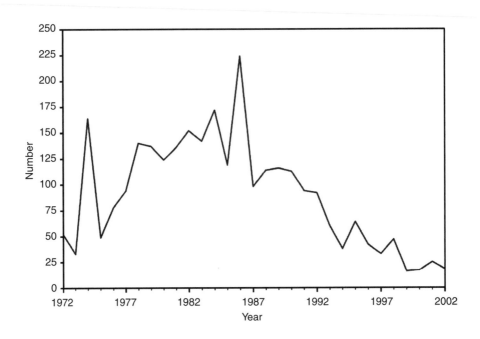

FIGURE 4-3 The graph shows the incidence of human cases of psittacosis in the United States between 1972 and 2002. As shown, the number of cases can fluctuate between 20 and 225 in any given year, probably due to the importation of infected exotic birds. (Figure courtesy of the Centers for Disease Control and Prevention.)

the conditions found in guano. As with most of these diseases, humans are an incidental, dead-end host. Human infection can result from transient exposure to infected birds or their droppings. Therefore, people often become infected without recalling having contact with birds. Infection occurs primarily through inhalation of aerosolized guano from infected birds. Other means of exposure include mouth-to-beak contact and direct transmission from infected bird feathers and tissues. Person-to-person and food-borne transmission have not been documented.

□ □ □ ▬▬▬▬▬▬▬▬▬▬▬▬▬▬▬▬▬▬▬▬▬▬▬▬▬

Critical Thinking

There is no evidence that any bioweapons program intended to use psittacosis or mass produce *Chlamydophila psittaci*. So, why did it make it to the Category B list?

▬▬▬▬▬▬▬▬▬▬▬▬▬▬▬▬▬▬▬▬▬▬▬▬▬ □ □ □

Clinical Presentation

The incubation period for psittacosis ranges from 1–4 weeks. However, most patients develop symptoms after 10 days. Psittacosis patients present with illness that ranges from mild to severe systemic illness with pneumonia. Pneumonia occurs most commonly in older adults. Psittacosis patients most often complain of fever, chills, headache, malaise, myalgia, nonproductive cough, difficulty breathing, and rash on the trunk of the body. This rash appears very much like the rash seen in typhoid fever patients. Some patients become lethargic and have sluggish speech. Other organ systems can be involved, which can lead to more serious conditions like heart complications, hepatitis, arthritis, conjunctivitis, encephalitis, and respiratory failure.

Diagnosis and Treatment

Chlamydophila psittaci can be cultured from respiratory secretions; however, very few laboratories can perform this very technical procedure and there are serious biosafety considerations. Serological tests, like complement fixation tests and microimmunofluorescence (MIF) can be quite helpful when used together with clinical presentation. In addition, an interview with the patient may help establish contact with a sick bird.

Antibiotic treatment with tetracycline is preferred for psittacosis. Patients should see improvement within 48–72 hours, but relapse may develop. Without specific antibiotic treatment, symptoms may resolve in weeks to months. The experienced case fatality rates with and without treatment is 1–5% and 10–40%, respectively.

Disease in Birds

Chlamydophila psittaci is an infection found most commonly in psittacine (parrot-like) birds, especially cockatiels and parakeets. The organism has also been found in ducks, turkeys, pigeons, chickens, gulls, and egrets. Outbreaks of parrot fever on duck and turkey farms have been directly tied to human cases of psittacosis.

Chlamydophila psittaci is shed in the feces and nasal discharges of infected birds. As with influenza virus, infected birds may appear to be healthy but are actually carrying and shedding *C. psittaci*. Latent infections of *C. psittaci* are common. Some birds may not develop active disease until several months to years after exposure. Morbidity and mortality vary with the species of bird and serotype of *C. psittaci*. Birds with parrot fever appear to be depressed or nervous and experience ruffled feathers, weakness, nasal discharge, respiratory distress, diarrhea, conjunctivitis, sinusitis, anorexia, and weight loss. Egg production is likely to decrease in sick birds. Diagnosis of infected birds is difficult and treatment is likely to be long term for pet birds or impractical for poultry. No vaccine is available for *C. psittaci*.

□ □ □ ▬▬▬▬▬▬▬▬▬▬▬▬▬▬▬▬▬▬▬▬▬▬▬▬▬▬

Psittacosis in Biowarfare

Chlamydia psittaci has previously been a component of several state-funded bioweapons research programs. Some characteristics that may make it a good potential bioweapon include its stability in the environment, ease for aerosolization, and worldwide prevalence.

The United States ended large-scale commercial importation of psittacine birds in 1993 with the implementation of the Wild Bird Conservation Act. However, importation on a limited basis continues. Bird smuggling is rare but remains a potential source of parrot fever and psittacosis. The Animal Plant Health Inspection Service (APHIS) of the USDA regulates the importation of birds and maintains treatment protocols under these regulations, but the regulations are not always sufficient to clear avian chlamydiosis from all birds.

▬▬▬▬▬▬▬▬▬▬▬▬▬▬▬▬▬▬▬▬▬▬▬▬▬▬ □ □ □

Viral Encephalitis

Viral encephalitis is an inflammation of the brain caused by a virus. Many viruses are capable of causing infections that lead to viral encephalitis. These include, but are not limited to, enterovirus, herpes simplex virus, varicella-zoster virus, Epstein-Barr virus, adenovirus, rubella, measles, and many of the arboviruses.

Arbovirus is shortened term for *ar*thropod-*bo*rne virus. Arboviruses are a large group of viruses that are transmitted by arthropods, most commonly blood-sucking insects and ticks. In the United States, arboviruses are spread mostly by mosquitoes. Birds are often the reservoir for these viruses. Mosquitoes and ticks act as the bridge between the bird reservoir and the secondary host, which is a horse, humans, or other animal. Humans are considered a dead-end host for these pathogens and are not considered part of the natural history of the diseases. Figure 4-4 offers a typical life cycle representation of an arbovirus.

Transmission for arboviruses begins when the female mosquito takes a blood meal from a reservoir vertebrate host, which in most cases is a bird. A viremia then sets in and is of a sufficient level and duration to affect other mosquitoes, thus propagating the cycle.

Arbovirus Transmission Cycle

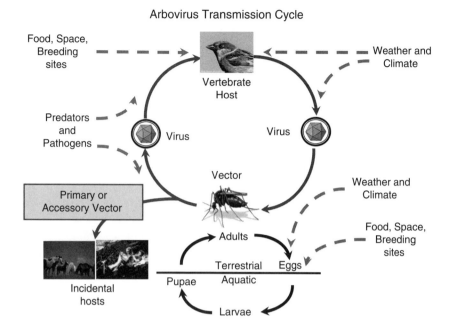

FIGURE 4-4 Arboviral encephalitides are maintained in nature by a number of reservoir hosts and vector. Their complex life cycles are influenced by many environmental factors that can dramatically affect the number of cases in birds, animals, and humans. (Image courtesy of the CDC Division of Vector Borne Infectious Diseases, Fort Collins, Colorado.)

The virus particles can then replicate in the salivary glands of the mosquito to be passed onto other vertebrate hosts or dead-end hosts, such as humans and horses, where overt disease occurs.

Once the viruses have gained access to the bloodstream, they multiply and head to the spinal cord and brain (central nervous system). Access to the brain is by blood or nerves. After breaching the blood-brain barrier, the viruses slip inside brain cells. This disrupts, damages, and ultimately ruptures the infected brain cells. Certain viruses have a preference for different areas of the brain. For example, the herpes simplex virus likes to target the temporal lobes located over each ear. The cells of the immune system rush to the brain and start attacking the viruses. This causes the characteristic brain swelling (cerebral edema). Both the infection and the attempts of the body to fight the infection are responsible for the symptoms of viral encephalitis.

For this chapter, we focus attention on only one cause of viral encephalitis, the Venezuelan equine encephalitis (VEE) virus. The reason for this is that VEE is one of the few viruses that the U.S. Biological Warfare program studied and considered for exploitation. In addition, the former Soviet Union program also worked with VEE for formulation and dissemination technologies.

History

Venezuelan equine encephalitis is a mosquito-borne viral disease that occurs throughout the Americas. As with other arboviruses, the disease cycles between mosquitoes and birds. A number of environmental factors contribute to the sporadic nature of this disease.

The VEE virus has a complex classification system due to its six subtypes (I–VI). From an epidemiological standpoint, this distinction is important. Some subtypes cause severe disease and epidemics. For instance, three of the six variants in subtype I have epidemic potential. Normal enzootic strains have a wide geographic distribution in the Americas; however, the pathogenic form has not been seen in the United States since 1971. Epidemic strains of VEE virus (I-A, I-B, and I-C) are known to cause disease in horses and humans. All other strains, referred to as *enzootic strains*, cause intermittent disease in humans.

Enzootic strains are routinely isolated from mosquitoes (mostly *Culex* species). These strains have a broad geographic distribution in the Americas and are maintained in a variety of rain-forest dwelling animals. Conversely, epidemic strains are transmitted by a wider array of mosquito species and had been amplified in horses and donkeys during outbreak situations. Strangely, none of these epidemic strains has been isolated from mosquitoes or vertebrate hosts since 1973.

The VEE virus was first isolated in 1938 from an infected horse's brain. Annual outbreaks in Colombia and Venezuela occurred through the 1960s. An epidemic in Venezuela that took place from 1962 to 1964 caused more than 23,000 human cases of VEE. In 1967, Columbia suffered a major epidemic, which caused approximately 220,000 human cases and more than 67,000 equine deaths. The largest recorded outbreak of VEE originated in Guatemala in 1969 and spread north to Texas over the course of a few years. This event led to the only known epidemic of VEE in the United States in 1971. The outbreak was due to subtype I-AB, which caused disease in horses and humans. Overall, from 1969 to 1971, human cases of VEE were in the thousands with more than 100,000 equine deaths.

In 1995, a major epizootic occurred in Venezuela and Columbia. Over an eight-month period, there were more than 100,000 human cases of the disease and an untold number of equine cases. In response to the outbreak, a massive mosquito eradication campaign was conducted with aerial spraying of pesticides. A good equine vaccine was not used early in the period that led up to the outbreak and could have prevented many of the equine cases (Pan American Health Organization, 1995).

Clinical Presentation

Infection in humans with VEE virus in adults usually leads to a low-mortality (<1%), influenza-like illness. The initial signs, lasting 24–48 hours, include fever, malaise, dizziness, chills, headaches, severe myalgia, arthralgia, nausea, and vomiting. Lethargy and anorexia can continue for 2–3 weeks. Severe illness in adults comes from neurological involvement due to swelling in and around the brain. A small percentage of patients (<15%) actually experience neurological problems such as photophobia, convulsions, stiff neck, and altered mental status. Some patients experience personality changes, fatigue, recurrent headaches, and altered senses; prognosis with the clinical disease is variable. Children infected by VEE virus experience severe encephalitis, where coma and death is a more likely outcome. Pregnant women infected with VEE can lead to death of the fetus in utero or stillbirth.

Diagnosis and Treatment

Diagnosis for VEE can be quite difficult. This often is accomplished through the clinical presentation coupled with serology by ELISA with paired serum samples from the patient. In addition, PCR assays have been developed by research laboratories and the LRN if clinicians submit cerebrospinal fluid for analysis.

Treatment for the most part involves supportive care, where the pain management and steroidal therapy provide relief. Acyclovir can also be given to interrupt viral replication. No FDA-approved vaccine is available for VEE virus. However, a live-attenuated vaccine for VEE was produced by the United States Army Medical Research Institute of Infectious Diseases in 1972. The vaccine remains in an experimental status and must be given under investigational new drug procedures with a written consent form.

Prevention

Effective VEE virus vaccines are available for horses. Prevention and control of mosquito-borne diseases involve source reduction, surveillance, biological control, chemical control, and educating the public on how to protect themselves with repellents and limiting their outdoor activities at night. In addition, most state and local governments have environmental surveillance programs that include testing for arboviruses. Often, these programs include serological testing of sentinel chicken flocks and mosquito trapping and testing to monitor disease prevalence and virus transmission. These are common practices for West Nile, Eastern equine encephalitis, Western equine encephalitis, and Saint Louis encephalitis viruses.

□ □ □ ▬▬▬▬▬▬▬▬▬▬▬▬▬▬▬▬▬▬▬▬▬▬▬▬▬▬▬▬▬▬▬▬▬▬▬

Venezuelan Equine Encephalitis in Biowarfare

If a bioterrorism attack were to occur using a viral encephalitis agent, experts feel the most likely agent for weaponization would be Venezuelan equine encephalitis virus. The virus particles would be aerosolized and disseminated, with human disease as the primary event. Horses would also be susceptible, but disease would most likely occur simultaneously without animals acting as sentinels. Disease symptoms in humans resemble the flu and would be hard to distinguish, so the basis of an outbreak would likely be a large number of sick individuals and horses in a given geographic area.

The human infective dose for VEE is considered to be 10–100 organisms, which is a principal reason that VEE is considered a militarily effective biowarfare agent. Neither the population density of infected mosquitoes nor the aerosol concentration of virus particles has to be great to allow significant transmission of VEE in a biowarfare attack. VEE particles are not considered stable in the environment and therefore are not as persistent as the bacteria responsible for Q fever, tularemia. or anthrax.

In 1969, the World Health Organization estimated that, if 50 kg of virulent VEE particles were aerosolized and disseminated efficiently over a city with 5 million people, 150,000 people would be exposed in a 1 km extent downwind from the release in approximately five to seven minutes. The result could be 30,000 illnesses and 300 deaths from this bioweapon.

▬▬▬▬▬▬▬▬▬▬▬▬▬▬▬▬▬▬▬▬▬▬▬▬▬▬▬▬▬▬▬▬▬ □ □ □

Ricin Poisoning

As stated in Chapter 2, biological toxins are produced by many bacteria, snakes, shellfish, molds, mushrooms, and plants. Many of these can be highly lethal, while some would serve mainly to incapacitate the victims and strain resources. One toxin in particular, ricin, has gotten a good deal of attention lately. It is a toxin very much in vogue these days due to its relative ease of production, at least in a crude form.

Ricin is one of the most lethal and easily produced plant toxins. The toxin is produced by the castor bean plant. Although the castor bean plant (*Ricinus communis*) produces a deadly toxin, it has been used mostly for good purposes. The plant grows to a height of eight feet and has a brightly colored, variegated leaf pattern (see Figure 4-5). These qualities allowed people to use it as an ornamental plant or border marker. For many years, castor beans have been harvested to make castor oil, which acts as a strong laxative.

Ricin is part of the waste "mash" produced when castor oil is made. The toxin is present in the entire plant but is concentrated in the beans. When extracted and purified, ricin can be formulated into a powder, mist, or pellet. Ricin is water soluble. Hence, ricin may be dissolved in water or weak acid. It is a very stable substance and is not affected greatly by extremes in temperature.

History

Because of its high toxicity and ease of production, ricin was considered for production and formulation by the United States during its biological weapons research program. In a classic case of international espionage in 1978, ricin was used to assassinate Georgi Markov, a Bulgarian defector. Reportedly, a small metal pellet containing ricin crystals was injected into Markov's calf muscle by a specially engineered weapon disguised as an umbrella. Markov died three days after the incident. Although the act was executed by Bulgarian government, the technology used to commit the act was supplied by the former Soviet Union.

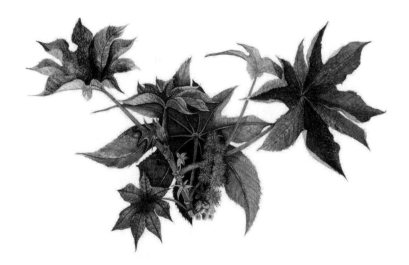

FIGURE 4-5 Castor bean plant and castor beans *(Ricinus communis)*. (Image courtesy of artist Lynne Railsback.)

In Minnesota, four members of the Patriots Council, an antigovernment extremist group, were arrested in 1991 for plotting to kill a U.S. marshal and some of his colleagues with ricin. The group planned to mix crude preparation of ricin with dimethylsulfoxide (DMSO) then apply it to surfaces of the marshal's car. The plan was discovered, and all four men were arrested. These four men were the first to be prosecuted in the United States under the Biological Weapons Anti-Terrorism Act of 1989.

In 2003, a rash of small-scale incidents in the United States involved ricin. Ricin was recovered from a package sent through a Greenville, South Carolina, post office and also turned up in a vial sent to the White House. In February 2004, a letter laced with ricin was discovered in Senate Majority Leader Bill Frist's office. Those responsible for these acts were never found, and no one was injured. These incidents, and others, are covered in Chapter 7, "Case Studies."

□ □ □ ▬▬▬▬▬▬▬▬▬▬▬▬▬▬▬▬▬▬▬▬▬▬▬▬▬

Critical Thinking

You can purchase castor beans from a number of seed catalogs. The plant grows to eight feet in height and makes a beautiful ornamental producing hundreds of seeds. With a few solvents and some basic chemistry equipment you can make a fairly pure extract of ricin from the seed mash. A number of references to making ricin are available on the Internet. Many biocrimes in the United States involve ricin. So, why is it legal at all to purchase castor beans? Surely, we can live without the plant.

▬▬▬▬▬▬▬▬▬▬▬▬▬▬▬▬▬▬▬▬▬▬▬▬▬ □ □ □

Poisoning

Toxins are neither infectious nor contagious. Therefore, person-to-person transmission is not a concern. Three routes of exposure are known to exist: inhalation, ingestion, and injection. Ricin irreversibly blocks protein synthesis at the cellular level. As little as 500 micrograms of ricin by injection would be enough to kill the average adult. A greater amount would be required to kill a human being by either inhalation or ingestion.

As with all things toxic, poisoning, or toxicosis, is dose dependent. The incubation period for ricin depends on how it enters the victim. If inhaled, poisoning takes about eight hours. If ingested, poisoning occurs in hours to days due to digestive processes and slow absorption through the gut. If ricin is injected under the skin, onset of poisoning could be immediate, depending on the location of injection and the dose of toxin injected.

Initial symptoms associated with inhalation of ricin toxin are weakness, fever, cough, nausea, muscle aches, chest pain, and cyanosis. Pulmonary edema occurs about 18–24 hours after inhalation, and severe respiratory distress and death from hypoxemia ensues the following day.

The seeds of the castor bean are quite attractive, which makes them useful in costume jewelry. Some seeds with a variegated pattern look like engorged ticks. Unfortunately, to small children they look good enough to eat, which is why they often become victims of castor bean poisoning. Within a few hours of ingestion, severe intestinal cramps along with nausea, vomiting, and headache occur. Following this, diarrhea, gastrointestinal bleeding, and dilation of the pupils ensues. Ultimately, victims will experience vascular collapse and die after about three days.

□ □ □ ▬▬▬▬▬▬▬▬▬▬▬▬▬▬▬▬▬▬▬▬▬▬▬▬▬▬▬▬▬

Ricin in Biowarfare

Because of ricin's extreme ease of production, wide availability, and potency, it is considered a potential agent for bioterrorism. A very crude preparation of ricin can be made by processing castor beans with a coffee bean grinder and an automatic drip coffeemaker.

▬▬▬▬▬▬▬▬▬▬▬▬▬▬▬▬▬▬▬▬▬▬▬▬▬▬▬▬ □ □ □

Diagnosis and Treatment

The diagnosis of ricin poisoning is often based on clinical symptoms coupled with detection of the toxin in serum or respiratory secretions. Since this is a toxin, DNA-based technologies are not useful. Ricin is extremely immunogenic; therefore. the toxin can be detected via serology. In addition, antigen-capture ELISA and immunohistochemistry applied to infected tissues can be very sensitive. Naturally, these established procedures can be performed only in state-of-the-art, certified laboratories like an LRN facility or specialized Department of Defense laboratory.

No treatment or vaccine is currently available for ricin poisoning. Supportive care is administered to the patient based on the route of exposure. This may include respiratory support for inhalational exposure or gastric lavage and the administration of cathartics to remove the toxin from the intestinal tract if ingestion is suspected.

Conclusion

Category B comprises quite a "mixed bag" of diseases and agents. All of the diseases covered here are zoonoses (brucellosis, glanders and melioidosis, psittacosis, and viral encephalitis). Clearly, all are serious problems complicated by intricate disease transmission dynamics and life cycles. Generally speaking, disease from these agents results in low mortality rates and long-term morbidity. The incidence of these diseases is relatively low to rare, which means that awareness among and recognition by clinicians may not be widespread, making diagnosis a challenge. Additionally, the ease with which one may obtain castor beans makes ricin an easy choice for the amateur bioterrorist. This may explain the rash of biocrimes involving ricin in the past few years. Regardless, all Category B agents have the potential to be exploited and could cause panic and social disruption.

Essential Termiology

- **Arbovirus**. An arthropod-borne virus, often transmitted by mosquitoes, with a complex life cycle involving mammalian reservoirs and hosts.

- **Brucellosis.** A zoonotic disease that normally affects cattle, goats, sheep, and swine; caused by numerous species of bacteria in the genus *Brucella*.
- **Glanders.** A zoonotic disease normally affecting horses, mules, and donkeys; caused by the bacterium *Burkholderia mallei*.
- **Melioidosis.** A zoonotic disease affecting a wide variety of animals and humans; caused by the bacterium *Burkholderia pseudomallei*. Normally found in the tropics, *B. pseudomallei* causes a disease similar to glanders but has a different ecology, where it is spread through contact with contaminated soil and water.
- **Q fever.** A zoonotic disease normally affecting sheep and cattle caused by the spore-forming rickettsia *Coxiella burnetii*.
- **Viral encephalitis.** A general term meaning "a swelling of the brain"; caused by a viral infection. A number of viruses, including many of the arboviruses, may cause this condition in humans. One of the most notable, when it comes to former bioweapons programs, is the Venezuelan equine encephalomyelitis virus.
- **Psittacosis.** The term used to describe human infection with *Chlamydophila psittaci*. When birds are infected with *Chlamydophila psittaci*, the term *avian chlamydiosis* is used. The disease in birds is also known as *parrot fever* and *ornithosis*.
- **Ricin.** A biological toxin derived from the castor bean plant (*Ricinus communis*).

Discussion Questions

- Describe the life cycle of an arbovirus? Which of the viral encephalitides has been exploited in former biowarfare programs?
- What is it about ricin that causes it to be used in so many recent biocrimes?
- What are the attributes of Category B agents? Apply each of the criteria to the diseases discussed in this chapter.
- In what ways are *Brucella* normally transmitted to humans?
- In what ways would an intentional outbreak of Q fever overwhelm the medical and public health communities?

Web Sites

Centers for Disease Control and Prevention, disease information: Brucellosis, available at www.cdc.gov/ncidod/dbmd/diseaseinfo/brucellosis_g.htm.

Centers for Disease Control and Prevention, disease information: Glanders, available at www.cdc.gov/ncidod/dbmd/diseaseinfo/glanders_g.htm.

Centers for Disease Control and Prevention, disease information: Melioidosis, available at www.cdc.gov/ncidod/dbmd/diseaseinfo/melioidosis_g.htm.

Centers for Disease Control and Prevention, Viral and Rickettsial Zoonoses Branch: Q fever, available at www.cdc.gov/ncidod/dvrd/qfever/index.htm.

Centers for Disease Control and Prevention, disease information: Psittacosis, available at www.cdc.gov/ncidod/dbmd/diseaseinfo/psittacosis_t.htm.

Centers for Disease Control and Prevention, Division of Vector Borne Infectious Diseases, Disease information: Arboviral Encephalitides, available at www.cdc.gov/ncidod/dvbid/arbor/arbdet.htm.

Centers for Disease Control and Prevention, emergency preparedness and response: Facts about ricin, available at www.bt.cdc.gov/agent/ricin/facts.asp.

References

Avian chlamydiosis. 1996. In: *Whiteman and Bickford's Avian Disease Manual*, 4th ed., ed. B. R. Charlton et al., pp. 68–71. Kennett Square, PA: American Association of Avian Pathologists.

Cutler, S. J., A. M. Whatmore, and N. J. Commander. 2005. Brucellosis: New aspects of an old disease. *Journal of Applied Microbiology* 98:1270–1281.

Derrick, E. H. 1937. "Q" fever, a new fever entity: clinical features, diagnosis, and laboratory investigation. *Medical Journal of Australia* 2:281–299.

Doganay, M., and B. Aygen. 2003. Human brucellosis—An overview. *International Journal of Infectious Diseases* 7:173–182.

Godoy, D., G. Randle, A. Simpson, D. Aanensen, T. Pitt, R. Kinoshita, and B. Spratt. 2003. Multilocus sequence typing and evolutionary relationships among the causative agents of melioidosis and glanders, *Burkholderia pseudomallei* and *Burkholderia mallei*. *Journal of Clinical Microbiology* 41:2068–2079.

Hippocrates. 400 BC. *Of the Epidemics*, trans. Francis Adams, available at http://etext.library.adelaide.edu.au/mirror/classics.mit.edu/Hippocrates/epidemics.html.

Johnston, W., M. Eidson, K. Smith, and M. Stobierski. 1999. Compendium of chlamydiosis (psittacosis) control, 1999. Psittacosis Compendium Committee, National Association of State Public Health Veterinarians. *Journal of the American Veterinary Medical Association* 214, no. 5:640–646.

Maurin, M., and D. Raoult. 1999. Q fever. *Clinical Microbiology Reviews* 12:518–553.

Miller, J., S. Engelberg, and W. Broad. 2001. *Germs: Biological Weapons and America's Secret War*. New York: Simon and Schuster.

Moore, J., and J. Elborn. 2003. *Burkholderia cepacia* and cystic fibrosis [online]. Northern Ireland Public Health Laboratory, Northern Ireland Regional Adult Cystic Fibrosis Centre, Belfast City Hospital, Northern Ireland, United Kingdom, available at www.cysticfibrosismedicine.com.

Nicoletti, P. 1992. The control of brucellosis—A veterinary responsibility. *Saudi Medical Journal* 13:10–13.

Pan American Health Organization. 1995. Brote de encefhalitis equine venezolana, 1995 [Outbreak of Venezuelan equine encephalitis, 1995]. *Bol Epidemiol* 16, no. 4:9–13.

Pappas, G., P. Papadimitriou, N. Akritidis, L. Christou, and E. Tsianos. 2006. The new global map of human brucellosis. *Lancet, Journal of Infectious Diseases* 6:91–99.

Reimer, L. 1993. Q fever. *Clincal Microbiology Reviews* 6:193–198.

Riedel, S. 2004. Biological warfare and bioterrorism: A historical review. *Baylor University Medical Center Proceedings* 17:400–406.

Ryan, K. J., and C. G. Ray, eds. 2004. In: *Sherris Medical Microbiology*, 4th ed. New York: McGraw Hill.

Smith, K., K. Bradley, M. Stobierski, and L. Tengelsen. 2005. Compendium of measures to control Chlamydophila psittaci (formerly Chlamydia psittaci) infection among humans (psittacosis) and pet birds, 2005. *Journal of the American Veterinary Medical Association* 226:532–539.

Vassalo, D. 1992. The corps disease: brucellosis and its historical association with the Royal Army Medical Corps. *Journal of the Royal Army Medical Corps* 138:148–150.

Vella, E. E. 1964. The British Army Medical Service and Malta fever. *Military Medicine* 128:1076–1090.

Yagupsky, P., and E. Baron. 2005. Laboratory exposures to *Brucellae* and implications for bioterrorism. *Emerging Infectious Diseases* [serial on the Internet], available at www.cdc.gov/ncidod/EID/vol11no08/04-1197.htm.

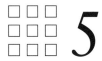

Category C Diseases and Agents

Where the telescope ends, the microscope begins. Which of the two has the grander view?
—Victor Hugo

Objectives

The study of this chapter will enable you to

1. List and explain the criteria used to define Category C agents.
2. Describe the signs and symptoms of Nipah virus fever, hantavirus, West Nile fever, and SARS.
3. Describe the clinical manifestations of Nipah virus fever, hantavirus, West Nile fever, and SARS.
4. Understand the challenges that public health officials and emergency management practitioners face when an intentional release of a Category C agent occurs in their community.

Key Terms

Category C, emerging diseases, Nipah virus fever, hantavirus, West Nile fever, SARS, emerging disease.

Introduction

Category C is comprised of newly **emerging diseases** and pathogens. No disease outbreak or epidemic escapes media coverage, whether it is an enteric disease due to contaminated lettuce, food-borne botulism, or the threat of "bird flu." We seem to be living in a world that is out of balance, as Laurie Garrett points out in her thought-provoking book *The Coming Plague* (1995). Our era may very well be characterized by eruptions of new diseases, epidemics of old diseases moving into new areas, diseases that are sparked by advances in technology, and diseases that come to us from insects and animals as civilization invades ecologies where humans have not trodden before (Garrett, 1995). Although these encounters have been occurring throughout history, technology now enables us to define the problems with great acuity. Our ability to determine the causal relationship between pathogen, host, and disease relies heavily on state-of-the-art technologies brought to us by advances in science and engineering. Still, to this day, the microscope remains a primary tool in the tool box. Moreover, electron microscopy provides researchers with high-powered visual proof of the existence of the pathogens that cause disease (Figure 5-1).

The Category C list changes with the world disease outbreak situation. Bioterrorism coordinators, emergency managers, and public health officials should periodically check the CDC web site for updates. Consider how much attention has been brought to the emergence and spread of the deadly H5N1 influenza virus, also known as *bird flu*. In a 10 year period, there have been a little more than 300 confirmed cases of bird flu in humans. However, nearly 60% of those human cases resulted in death and approximately 200 million birds have either died directly from the illness or indirectly from the control efforts aimed at "stamping out" the problem. Public health officials fear that H5N1 may spark the next pandemic. Bird flu due to the H5N1 virus is covered in Chapters 8 and 9, due to the effect that this outbreak has had on the poultry industry.

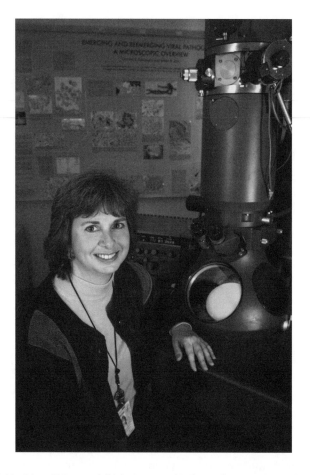

FIGURE 5-1 Cynthia Goldsmith, a CDC research biologist, seated in front of a transmission electron microscope. During the last 20 years at the CDC, Ms. Goldsmith's work as an electron microscopist has repeatedly played a key role in the rapid identification of emerging pathogens, including hantavirus, Nipah virus, and SARS coronavirus. (Courtesy of U.S. Health and Human Services, Public Health Image Library, Image No. 7274.)

A would-be terrorist or rogue state might take advantage of any emerging pathogen or situation to create added fear, panic, and social disruption. The potential exploitation of an emerging pathogen is the reason why Category C exists. Chapter 5 explores four examples of emerging disease pathogens that have occurred in the past 10 years: Nipah virus, hantavirus, West Nile virus, and SARS virus.

Nipah Virus

In 1998, a mysterious outbreak in the peninsular region of Malaysia caught public health officials by surprise (Centers for Disease Control and Prevention, 1999). The outbreak took place over an eight-month period. When it was over, more than 1 million pigs had to be destroyed. Moreover, there were 257 human cases from the same pathogen, which caused 105 deaths (a 41% case fatality rate). Most human cases were from people employed in the swine industry who had direct contact with live pigs (Parashar et al., 2000). The outbreak had a profound psychological and economic impact on the country.

The outbreak was due to Nipah virus, a pathogen completely unknown to scientists before this outbreak (see Figure 5-2). The pathogen was fully characterized by molecular methods as a paramyxovirus in the genus *Henipavirus* (Wong et al., 2002). Nipah virus is very similar to another recently emergent pathogen, Hendra virus, which causes severe respiratory and encephalitic disease in horses and humans.

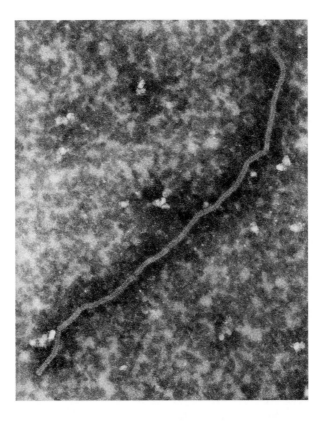

FIGURE 5-2 Under a highly magnified view of 168,000×, this transmission electron micrographic image revealed ultrastructural details of a Nipah virus nucleocapsid, a virus named for the location in Malaysia where it was first isolated. (Courtesy of U.S. Health and Human Services, Public Health Image Library, Image No. 8256.)

Nipah virus causes severe, rapidly progressive encephalitis in humans. In pigs, Nipah virus causes severe respiratory illness with neurological complications. Transmission of the virus to humans is associated with close contact to infected pigs. Survivability of Nipah virus outside the host has not been determined.

In September 1998, the Malaysian Ministry of Health (MOH) began to receive reports from three geographic locations of a number of human cases of febrile encephalitis with high mortality. Initially, MOH authorities believed the outbreak was due to Japanese encephalitis (JE) virus, a mosquito-borne RNA virus. However, JE vaccination and mosquito control efforts conducted over several months failed to halt the epidemic. Numerous features of this outbreak's epidemiology were inconsistent with past JE outbreaks. Remarkably, researchers noted that human case patients had an association with infected animals from a concurrent and severe outbreak of respiratory disease in pigs and that there was a notable absence of illness in children. Subsequently, serological testing coupled with epidemiological findings showed that the Malaysians were not dealing with JE. Tissue culture isolation eventually led them to the actual etiologic agent of the outbreak (Chua et al., 1999). Nipah virus gets its name from the village (Sungai Nipah) where the first cases were reported. In March 1999, a related outbreak occurred in Singapore, where abattoir workers were exposed to swine imported from Malaysia. The outbreak was quickly identified and stamped out.

Transmission

The natural cycle of transmission of Nipah virus involves flying foxes (fruit bats, *Pteropus*) as reservoirs and pigs as amplifying hosts (Calisher et al., 2006). Hendra virus also is found in fruit bats. Many species of fruit bats are found in Malaysia. Two species of flying fox, the island flying fox (*Pteropus hypomelanus*) and Malayan flying fox (*Pteropus vampyrus*), have been shown to be asymptomatic carriers of the virus. No secondary hosts have been implicated.

Researchers have not yet determined how Nipah virus is transmitted from bats to pigs. They suspect that fruit trees close to pig pens are foraged by the bats and the virus is spread by this close proximity (urine or saliva on partially eaten fruit). Most human cases (93%) had direct contact with pigs or secondary contact with body fluids, urine or feces (Calisher et al., 2006). Person-to-person transmission has not been established or related to any cases from the 1998–1999 outbreak.

In the Malaysian outbreak of Nipah virus, the contagion was rapidly spread from farm to farm by the movement of infected pigs. Malaysia's domestic pig population prior to the outbreak was 2.4 million. The total annual value was estimated to be about $400 million, with a total export value of $100 million (U.S. dollars). As a result of the outbreak, approximately 1.1 million pigs were culled to prevent the spread of the disease. This alone resulted in an estimated loss of $217 million. During the outbreak, pork consumption in Malaysia dropped by almost 80% (Food and Agriculture Organization of the United Nations, 2002).

In 2004 an outbreak of Nipah virus occurred in Bangladesh. Only 34 human cases were identified; however, more than 75% of the case patients died (Hsu et al., 2004). Another outbreak of Nipah virus occurred in early 2005 in the Tangail District of Bangladesh, when 13 people became ill and lost consciousness after drinking palm fruit juice. The fruit may have been contaminated with infected fruit bat droppings. Blood samples from case patients were sent to the CDC to confirm Nipah virus infection; one was confirmed positive (Luby et al., 2006).

Clinical Presentation, Diagnosis, and Treatment

The incubation period for Nipah virus in humans is believed to be 3–14 days. Initial symptoms are fever and headache. Nipah virus produces widespread effects and induces necrosis of endothelial cells in vasculature and neuronal damages. Subsequently, case patients experience dizziness, drowsiness, disorientation, and vomiting. Endothelial cells are involved in vascular permeability and damage to the cells leads to vessel leaking and ultimately to hypovolemic shock. The most severely affected develop encephalitis, seizures, and coma. Complications noted during the Malaysian outbreak included septicemia, intestinal bleeding, and renal impairment (Wong et al., 2002).

Laboratory diagnostic methods for Nipah virus infections now include serology, histopathology, immunohistochemistry, real-time PCR, and virus isolation. The virus is classified BSL-4. There is no cure for Nipah; however, a vaccine is in development. Current treatment involves supportive care.

Nipah Virus and Biowarfare

Nipah virus has been listed by the Centers for Disease Control and Prevention as a Category C potential bioterrorist agent. This is described as an emerging pathogen that has a potentially high morbidity and mortality as well as a major health impact. Currently, spread of the disease involves close contact with pigs. However, aerosolization may be a possible bioterrorist method of dispersal. Additionally, the potential for this virus to infect a wide range of hosts and produce significant mortality in humans makes this emerging virus one of public health concern. Due to the need to cull infected pigs, attack with this agent could produce a great economic impact to a nation's pork industry. During the Nipah outbreak in Malaysia, widespread panic and fear occurred until the outbreak was brought under control.

Hantavirus

An outbreak of a cluster of serious febrile illness occurred in New Mexico in 1993. A task force of scientists, public health experts, and epidemiologists discovered that the outbreak was due to hantavirus. **Hantavirus** is the causative agent of hantavirus pulmonary syndrome (HPS) and hemorrhagic fever with renal syndrome (HFRS) in humans (Duchin et al., 1994). From what we know now, this disease agent occurs naturally throughout most of North and South America, it is airborne, and in the absence of prompt medical attention, infections are usually fatal. This agent serves as a perfect example of a pathogen that makes a dramatic entry into modern-day society, bringing with it numerous challenges. For its attributes and its sudden arrival, hantaviruses were placed in Department of Health and Human Services Category C.

Hantavirus is a three-segmented RNA virus in the family Bunyaviridae. A number of rodent species act as the reservoir for these viruses in nature. Rodents transmit the disease horizontally within their species and vertically to humans through aerosolized virus particles from their dried feces and urine (LeDuc, Childs, and Glass, 1992). The hantavirus-caused diseases HFRS and HPS are considered to be pan-American zoonoses. More than 25 antigenically different viral species make up this group. Table 5-1 provides a breakdown of hantavirus by type, endemic region, and rodent host.

Hantaviruses are encapsulated in a lipid envelope; therefore, they are easily destroyed by common disinfectants, such as acetone, iodine, ethanol, and chlorine (Kraus et al., 2005). In addition, hantaviruses are deactivated by UV light, low pH, and temperatures above $37°C$ ($98.6°F$).

Hantaviruses previously recognized as causing HFRS in the Old World are Dobrava, Hantaan, Puumala, and Seoul. Infected rodents remain so for life, yet they are often unaffected by the virus and will transmit it among themselves. It is unknown whether animals other than the natural rodent hosts are epidemiologically important. Many other hantaviruses have been isolated and characterized but not linked to human illness. Most human infections with hantavirus in North America are associated with rodents of the subfamily *Sigmodontinae* (Childs et al., 1994). As many as three hantaviruses have been found circulating in one location; each with its own rodent reservoir. Rodents other than the primary reservoirs may play an important role as a carrier (a common reservoir for hantavirus is shown in Figure 5-3).

History

Disease outbreaks that occurred during the American Civil War are now believed to have been due to hantavirus. In addition, there are records of HFRS from both world wars.

Table 5-1 Hantavirus by Type, Endemic Region, and Host Species

Hantavirus Type	Endemic Region	Rodent Host Species
Andes	Argentina, Chile	*Oligoryzomys longicaudatus* (long-tailed pygmy rice rat)
Bayou	Southeastern United States	*Oryzomys palustris* (rice rat)
Black Creek Canal	Southeastern United States	*Sigmodon hispidus* (cotton rat)
Dobrava	Europe, Balkans	*A. agrarius, A. flavicollis* (yellow neck mouse)
Hantaan	Asia, Far East Russia	*Apodemus agrarius* (striped field mouse)
Hu39694	Central Argentina	Unknown
Juquitiba	Brazil	Unknown
Laguna Negra	Paraguay, Bolivia	*Calomys laucha*
Lechiguanas	Central Argentina	*O. flavescens*
Monongahela	Eastern United States, Canada	*Peromyscus maniculatus* (deer mouse)
New York	Eastern United States, Canada	*Peromyscus leucopus* (white-footed mouse)
Oran	Northwestern Argentina	*O. longicaudatus*
Puumala	Europe	*Clethrionomys glareolus* (red bank vole)
Seoul	Worldwide	*Rattus norvegicus, R. rattus* (Norway brown rat, roof rat)
Sin Nombre	Central and western United States, Canada	*Peromyscus maniculatus* (deer mouse)

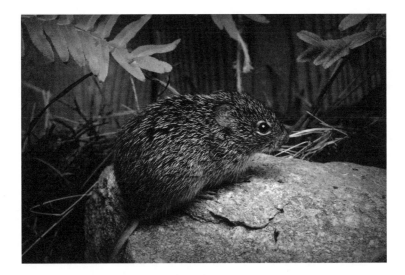

FIGURE 5-3 This is a cotton rat, *Sigmodon hispidus*, whose habitat includes the southeastern United States and Central and South America. The cotton rat is a hantavirus carrier that becomes a threat when it enters human habitation in rural and suburban areas. Hantavirus is a deadly disease transmitted by infected rodents through urine, droppings, or saliva. Humans can contract the disease when they breathe in aerosolized virus. All hantaviruses known to cause HPS are carried by New World rats and mice of the family Muridae, subfamily Sigmodontinae, which contains at least 430 species that are widespread throughout North and South America.

What is thought to be the first outbreak of hantavirus causing HFRS was recorded in Russia in 1913. Reportedly, Japanese troops in Manchuria experienced cases in 1932. In the early 1950s, Western physicians recorded more than 3,200 cases of an acute, debilitating, febrile illness in United Nations forces fighting in the Korean War. The illness, known as Korean hemorrhagic fever, affected soldiers living out of foxholes along the contested border between North and South Korea (Ricketts, 1954). Since the mortality rate was high (10–15%), the U.S. Army Medical Department formed the Hemorrhagic Fever Commission to conduct an epidemiological investigation. Results of the commission indicated that a field mouse (*Apodemus agrarius coreae*) was harboring the infectious agent. However, it was not until 1977 that the infectious agent was isolated and named *Hantaan* for the river that runs near the 38th parallel, which separates North and South Korea (Lee, Lee, and Johnson, 2004). The Hemorrhagic Fever Commission preserved more than 600 serum samples from 245 soldiers. Later, in 1990, the serum samples from these 245 soldiers were screened for antibody to the Hantaan virus. Almost 40 years after the outbreak, investigators detected an antibody to Hantaan virus in 94% of the samples. In 1979, a virus similar to Hantaan caused hemorrhagic fever in laboratory workers. This virus, named *Seoul virus* after the site of the initial studies, infected Norway rats and roof rats shipped to Japan and Europe. Shipping these laboratory animals led to the dissemination of the Seoul virus.

Four Corners Outbreak

In 1993, an outbreak of illness resulted in a number of fatalities on the Navajo Nation Indian Reservation in New Mexico. As the outbreak spread, cases were distributed around the Four Corners region of the United States (Chapman and Khabbaz, 1994). The region gets its name from the perfectly formed grid square that marks the boundary between the states of Arizona, Colorado, New Mexico, and Utah. These cases, later described as hantavirus pulmonary syndrome, were attributed to a new species of hantavirus. Actually, nothing was new about it. The virus had probably been in the region for many years but had not been the cause of so much notable human illness in the past.

Several young Navajo tribal members presented to the Indian Health Service physicians with sudden onset of respiratory failure in May 1993. By June of that year, 12 people had succumbed to the illness. Initially, the illness was diagnosed as unexplained acute respiratory distress syndrome. Patients presented with abrupt fever, severe headache, myalgia, and cough, followed by rapidly progressive pulmonary edema (Stelzel, 1996). Within 2–10 days, this condition led to respiratory failure, hypotension, and death. New Mexico Public Health officials teamed with CDC investigators to set up surveillance and laboratory testing. The team found that serum from the patients showed cross-reactive antibodies to Hantaan, Seoul, and Puumala virus antigens. However, the condition in these patients had developed into a pulmonary form unlike any other clinical presentation of hantavirus infection. The investigation also focused on the wildlife and domestic animals in the area of the outbreak (Calisher et al., 1999). Epidemiologists were quick to discover that the virus was being spread through the dried feces and urine of *Peromyscus* mice. Unfortunately, the Navajo believe that mice are responsible for bringing seeds to the earth, which enable humans to survive. The fact that mice are highly respected in Navajo culture made disease control efforts difficult. Tribal members had to accept all forms of rodent population management efforts, which include trapping, housecleaning, and reduction of harborage.

Outbreaks of hantavirus-related diseases are often attributed to weather patterns. Drought causes plants to die, which leads to a decrease in rodent populations. Conversely, heavy snowfall and spring rains allows plants to flourish and rodent populations to surge. These surges in the rodent population cause rodents to compete for food and protection in the dryer months that follow. The competition puts pressure on some infected rodents, forcing them into peridomestic environments, putting more people at risk for infection. Hantavirus pulmonary syndrome is most common in spring and summer months, when rodents are most active. Although the overall risk for HPS in endemic areas is relatively low, infections are associated with an increased population of rodents in and around the house. Activities that put people in contact with rodent droppings, urine, or nesting materials place the individual at higher risk for infection. Indoor exposures have been linked to rodents in the home or near dwellings, especially in colder months. Cleaning buildings that have been closed up for a period of time, such as cabins, barns, and storage facilities, also increases the risk of exposure.

Persons living in squalid housing conditions, employed in agricultural, and wilderness camping or other outdoor activity in endemic areas are at greater risk for hantavirus infections. Hikers and campers may be exposed when they use infested trail shelters or camp near rodent harborage. Construction and utility workers can be exposed when they work in crawl spaces under houses that may have a rodent population. Research shows that many HPS case patients acquired the virus after having been in frequent contact with rodents or their droppings for long periods (Centers for Disease Control and Prevention, Special Pathogens Branch, 2007).

Worldwide, approximately 150,000 hospitalizations due to hemorrhagic fever with renal syndrome are reported each year. Most cases come from China, where hantavirus was first recognized in 1931. Approximately 500 cases of Korean hemorrhagic fever are reported annually from South Korea. Many HFRS outbreaks occurring in Asia and Europe are due to people planting and harvesting crops having contact with field rodents.

Transmission

Normally, humans become infected with hantavirus by the inhalation of aerosolized virus particles from rodent excreta. Transmission of hantavirus begins with a chronically infected rodent. Horizontal transmission occurs between rodents of the same species. Infections in rodents are asymptomatic and not deleterious to the rodent, making them ideal reservoirs. Rodents shed the virus in their urine, feces, and saliva. Humans become infected when they disturb the infected rodent's environment and breathe the infected particles, a process called *aerosolization*. Although less likely, transmission may occur through breaks in the skin. Virus particles may contaminate food sources and people may become infected through consumption. Very rarely, a bite from an infected rodent may cause disease. Person-to-person transmission of hantaviruses have not been reported. Several laboratory-acquired cases of HFRS have been reported. Hantaviruses are categorized as BSL-4 agents when propagating them in culture or passing them through laboratory animals known to be efficient reservoirs.

Clinical Presentation, Diagnosis, and Treatment

The incubation period for hantavirus infection is believed to be 14–17 days. Initially, HPS case patients experience headache, fatigue, fever, increased respiratory and heart rates, and myalgia of the large muscles in the thighs, hips, back, and shoulders. Roughly half of all patients experience dizziness, chills, and various gastrointestinal symptoms, such as nausea, vomiting, diarrhea, and abdominal pain.

Four to ten days after the initial presentation, patients begin to experience coughing, rales, and shortness of breath due to severe hypotension and rapidly progressive pulmonary edema, requiring immediate hospitalization and ventilation. Approximately 40% of HPS case patients die within the first 48 hours due to hypoxia and shock.

The CDC maintains a national surveillance program for hantavirus pulmonary syndrome. To assist physicians with the recognition of this illness, a specific case definition for HPS was published: a previously healthy person presenting with a febrile illness with a temperature at or above 101°F (38.3°C), unexplained acute respiratory distress syndrome, radiographic evidence of bilateral interstitial infiltrate that develops within one week of hospitalization, and respiratory compromise that requires supplemental oxygen. If sudden death occurs before supplemental oxygen and noncardiogenic pulmonary edema is present on autopsy without an identifiable, specific cause of death, diagnosis can be made (Centers for Disease Control and Prevention, 1997).

Confirmatory diagnosis of HPS requires meeting specific inclusion and exclusion criteria plus laboratory confirmation. The CDC uses ELISA to detect the presence of hantavirus specific immunoglobulin M (IgM) in acute-phase serum or a fourfold rise in titers of immunoglobulin G (IgG) from acute- and convalescent-phase sera. Immunohistochemistry can be used on formalin fixed tissues to detect hantavirus antigen when serum is unavailable. Virus detection by PCR or isolation from whole blood or serum may also be useful.

Treatment of HPS requires early and aggressive intensive care, focusing on oxygenation of the blood, electrolyte balance, and maintaining blood pressure. There was a grave prognosis for many of the initial victims of the Four Corners Outbreak because health-care providers did not know what they were dealing with. Now, history of exposure leads physicians in endemic areas to a more rapid diagnosis. Early aggressive supportive care is needed for a successful resolution of symptoms. Without treatment, the prognosis for HPS is grave. With supportive care and symptom-targeted therapy, patients can recover from the disease. Chronic lung and heart damage may result depending on the aggressiveness of supportive care.

West Nile Virus

West Nile virus (WNV) is a single-stranded RNA virus in the genus *Flavivirus* (family Flaviviridae). West Nile virus is a member of the Japanese encephalitis virus antigenic complex of mosquito-borne flaviviruses. Also included in this complex is Saint Louis encephalitis virus, Kunjin virus, and Murray Valley encephalitis virus.

West Nile virus was initially isolated in 1937 from a febrile patient in the West Nile district of Uganda. Since then, WNV has been isolated from mosquitoes, humans, birds, and other vertebrates in Africa, Eastern Europe, western Asia, and the Middle East (Murgue, Zeller, and Deubel, 2002). Over the last 50 years, there have been several significant outbreaks of West Nile fever. Studies conducted in Egypt in the 1950s showed that the natural history of this disease can vary dramatically. At one extreme are areas where WNV circulates routinely with uncomplicated West Nile fever manifesting as a mild and common childhood disease, which is easily confused with other febrile conditions. In this situation, the heightened infection rate improves background immunity and increases with age. Hence, West Nile fever epidemics and West Nile encephalitis are rare. The other extreme exists in industrialized urban areas, where little or no previous WNV activity has occurred. Here, aging and immunologically naive populations are likely to encounter WNV for the first time. This leads to West Nile fever epidemics with numerous cases of West Nile encephalitis (Knudsen, Andersen, and Kronborg, 2003).

There have been many West Nile outbreaks throughout the world. Like Egypt, Israel experienced outbreaks in the 1950s. In 1957, nursing homes in Israel reported severe neurologic disease and death associated with West Nile fever. An outbreak in Romania is believed to be the catalyst for several outbreaks in large industrialized urban areas.

West Nile was first discovered in the United States in 1999. Sixty-two cases and seven deaths (11% case fatality rate) resulted from it in New York City and the surrounding area. Horses, crows, and exotic birds from a zoo were also found to be infected. Initially, Saint Louis encephalitis virus was believed to be the cause of the human infections until WNV was isolated from both the human and animal specimens. This discovery marked the first appearance of WNV in the Western Hemisphere (Jia et al., 1999).

Naturally, there has been some speculation as to how WNV was introduced into the United States. No one really knows for sure. However, the isolates characterized from the 1999 outbreak were shown to be antigenically similar to a strain that circulated in Israel from 1997 to 2000 (Ebel et al., 2001). In 2002, officials at the CDC affirmed that they provided scientists in Iraq with WNV isolates in the 1980s and 1990s. This has led some to believe that the introduction was intentional. The more plausible explanation for a mosquito-borne disease such as this is that the introduction was accidental. Perhaps infected mosquitoes or a reservoir host gained access to the United States via international transportation or trade.

Table 5-2 Number of Confirmed Human Cases and Fatalities from West Nile Fever in the United States, 1999–2006

	1999	2000	2001	2002	2003	2004	2005	2006
Cases	62	21	66	4156	9862	2539	3000	4269
Deaths	7	2	9	284	264	100	119	177

Source: All data come from CDC, Division of Vector-Borne Diseases West Nile Virus Statistics, Surveillance and Control web site available at www.cdc.gov/ncidod/dvbid/westnile/surv&control.htm.

Since the first detected case in 1999, the number of cases and deaths in humans has increased dramatically almost every year. Table 5-2 presents a summary of West Nile cases in the United States reported between 1999 and 2006.

Horses are affected by WNV infections more often than any other domestic animals. In 2003, 4,554 horses were diagnosed with clinically apparent WNV infection. Ravens, jays, and crows (corvids; family *Corvidae*) serve as a reservoir for WNV. Certain female mosquito species that feed primarily on birds (ornithophilic) enable maintenance of WNV in avian hosts. Other female mosquito species that are not so particular in their blood feeding take up the virus from infected birds and pass them along to other animals. Reservoir competency and field studies suggest that horses or other mammals do not serve as reservoirs for infection, which make them incidental hosts (McLean et al., 2001).

☐ ☐ ☐ ▄▄▄▄▄▄▄▄▄▄▄▄▄▄▄▄▄▄▄▄▄▄▄▄▄▄▄▄▄▄▄▄

Critical Thinking

West Nile fever burned like a slow-moving wildfire across the United States from New York City to the California coastline in approximately four years. Clinicians, public health officials, mosquito control specialists, and animal health professionals all had to come together to mitigate the impact of this emerging disease in the United States. Although much has been done, this serious disease appears to have a foothold on U.S. soil, and cases have increased dramatically from 2006–2007. When the outbreak was first realized in 1999, some government officials were left to wonder how the pathogen made entry into the United States. Could it have been due to an intentional act?

▄▄▄▄▄▄▄▄▄▄▄▄▄▄▄▄▄▄▄▄▄▄▄▄▄▄▄▄▄▄▄▄ ☐ ☐ ☐

Transmission

Worldwide, many different species of mosquitoes have been found to transmit WNV. West Nile virus has been isolated from ticks in Eurasia, but their role in natural transmission of the virus remains elusive. In North America, WNV has been detected in more than 40 different species of mosquitoes. Mosquitoes in the genus *Culex* are the most important vectors for maintaining WNV in nature, but no one knows which species are most responsible for transmission to humans.

As to how WNV persists in the environment is not exactly known. However, studies have shown that several possible mechanisms may work together to provide the opportunities necessary for the virus to survive and thrive. Environmental surveillance studies conducted in New York City post 1999 showed that *Culex* mosquitoes were capable of overwintering in the NYC sewer system. Laboratory studies have shown that transovarial transmission of WNV is possible with *Culex vishnui* mosquitoes. Studies done with birds indicate that contact transmission between birds may occur and that migratory birds may play a role in transporting WNV and its vectors to unaffected regions (Centers for Disease Control abnd Prevention, 2000).

Laboratory-acquired infections have occurred with WNV. In 2002, the CDC documented West Nile fever in two laboratory workers. The first became infected through a wound sustained from a scalpel while removing the brain from an infected blue jay. The second case was from a needle stick to a worker harvesting WNV-infected mouse brains. In 2002, West Nile virus was found to be present in the blood supply. Twenty-three cases of WNV infection were due to infected blood components from 16 WNV-viremic blood donors. This finding prompted blood collection agencies to begin screening blood donations. The following year, 737 donor samples were found to be WNV positive, prompting blood bank officials to discard their donations. Despite the screening, two cases of confirmed blood-transfusion-associated West Nile fever were documented in 2003. Nationwide blood screening for WNV has been successful in preventing transfusion-transmitted WNV (Stramer et al., 2005). However, as with all blood donation screening, infections can be transmitted to transfusion recipients on rare occasions despite negative donor test results. Although WNV transmission by blood transfusion is rare, the few cases seen since 2002 underscore the importance of clinical recognition, effective WNV blood screening strategies, and investigation coordination (Pealer et al., 2003).

In August 2002, four patients receiving organ transplants from one organ donor were diagnosed with WNV infection. One of the transplant recipients subsequently died from the infection. The organ donor had received blood products from 63 blood donors to help combat injuries sustained in an accident. Ironically, the last blood transfusion received had been from a WNV-viremic blood donor. Although believed to be rare, transplacental transmission of WNV is possible, with one confirmed case taking place in 2002.

Clinical Presentation, Diagnosis, and Treatment

The incubation period for WNV is approximately 3–14 days. Epidemiologists believe that about 80% of people infected with WNV are asymptomatic. Approximately 20% of those infected develop a mild illness, termed *West Nile fever*. Uncomplicated West Nile fever typically begins with sudden onset of fever, headache, lymphadenopathy, and myalgia, often accompanied by gastrointestinal symptoms. The acute illness usually lasts 3–6 days, but prolonged fatigue is common. In earlier epidemics where West Nile fever cases predominated, nearly half of all case patients presented with a maculopapular rash.

Less than 1% of WNV infections result in severe neurological disease. The more severe form of the disease is referred to as West Nile encephalitis, West Nile meningitis or West Nile meningoencephalitis. *Encephalitis* refers to an inflammation of the brain, *meningitis* to an inflammation of the membrane around the brain and the spinal cord, and *meningoencephalitis* to inflammation of the brain and the membrane surrounding it. The symptoms of these severe infections include headache, high fever, neck stiffness, stupor, disorientation, coma, tremors, convulsions, muscle weakness, and paralysis. Severe neurological disease due to WNV infection may occur in patients of all age groups. Year-round transmission is possible in some areas.

SARS Virus

Severe acute respiratory syndrome (SARS) appeared as an outbreak in China very suddenly in 2003. SARS serves as an example of a Category C disease due to the many challenges government agencies faced from a newly emerging disease, which seemingly came out of nowhere. What caused it was never seen before coronavirus (Figure 5-4). The coronavirus that causes SARS is highly infectious. Some of the patients from this outbreak were referred to as *superspreaders* because they shed so much virus they infected many other people. The initial outbreak that had the world's attention occurred in May 2003 in Hong Kong, but an epidemiological investigation showed the true origin led back to China's Guangdong Province.

Guangdong is one of the more prosperous areas of China. It can be characterized as an area dotted with industrial complexes surrounded by fertile farmlands, where people work and live in close proximity to their animals. Animals are an important part of life in Guangdong. In fact, much of South China is known for its live animal markets. In this region, the Chinese believe that eating freshly killed wild animals promotes vitality and good health. In the live animal markets, you may purchase cats, dogs, snakes, bats, and civets. Once you make your purchase the animal is butchered for the customer to take home.

SARS is believed to have developed here in the live markets or farm settings of Guangdong province. On November 16, 2002, a 45-year-old man in Foshan, a Guangdong city of 3.4 million, became ill with an unusual respiratory illness (Knobler et al., 2004). No one knows exactly where or how he contracted the illness. He had no travel history, but he had recently prepared chicken, cat, and snake for household meals. An epidemiological investigation showed that many of the earliest SARS case patients had possible associations with the use of wild animal food sources. The man, a local leader in

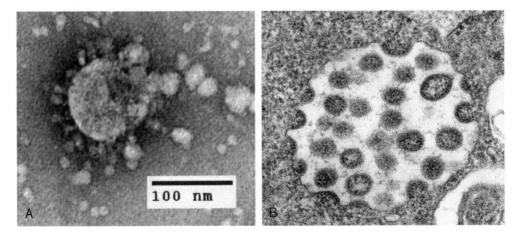

FIGURE 5-4 The SARS coronavirus in these transmission electron microscope photographs shows the gross external structure (A) and a number of virions (B) inside an infected cell. (Images provided courtesy of Cynthia Goldsmith, CDC electron microscopist.)

the province, was married with four children. Within weeks, his wife, a niece, an aunt, and her husband also became ill (Xu et al., 2004). The initial case patient and his four family members are thought to have been the first cluster of a disease that infected 8,096 people around the world and killed 774 before ebbing in the summer of 2003 (9.5% case fatality rate). Guangdong was especially hard-hit, accounting for more than 1,500 probable cases and 58 deaths.

It took months after this first known infection for health authorities throughout the world to identify the disease as something new, learn its characteristics, and determine how to deal with it (Goldsmith et al., 2004). In the early days of SARS, little was known by anyone anywhere about this mysterious disease. Medical workers had no diagnostic criteria and no clinical test, and the incubation period was unknown. The method of transmission was uncertain, as was the effectiveness of protective equipment and safety requirements. SARS spread from Foshan into other areas of Guangdong. By January 2003, it was seen in Guangzhou, the provincial capital, where workers in the health industry began to fall ill.

SARS was a tragedy. In the space of a few months, the deadly virus emerged from the jungles of central China and moved to several other countries by various means of transportation. In Canada, SARS caused severe illness in more than 3,300 people. Southern Ontario was the worst-affected jurisdiction outside Asia, with SARS infecting 375 people and killing 44 (SARS Commission, 2006).

It caused untold suffering to its victims and their families, forced thousands into quarantine, brought the health system in the Greater Toronto Area and other parts of the province to its knees, and seriously affected health systems in other parts of the country. In addition, travel advisories issued by the World Health Organization and the CDC, advising people to avoid all travel to Ontario, caused the local economy there to suffer great losses. Nurses lived daily with the fear that they would die or infect their families with a fatal disease. Respiratory technicians, doctors, hospital workers, paramedics, and home care workers lived with the same fear. Of the almost 375 people who contracted SARS in Ontario, 72% were infected in a heath-care setting. Of this group, 45% were health workers (McDonald et al., 2004). Most of these workers were nurses whose jobs brought them into the closest contact with sick patients. This does not show the full burden of SARS on nurses and paramedics and other health workers. In many cases nurses sick with undetected SARS brought illness, and in some cases death, home to their families (SARS Commission, 2006).

SARS and Public Health

As mysteriously as it appeared, the deadly SARS virus was contained and put to rest. Hundreds of cases were dealt with in several countries connected by international travel routes to China. Case fatality rates were very high. Infection control procedures, isolation, and quarantine all were needed to contain the problem. Yet, the global public health community managed to muster an amazing effort, which now speaks volumes about the importance of public health education, surveillance, and modern technology. Is this indicative of how all new emerging disease threats will be handled?

Lessons Learned with SARS

- Despite the unwillingness of the Chinese government to share information from the initial cases in this outbreak, the world health community collaborated in an unprecedented manner. A consortium of laboratories managed to sequence the genome of this newly discovered pathogen in a few days to develop rapid diagnostic and surveillance tools.

- International travel played a tremendous role in the spread of SARS. This shows us that the "connectedness" of our cities and populations can spread a deadly pathogen from one side of the world to the other in hours.

- Health-care facilities played an important role in the epidemiology of SARS. Patients infected with the SARS-coronavirus disease are likely to present to health-care facilities. If unrecognized as SARS, these patients may transmit SARS to health-care workers and other patients. Health-care workers accounted for a significant percentage of cases in most major SARS outbreaks reported.

- Is coronavirus just a relic, a coincidence? Some people with the disease were not presenting with antibodies to coronavirus, while there were some people showing no signs of the disease that were positive for antibodies to coronavirus. This finding is still very puzzling to many. Because the outbreak was so short-lived, we do not know how this disease might affect a large population or what role asymptomatic or subclinical patients play in the dynamics of disease transmission.

- AIDS patients did not seem to be affected by the SARS coronavirus. That fact is very puzzling to researchers.

Conclusion

Emerging diseases present a very unique challenge to public health officials and infectious disease specialists. Perhaps they have been with us for millions of years, lurking in a dark corner of the environment, waiting for an opportunity to jump from their natural cycle of transmission to a human host. Or, they may represent something totally new. Regardless of their origin, an emerging disease pathogen must be characterized quickly by molecular biologists and microbiologists. The dynamics of disease transmission must be investigated by teams of epidemiologists. Treatment regimens must be formulated by clinicians working on the front lines of the outbreak. Disease prevention strategies and risk communications must be quickly formulated by public health officials. Finally, media attention for emerging disease outbreaks forces government officials at all levels to address the problem with planning and preparedness activities aimed at preserving the health of the public. Category C agents may be exploited in much the same way that hoax powder incidents followed the 2001 Amerithrax event. In addition, terrorist groups and rogue states might take advantage of the emergence of one of these special pathogens to intentionally introduce an emerging disease into an area, thereby causing fear, panic, and social disruption.

Essential Terminology

- **Emerging disease.** Any disease, of various cause, that has newly appeared or is rapidly expanding its range in the human species.

- **Nipah virus fever.** A febrile illness caused by Nipah virus, a virus in the genus henipavirus of the family Paramyxoviridae. Henipaviruses are characterized by their large size, natural occurrence in Pteropid fruit bats, and recent emergence as zoonotic pathogens capable of causing illness and death in domestic animals and humans.

- **Hantavirus.** One of the four genera of the family Bunyaviridae. Hantaviruses are spread by rodents and target the kidneys, lungs or pulmonary system, and heart. The word *hantavirus* is derived from the Hantaan River, where the Hantaan virus (the etiologic agent of Korean hemorrhagic fever) was first isolated. The disease associated with Hantaan virus is called *Korean hemorrhagic fever* or *hemorrhagic fever with renal syndrome* (HFRS).

- **West Nile fever.** A febrile illness caused by West Nile virus, which is transmitted from birds to people through the bite of an infected *Culex* mosquito. The virus is closely related to other flaviviruses including those responsible for St. Louis encephalitis, Japanese encephalitis, and Murray Valley encephalitis.

- **SARS.** An acronym for *severe acute respiratory syndrome*, which is an atypical form of pneumonia. It first appeared in November 2002 in Guangdong Province, China. SARS is caused by the SARS coronavirus (SARS-CoV), a novel coronavirus.

Web Sites

Food and Agriculture Organization (FAO), Manual for Diagnosis of Nipah Virus Infection, available at www.fao.org/DOCREP/005/AC449E/AC449E00.htm.

World Health Organization, Nipah Virus Overview, available at www.who.int/mediacentre/factsheets/fs262/en/index.html.

Centers for Disease Control and Prevention, Special Pathogens Branch, All About Hantavirus, available at www.cdc.gov/ncidod/diseases/hanta/hps/noframes/phys/clinical.htm.

This URL allows you to view an excellent film about SARS from CDC Public Health Grand Rounds. It will point out, through the experiences of the public health community of Toronto, Canada, just how tough it was to control this outbreak; available at www.publichealthgrandrounds.unc.edu/sars/index.htm.

Centers for Disease Control and Prevention, Division of Vector-Borne Diseases, West Nile Virus home page, available at www.cdc.gov/ncidod/dvbid/westnile.

References

Calisher, C., J. Childs, H. Field, K. Holmes, and T. Schountz. 2006. Bats: Important reservoir hosts of emerging viruses. *Clinical Microbiology Reviews* 19:531–545.

Calisher, C., W. Sweeney, J. Mills, and B. Beaty. 1999. Natural history of Sin Nombre virus in western Colorado. *Emerging Infectious Diseases* 5:126–134.

Centers for Disease Control and Prevention. 1997. Case definitions for infectious conditions under public health surveillance. *Morbidity and Mortality Weekly Report* 46, no. RR10 (May 02):1–55.

Centers for Disease Control and Prevention. 1999. Outbreak of Hendra-like virus—Malaysia and Singapore, 1998–1999. *Morbidity and Mortality Weekly Report* 48:265–269.

Centers for Disease Control and Prevention. 2000. Update: Surveillance for West Nile virus in over-wintering mosquitoes—New York, 2000. *MMWR Morbidity and Mortality Weekly Report* 49, (March 10):178–179.

Centers for Disease Control and Prevention. 2007. Special Pathogens Branch. All About Hanta-viruses available at www.cdc.gov/Ncidod/diseases/hanta/hps/noframes/at_risk.htm.

Chapman, L., and R. Khabbaz. 1994. Etiology and epidemiology of the Four Corners hantavirus outbreak. *Infectious Agents of Disease* 3:234–244.

Childs, J., T. Ksiazek, C. Spiropoulou, J. Krebs, S. Morzunov, G. Maupin, K. Gage, P. Rollin, J. Sarisky, R. Enscore, et al. 1994. Serologic and genetic identification of *Peromyscus maniculatus* as the primary rodent reservoir for a new hantavirus in the southwestern United States. *Journal of Infectious Diseases* 169:1271–1280.

Chua, K. B., K. Goh, K. Wong, A. Kamarulzaman, P. Tan, T. Ksiazek, S. Zaki, G. Paul, S. Lam, and C. Tan. 1999. Fatal encephalitis due to Nipah virus among pig-farmers in Malaysia. *Lancet* 354:1257–1259.

Duchin, J., F. Koster, C. Peters, G. Simpson, B. Tempest, S. Zaki, T. Ksiazek, P. Rollin, S. Nichol, E. Umland, et al. 1994. Hantavirus pulmonary syndrome: a clinical description of 17 patients with a newly recognized disease. *New England Journal of Medicine* 330:949–955.

Ebel, G., A. Dupuis, K. Ngo, D. Nicholas, E. Kauffman, S. Jones, D. Young, J. Maffei, P. Shi, K. Bernard, and L. Kramer. 2001. Partial genetic characterization of West Nile virus strains, New York State, 2000. *Emerging Infectious Diseases* 7, no. 4 (July–August):650–653.

Food and Agriculture Organization of the United Nations. 2002. Regional Office for Asia and the Pacific Animal Production (RAP) and Health Commission for Asia and the Pacific. *Manual on the Diagnosis of Nipah Virus Infection in Animals*. RAP publication no. 2002/01. Rome: Regional Office for Asia and the Pacific Animal Production.

Garrett, L. 1995. *The Coming Plague: Newly Emerging Diseases in a World out of Balance*. New York: Farrar, Straus and Giroux.

Goldsmith, C., K. Tatti, T. Ksiazek, P. Rollin, J. Comer, W. Lee, et al. 2004. Ultrastructural charac-terization of SARS coronavirus. *Emerging Infectious Diseases* [serial online] (February), avail-able at www.cdc.gov/ncidod/EID/vol10no2/03-0913.htm.

Hsu, V., M. Hossain, U. Parashar, M. Ali, T. Ksiazek, I. Kuzmin, et al. 2004. Nipah virus encepha-litis reemergence, Bangladesh. *Emerging Infectious Diseases* [serial online] (December), avail-able at www.cdc.gov/ncidod/EID/vol10no12/04-0701.htm.

Jia, X., T. Briese, I. Jordan, A. Rambaut, H. Chi, J. Mackenzie, R. Hall, J. Scherret, and W. Lipkin. 1999. Genetic analysis of West Nile New York 1999 encephalitis virus. *Lancet* 354:1971–1972.

Knobler, S., A. Mahoud, S. Lemon, A. Mack, L. Sivitz, and K. Oberholtzer, eds. 2004. *Learning from SARS: Preparing for the Next Disease Outbreak*. Workshop summary, Forum on Microbial Threats, Board on Global Health, Institute of Medicine of the National Academies, Washington, DC: National Academies Press.

Knudsen, T., O. Andersen, and G. Kronborg. 2003. Death from the Nile crosses the Atlantic: The West Nile Fever story. *Scandinavian Journal of Infectious Disease* 35:820–825.

Kraus, A., C. Priemer, H. Heider, D. Kruger, and R. Ulrich. 2005. Inactivation of Hantaan virus-containing samples for subsequent investigations outside biosafety level 3 facilities. *Intervirology* 48:255–261.

LeDuc, J., J. Childs, and G. Glass. 1992. The hantaviruses, etiologic agents of hemorrhagic fever with renal syndrome: a possible cause of hypertension and chronic renal disease in the United States. *Annual Review of Public Health* 13:79–98.

Lee, H., P. Lee, and K. Johnson. 2004. Isolation of the etiologic agent of Korean hemorrhagic fever. *Journal of Infectious Diseases* 190:1708–1710.

Luby, S., M. Rahman, M. Hossain, L. Blum, M. Husain, E. Gurley, et al. 2006. Foodborne transmission of Nipah virus, Bangladesh. *Emerging Infectious Diseases* [serial online] (December), available from www.cdc.gov/ncidod/EID/vol12no12/06-0732.htm.

McDonald, L., A. Simor, I. Su, S. Malone, M. Ofner, K. Chen, et al. 2004. SARS in healthcare facilities, Toronto and Taiwan. *Emerging Infectious Diseases* [serial online] (May), available at www.cdc.gov/ncidod/EID/vol10no5/03-0791.htm.

McLean, R., S. Ubico, D. Docherty, W. Hansen, L. Sileo, and T. McNamara. 2001. West Nile virus transmission and ecology in birds. *Annals of the New York Academy of Science* 951:54–57.

Murgue, B., H. Zeller, and V. Deubel. 2002. The ecology and epidemiology of West Nile virus in Africa, Europe and Asia. *Current Topics in Microbiology and Immunology* 267:195–221.

Parashar, U., L. Sunn, F. Ong, A. Mounts, M. Arif, et al. 2000. Case-control study of risk factors for human infection with a new zoonotic paramyxovirus, Nipah virus, during a 1998–1999 outbreak of severe encephalitis in Malaysia. *Journal of Infectious Diseases* 181:1755–1759.

Pealer, L., A. Marfin, L. Petersen, R. Lanciotti, P. Page, S. Stramer, M. Stobierski, K. Signs, B. Newman, H. Kapoor, J. Goodman, M. Chamberland, and West Nile Virus Transmission Investigation Team. 2003. Transmission of West Nile virus through blood transfusion in the United States in 2002. *New England Journal of Medicine* 349:1236–1245.

Ricketts, E. 1954. Report of the clinical and physiological research at Hemorrhagic Fever Center, Korea, fall of 1953. *Medical Bulletin of the United States* 2:29–31.

SARS Commission. 2006. *Final Report, vol. 2, Spring of Fear. The Story of SARS.* Toronto, Canada: SARS Commission.

Stelzel, W. 1996. Hantavirus pulmonary syndrome: Epidemiology, prevention, and case presentation of a new viral strain. *Nurse Practitioner* 21:89–90.

Stramer, S., C. Fang, G. Foster, et al. 2005. West Nile virus among blood donors in the United States, 2003 and 2004. *New England Journal of Medicine* 353:451–459.

Wong, K., W. Shieh, S. Kumar, K. Norain, W. Abdullah, J. Guarner, C. Goldsmith, K. Chua, S. Lam, C. Tan, K. Goh, H. Chong, R. Jusoh, P. Rollin, T. Ksiazek, S. Zaki, and the Nipah Virus Pathology Working Group. 2002. Nipah virus infection pathology and pathogenesis of an emerging paramyxoviral zoonosis. *American Journal of Pathology* 161:2153–2167.

Xu, R-H, J-F He, M. R. Evans, G-W Peng, H. E. Field, D-W Yu, et al. 2004. Epidemiologic clues to SARS origin in China. *Emerging Infectious Diseases* [serial online] (June), available at www. cdc.gov/ncidod/EID/vol10no6/03-0852.htm.

Recognize, Avoid, Isolate, and Notify

The most dangerous situation is where you're facing peril but you're not aware of it.
—Rudolph Giuliani

Objectives

The study of this chapter will enable you to

1. List and discuss the components of RAIN.
2. Discuss how individuals or responders might recognize biothreat agents or the diseases they cause.
3. Describe methodologies used to detect biological agents in the field.
4. Discuss the limitations of field tools for biothreat pathogen detection.
5. Discuss methods and strategies to avoid biological contamination.
6. Discuss methods and strategies to isolate biological agents or contagious persons or animals from others.
7. Discuss notification procedures and considerations once biological agents have been disseminated or enter a population of people or animals.

Key Terms

First responder, first receiver, RAIN (recognize, avoid, isolate, notify), gold standard, accuracy, sensitivity, specificity.

Introduction

In the late 1990s, there was a renewed awareness of the threat posed to Western civilization from weapons of mass destruction. Much of the incentive for bolstering the nation's preparedness posture came from political reaction to several key events. Three specific events that took place in the year 1995 are noteworthy. First, on March 20, the terrorist cult Aum Shinrikyo staged an attack on the Tokyo subway system with sarin nerve gas.

Second, on April 19, Timothy McVeigh bombed the Alfred P. Murrah Federal Building in Oklahoma City. Third, white supremacist Larry Wayne Harris was arrested by the FBI for purchasing cultures of *Yersinia pestis* (plague bacterium) from the American Type Culture Collection (Chantilly, Virginia) under false pretenses. It is not exactly clear what he intended to use them for, but the mail and wire fraud he committed was sufficient reason to arrest and convict him. Notwithstanding, the dissolution of the Soviet Union in 1991 meant that stockpiles of chemical, biological, and nuclear weapons were now in the hands of some unstable, independent states. Political and economic turmoil in these former Soviet states put the status of their biological weapons in question. It caused many U.S. government officials to ask questions like these: Were all Soviet biological weapons secure and accounted for? Could Soviet bioweapon stocks fall into the hands of a terrorist group or rogue states?

The Nunn-Lugar-Domenici (NLD) Defense against Weapons of Mass Destruction Act of 1996 (Public Law 104-201) mandated training for the 120 most populous cities in the United States (Socher and Leap, 2005). In the 1998 Appropriations Act (Public Law 105-119), members of Congress expressed their concern for the potentially catastrophic effects of a chemical or biological act of terrorism. Congress stated that, while the federal government plays an important role in preventing and responding to these types of threats, state and local public safety personnel are typically *first to respond* to the scene when such incidents occur (GAO Report, 1999). As a result, Congress authorized the Attorney General to assist state and local public safety personnel (now known primarily as **first responders**) in acquiring the specialized training and equipment necessary to safely respond to and manage terrorist incidents involving weapons of mass destruction (WMD). On April 30, 1998, the Attorney General delegated authority to the Justice Department's Office of Justice Programs to develop and administer training and equipment assistance programs for state and local emergency response agencies to better prepare them against this threat. To execute this mission, the Office of Justice Programs established the Office for Domestic Preparedness to develop and administer a national Domestic Preparedness Program (1999).

Community Response Organizations

A community's ability to analyze and assess the terrorist WMD threat, and its vulnerability to that threat, is the first step in developing a contingency plan. Every community should have an Emergency Response Plan to minimize the catastrophic impact of a terrorist WMD attack by addressing the complexities of such an attack.

The term *hazardous substance* refers to any substance that results or may result in adverse effects on the health or safety of employees. This includes substances defined under Section 101(14) of the Comprehensive Environmental Response, Compensation, and Liability Act (CERCLA) of 1980: biological or disease-causing agents that may reasonably be anticipated to cause death, disease, or other health problems; any substance listed by the U.S. Department of Transportation as hazardous material under 49 CFR 172.101 and appendices; and substances classified as hazardous waste.

"Emergency response or responding to emergencies means a response effort by employees from outside the immediate release area or by other designated responders (i.e., mutual aid groups, local fire departments, etc.) to an occurrence which results, or is likely to result, in an uncontrolled release of a hazardous substance. Responses to incidental releases of hazardous substances where the substance can be absorbed, neutralized, or otherwise controlled at the time of release by employees in the immediate release area, or by maintenance personnel are not considered to be emergency responses within the scope of this standard. Responses to releases of hazardous substances where there is no potential safety or health hazard (i.e., fire, explosion, or chemical exposure) are not considered to be emergency responses." (Standards, 29 Code of Federal Regulations [CFR], 1910.120(a)(3)).

When it comes to dealing with hazardous materials, such as chemical, biological, radiological/nuclear, and explosive (CBRNE), responders function at various levels. These performance levels and their requisite training are specified in 29 CFR, 1910.120. They are as follows:

- *First responder awareness level* are "individuals who are likely to witness or discover a hazardous substance release and who have been trained to initiate an emergency response sequence by notifying the proper authorities of the release. They would take no further action beyond notifying the authorities of the release" [1910.120(q)(6)(i)].

- *First responder operations level* are "individuals who respond to releases or potential releases of hazardous substances as part of the initial response to the site for the purpose of protecting nearby persons, property, or the environment from the effects of the release. They are trained to respond in a defensive fashion without actually trying to stop the release. Their function is to contain the release from a safe distance, keep it from spreading, and prevent exposures" [1910.120(q)(6)(ii)].

- *Hazardous materials technicians* are "individuals who respond to releases or potential releases for the purpose of stopping the release. They assume a more aggressive role than a first responder at the operations level in that they will approach the point of release in order to plug, patch or otherwise stop the release of a hazardous substance" [1910.120(q)(6)(iii)].

- *Hazardous materials specialists* are "individuals who respond with and provide support to hazardous materials technicians. Their duties parallel those of the hazardous materials technician, however, those duties require a more directed or specific knowledge of the various substances they may be called upon to contain. The hazardous materials specialist would also act as the site liaison with Federal, state, local and other government authorities in regards to site activities" [1910.120(q)(6)(iv)].

- *On scene incident commanders* are "individuals who assume control of the incident scene and be responsible for responder safety and operational structure in accordance with the National Incident Management System (NIMS) and the principles of Incident Command System (ICS). These individuals will be trained on all aspects of the threat beyond the first responder awareness level and up to the first responder operations level" [1910.120(q)(6)(v)].

Health-care workers risk occupational exposures to chemical, biological, or radiological materials when a hospital receives contaminated patients, particularly during mass casualty incidents. These hospital employees, who may be termed **first receivers**, work at a site remote from the location where the hazardous substance release occurred. This means that their exposures are limited to the substances transported to the hospital on victims' skin, hair, clothing, or personal effects (Horton, Berkowitz, and Kaye, 2003).

The location and limited source of contaminant distinguishes first receivers from other first responders (e.g., firefighters, law enforcement, paramedics, etc.), who typically respond to the incident site (Occupational Safety and Health Administration, 2005).

The Concept of RAIN

The ranks of responders are mostly comprised of individuals trained to the awareness level. Responders at this level are not qualified or certified to perform ongoing operations or support at the scene of a WMD incident (OSHA 1910.120.(q)(6)(i)). Therefore, the key of awareness training programs should be to convey information in such a way as to give first responders and first receivers a keen sense of awareness and a commonsense framework for what to do when they believe that hazardous materials have been released.

Based on the volumes of information available about biological agents, knowledge and skills stressed in training programs should be applied so that individuals are prepared to respond rapidly. They must recognize the potential hazard, avoid becoming contaminated, isolate the area, and make appropriate notifications. Accordingly, the acronym **RAIN** (recognition, avoidance, isolation, and notification) may be used by responders and receivers to quickly gather and process information and to synthesize the information to facilitate life and safety actions in a WMD incident. This concept and acronym was devised by preparedness trainers in the development training guidelines and curriculum for the original (1999) Domestic Preparedness program's awareness level training (Socher and Leap, 2005).

In brief, the concept of RAIN may be applied by individuals in the following manner:

- **Recognize** the hazard or threat (What do I see, hear, or smell that indicates a biological threat is present?). The goal is to get first responders and first receivers to rapidly interpret and mentally process a suspicious event for what it is.
- **Avoid** the hazard, contamination, or injury (What do I stay away from?). What actions must responders and receivers take to avoid liquids, powders, clouds, or vapors that are potentially harmful to them? The concept of *time, distance*, and *shielding* (TDS) concerns avoiding exposure *time* to the threat, putting *distance* between people and the threat, and *shielding* with protective equipment or barriers. The concept of TDS is often applied for radiological hazards, but it has merit also with biological materials, assuming one is aware of the release site.
- **Isolate** the hazard area (Whom do I protect?). What actions are necessary for responders and receivers to isolate or reduce exposure to contamination or threat, attempt to remove other people who may be in the contaminated area, and keep people from going into the contaminated area?
- **Notify** the appropriate support (Whom do I call?). What actions are needed to notify the proper authorities and agencies, giving them as much information as possible about the event?

Recognition

The insidious nature of biological weaponry contributes to the difficulty we currently face in attempting to recognize when a biological threat exists. Recall that, in many cases, only small amounts of viable, formulated materials are needed to perpetrate biological attacks. Most biological agents have an incubation period before outward signs of disease become apparent in their victims. In addition, the onset of symptoms is often so nonspecific (flulike illness) that one would probably not recognize them as something out of the ordinary. Since there is a high probability that a biological agent may not be discovered until days after the actual event, there may be no first response. Actually, the first real indications of a biological incident will probably come from 911 operators, Emergency Medical Service personnel, and the medical community—especially the emergency departments in local hospitals. Alert and trained emergency response personnel can be the first line of defense by reporting suspicious items or actions and recognizing unusual trends in people, animals, or certain areas.

A number of associated signs and symptoms occurring in a specific area or community tying together many people—numerous calls to 911 (people asking for assistance and reporting high fevers, vomiting, etc.) or a sudden rush of people showing up at urgent care facilities or emergency rooms—should alert the medical community that a biological event may have occurred. Recognizing these clues or patterns may alert responders or public health officials to interview patients, family members, and possible contacts. Questions asked could focus on recent travel history, personal associations, employment, and attendance at community events.

For obvious reasons, intentional releases of biological agents are likely to be done covertly. However, outward warning signs or clues may alert the responder to the possible presence of biological agents both prior to an incident and at the scene. The incident may come with verbal or written threats issued prior to an attack. Old war stocks of formulated biothreat agents may be contained in bomblets that do not produce much blast or fire damage. Hence, a low explosive device releasing a powdery substance or mist may be indicative of a bioweapons release. An abandoned spray device that seems out of place may be a clue that a biothreat agent has been delivered. Responders may come upon a scene of a clandestine laboratory where biological agents were being prepared as evidenced by containers from laboratory or biological supply houses. In addition, biosafety cabinets, incubators, active cultures and stocks of culture medium associated with an unauthorized bio-production facility might be discovered.

□ □ □ ▬▬▬▬▬▬▬▬▬▬▬▬▬▬▬▬▬▬▬▬▬▬▬▬▬▬▬▬▬▬▬▬▬▬

Indications of Possible Biowarfare Attack

- The discovery of a disease due to a pathogen that does not occur naturally in a given geographic area.
- Multiple disease entities in the same patients, indicating that mixed agents have been used in the attack.
- Large numbers of both military and civilian casualties, when such populations inhabit the same area.
- Data from a biosensor suggesting a massive point-source outbreak.
- Large outbreak of disease due to an apparent inhalation route of infection.
- High percentage morbidity and mortality relative to the at-risk population.
- Illness limited to fairly localized or circumscribed geographical areas.

- Low attack rates in personnel who work in areas with filtered air supplies or closed ventilation systems.
- Sentinel dead animals of multiple species.
- Absence of a competent natural vector in the area of outbreak (for a biological agent that is vector borne in nature).

Source: S. L. Wiener and J. Barrett. Biological warfare defense. In: *Trauma Management for Civilian and Military Physicians*, pp. 508–509. Philadelphia: W.B. Saunders, 1989.

Sampling and Detection Methods

Agent Detection Technologies

The means to detect and identify biological incidents is much smaller than current capabilities for chemical and radiological detection. Typically, samples are collected on site, observing rules of evidence and maintaining a chain of custody (Figure 6-1). The samples are taken to a highly sophisticated laboratory, where they are analyzed with

	Diseased D+	Diseased-free D−	
Test Postive T+	True Positive	False Positive	Positive Predictive Value
Test Negative T−	False Negative	True Negative	Negative Predictive Value
	Sensitivity	Specificity	

Sensitivity = TP/(TP+FN)
(True positive rate)

Specificity = TN/(TN+FP)
(True negative rate)

Positive Predictive Value (PPV) = TP/(TP+FP)

Negative Predictive Value (NPV) = TN/(TN+FN)

FIGURE 6-1 Joint Biological Agent Identification and Diagnostic System test participants collect samples of suspect biological warfare agents from the field during a joint two-week operational test at Brooks City Base, San Antonio, Texas. Biosampling protocols and test procedures for sample processing are critical to the accurate identification of biothreat organisms. (Image courtesy of the United States Army.)

various techniques that include bioassay, immunoassay, nucleic-acid assay, and the culture of living organisms.

On-site detection of biological agents is currently not practical for most responders. This section briefly introduces the reader to some primary technologies used in pathogen and toxin detection. Before we proceed into the details, we spend some time on the problems associated with agent sampling and detection. All too often, important principles and limitations are overlooked by the professionals that rely on the "tools of the trade."

A number of complexities are related to agent detection and the technologies employed to accomplish this. First, we may need to determine if an agent is present in our environment (i.e., on an object, in the soil or water, etc.) or if the agent is the cause of disease-related signs and symptoms. These are two very different problems governed by dramatically different rules and regulations. Therefore, in our treatment of this subject, we split the discussion into clinical and environmental methods.

Sampling Methods

Before we can perform an appropriate test we must take a good sample. In other words, *do not take bad samples to good tests.* Never underestimate the importance of this statement. Sampling efficiency needs to be as high as possible, and methods must be validated for sampling and testing collective schemes. Materials used in the sampling tools and procedures may not be compatible with the detection methods. For instance, a certain buffer may degrade or alter the substance or agent we are trying to detect. In addition, the material used to retrieve the sample from a surface may retain most of the agent but not allow it to go into solution after retrieval. Regardless of the physical and chemical considerations, *studies are necessary* to determine the efficiency of sampling and detection combinations. Lead agencies in the federal government (CDC, DOD, FBI, etc.) have validated protocols and devices for performing sampling of biothreat agents and taking clinical samples from patients. Different sampling methods may be, and often are, required for different assays.

When it comes to environmental and clinical sampling, methods are dramatically different. In addition, often a number of critical steps in sample preparation are necessary before a sample is subjected to a test method. It would not be practical here to go into all the methods of sampling and preparation. Suffice it to say, we are dealing with some very complicated issues. Ideally, the samples we take would be sterile and free of all inhibitors. In reality, that is seldom the case. Sample matrices can be very complex. Take water, for example. There are many types of water. Detection of an agent in distilled water using a nucleic acid–based test may not be possible if the agent was in treated water, wastewater, rainwater, or recycled water. Likewise, taking a stool sample presents different challenges than taking a blood sample. A variety of challenges are present in both samples. With stool, you have to isolate your agent from a long list of other organisms. In addition, a number of inhibitors in the stool can undermine the performance of test reagents. The same holds true for blood. You may have to remove red blood cells from your sample. The heme group in a red blood cell might inhibit some test reagents. Your agent may be an intracellular pathogen. How will you get the agent out of the macrophage and make it available to the assay? This is where sample preparation comes in.

☐ ☐ ☐ ━━━

Critical Thinking

What confounding factors might affect the taking of an environmental sample? What is meant by the statement: *Never take bad samples to a good test.*

━━━ ☐ ☐ ☐

It can be very difficult to take a good sample. What you do with that sample before you subject it to testing is called *sample preparation*. Some nucleic acid-based tests require several hours of technical and laborious extraction procedures. All this adds to the complexity of the test. Very few procedures can be performed in the field by unskilled personnel. For this reason Health and Human Services issued a statement in 2002 advising against the use of rapid anthrax tests for first responders.

With respect to environmental detection, we will cover only the most relevant aspects of biothreat pathogen detection in an environmental setting. This includes all things outside of sampling and testing a patient. To the professionals that do this as a part of their jobs, this might be the surface of an object, a suspicious package, or air, water or the soil near a dead animal, to name just a few.

Clinical samples are complicated matrices. Environmental samples can be even more variable. As previously mentioned, there are many types of water. The same applies for soil. In addition, environmental samples may contain pollutants, heavy metals, and organic compounds (e.g., humic acids) that can defeat the sampling and testing methods. We explore some of the more common methods for testing a sample. Included is a look at some of the more advanced technologies and a discussion of the dipstick assays.

Nothing beats getting an isolate from the environment. Therefore, *culturing remains the gold standard in many environmental testing programs*. For the most part, other technologies are an inference to the presence of the pathogen. With culturing isolates, we get a result that can be seen, and then we have the ability to run a battery of physical and chemical tests. Bioforensic and epidemiologic investigations often include a picture of the organism either on a Petri dish or the surface of a microscope slide. This illustrates the importance of obtaining a laboratory isolate. Furthermore, if we have the pathogen in pure culture, we can perform a number of genetic tests that may help with attributing the offending organism to a source at the completion of that investigation. In fact, a new federal organization that deals in "bioforensics" has been established at Fort Detrick, Maryland, to aid the FBI, CDC, and Department of Defense in their investigations for potential acts of bioterrorism.

Test Accuracy

We should not assume that a test method is completely accurate. **Accuracy** is the degree of sensitivity and specificity at which a diagnostic test performs. In fact, test performance, or accuracy, is defined by a number of important terms (Douglass, 1993). The hallmark by which we measure these tools is often its performance compared to a **gold standard** or reference method of choice. When the agent is present and the test detects it, we call that a *true positive*. When the agent is absent and the test indicates the same, we refer to that as a *true negative*. When the agent is present and the test fails to detect it, we call that a *false negative*. When the test indicates positive and the agent is absent, we call that a *false*

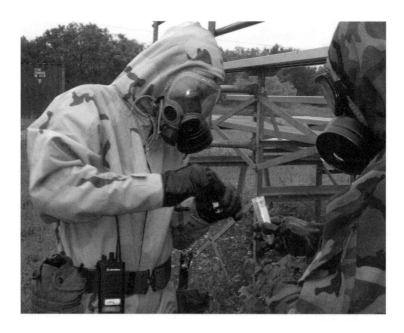

FIGURE 6-2 Indices used to determine the accuracy of a diagnostic test.

positive. The correct use of these terms is important. The matrix in Figure 6-2 shows how all performance indices are calculated in a simple scheme.

Moreover, we need to understand the implications of an incorrect result. False negatives can lead to a missed diagnosis and lack of proper treatment. With an environmental test, a false negative could lead an incident commander to declare an area "all clear" and put people back at risk. False positives could result in someone being inappropriately or needlessly treated for a disease. With an environmental test, this could lead to hundreds of people being needlessly put on prophylaxis, as occurred in 2001 in New York City during the anthrax scare.

Sensitivity is the probability that a test will produce a true positive result when the agent is present in a sample. This is often determined by direct comparison to a reference method or "gold standard." So, let us say that a test indicates positive 52 times out of 100 positive samples. The sensitivity in this example is only 52%. You would be almost better off to flip a coin to make a determination. **Specificity** is the probability that a test will produce a true negative result when used on a sample that does not contain the agent. This is also determined by comparison to a reference or gold standard. When it comes to biothreat agent detection, test validation is often performed with a panel of different strains of the same agent and a number of related and unrelated organisms (referred to as *nearest neighbor testing*). So, as an example let us take a field test for *Bacillus anthracis (Ba)* spores; here, a thorough validation testing program would include a sensitivity panel of approximately 100 strains of *Ba* and our specificity panel would include nonpathogenic strains of *Ba*, other bacilli, a wide array of other bacteria, and perhaps some common substances used as hoax powders.

Some other indices commonly used in assay performance are *positive predictive* and *negative predictive values* (PPV and NPV, respectively). PPV is the probability that the agent is present when a positive test result is observed. Conversely, NPV is the probability that the agent is absent when a negative test result is observed. These indices can be very useful when considering consequence management options.

Some Common Test Methodologies

Wicking Assays

Wicking assays, or dipsticks, are immunochromatographic tests that work very simply and practically. This can be very advantageous for test needs in a field setting. Wicking assays, first described in the late 1960s, were originally developed to assess the presence of specific serum proteins. A good example of these that we can all relate to is the EPT, or early pregnancy test. Two lines present on an EPT test strip normally indicate pregnancy is likely with 99.9% accuracy. Over the past decade, many wicking assays were developed for the diagnosis of infectious diseases, cancer, cardiovascular problems, pancreatitis, and illicit drug use. Other promising areas for the use of such assays are drug monitoring, food safety, environmental monitoring, and veterinary medicine. Assays using this format take approximately 15 minutes to run and are simple to use, requiring only the dilution of the test agent in a sample buffer and applying several drops to the test strip. Dipstick devices normally employ a colloidal gold (or other)-labeled antibody dried onto a filter pad affixed to a nitrocellulose strip. A capture antibody is applied in a line on the strip and dried. To perform the test, a specimen is suspended in buffer and added to the pad containing the colloidal gold-labeled antibody. The antibody specifically binds to antigen present in the specimen, and the resulting complex wicks down the membrane where it binds to the capture antibody. A positive reaction is visualized as a red line created by the bound colloidal gold. Similar assays using different detection systems have been developed, including those based on latex particles and phosphatases.

The present generation of handheld assays has several limitations. Normally, only one agent is detected per assay strip. Therefore, if an unknown sample needs to be characterized, several handheld assays may be required to obtain a presumptive identification. The second limitation is that each of the assays has varying sensitivity levels to their respective target agents. Assays for bacterial agents tend to be the most sensitive, able to detect from 20,000 to 200,000 cells per milliliter (ml), while those for toxins have sensitivities ranging from 50 picograms to 50 nanograms per ml. Assays specific for viruses usually have the lowest sensitivities, ranging from 20,000 to 2 million virus particles per ml. Third, since these assays are visualized as a red line created by the bound colloidal gold, the sensitivity is limited to what can be seen by the unaided and uncalibrated human eye. An arbitrary quantitation of the detection sensitivity of these assays is done by assigning a number between 0 and 5, with the increasing intensity of the red line assigned a higher value. In addition to the somewhat arbitrary nature of this process, numeric values can vary based on the skill of the technician responsible for validating a given lot of assays. Finally, there is a trade-off between sensitivity and specificity. Hence, the developer tweaking one of these assays may have to sacrifice specificity to make a more sensitive tool and vice versa.

Recent advances in detection and labeling technologies that, in some instances, would improve the sensitivities of assays by at least an order of magnitude and make detection quantitative not merely subjective may offset the disadvantages inherent to present handheld assays. To detect very low levels of antigen, which may be present at low concentrations in vivo or environmental samples, the sensitivity of conventional gold-labeled lateral flow assays can be enhanced up to one order of magnitude by using a silver enhancement step. Lateral flow assays are run, as just described, washed in a buffer solution, then immersed in a silver enhancer reagent for 5 minutes. This system has the advantage of greater sensitivity but does not need a specialized mechanism to read the assay, which is advantageous for use in a field setting.

Alternative approaches to antibody labeling coupled with specialized quantitative readers can also lead to significant improvements in the sensitivity of lateral flow immunoassays. For example, superparamagnetic nanoparticles comprising either iron oxide or iron oxide in a polysaccharide matrix can be used to label antibodies in place of gold. The labeled antibody-antigen mixture wicks up the membrane, as described, and is deposited at the site of the solid-phase antibody, and the magnetic flux is measured in the antigen capture zone. This technology has three advantages. First, the signal is permanent and can be read more than one time. Second, the signal is quantitative and can be assigned a value in millivolts. Third, the signal generated is comparable to the detection limits seen with the most sensitive radionucleotide labels.

Commercially Available Tests for Biowarfare Agents [[3]]

Imagine a scenario where first responders arrive at the scene of an incident involving a suspect powder. The scene is cleared and a HazMat technician dressed in a Level A ensemble goes into the building to take a sample. As he exits, the sample is rushed into an awaiting HazMat response unit for field testing. What are they using? What can they do with the results? These are good questions that deserve to be investigated at the local level. When you look at what is available on the market today you have to ask the question, What is the accuracy of these tools and who performed the scientific study to validate the claim? It is our opinion that the accuracy of many of these devices or field tests is either overstated by the manufacturer or unknown.

☐ ☐ ☐ ▬▬▬▬▬▬▬▬▬▬▬▬▬▬▬▬▬▬▬▬▬▬▬▬▬▬▬▬▬▬▬▬▬▬

Department of Health and Human Services Statement Issued July 2002

"The U.S. Department of Health and Human Services recommends against use by first responders of hand-held assays to evaluate and respond to an incident involving unknown powders suspected to be anthrax or other biological agents."

▬▬▬▬▬▬▬▬▬▬▬▬▬▬▬▬▬▬▬▬▬▬▬▬▬▬▬▬▬▬▬▬▬▬ ☐ ☐ ☐

The Association of Analytical Communities (AOAC) was contracted by the Department of Homeland Security to assess the accuracy of several commercially available assays for the detection of *Bacillus anthracis* spores. The study involved 12 centers and took more than a year to complete.

A visit to the AOAC web site (www.aoac.org/testkits/kits-bioterror.html) shows a listing of most commercially available assays for the biowarfare agents. The list states the name of the manufacturer, the name of the test, and the agent it supposedly detects. Also, there is a column for what "recognition" the assay has for substantiating its accuracy and validity. Only two of these tools have any "recognition."

Nucleic Acid-Based Methods

Polymerase chain reaction and real-time PCR show a lot of promise for use in the field. In fact, real-time PCR protocols are used throughout the CDC Laboratory Response Network to definitively detect biothreat pathogens, the SARS virus and highly pathogenic H5N1. A number of PCR assays and specific probe reagents were developed for several signature sequences for each pathogen. Three to five gene sequences are used for each of the agents. In this way, specificity is absolute for a positive identification.

Automated Systems

Automated systems are at the pinnacle of biothreat testing. Chapter 13 is dedicated to one of these systems, the biohazard detection system, which has been deployed throughout the U.S. Postal System. In addition, the BioWatch program has deployed sentinel systems that automatically collect air samples in a number of cities across the United States for further testing in an LRN laboratory.

Avoidance

The key to avoidance is personal protection and the establishment of protection zones. Safety considerations are imperative, not only for responders but for the general public. All personnel who enter the potentially contaminated area must follow local incident response procedures, if a plan exists.

□ □ □ ▬▬▬▬▬▬▬▬▬▬▬▬▬▬▬▬▬▬▬▬▬▬▬▬▬▬▬▬▬▬▬▬▬▬

Critical Thinking
What should a responder, or any individual, do when recognizing that something is suspicious or hazardous?

▬▬▬▬▬▬▬▬▬▬▬▬▬▬▬▬▬▬▬▬▬▬▬▬▬▬▬▬▬▬▬▬▬▬ □ □ □

The most critical vulnerability to be addressed during a biological material response is protection from small airborne particles. First responders dispatched to suspect biothreat events should be outfitted with personal protective equipment (PPE) that includes negative pressure air-purifying respirators with OSHA approved CBRNE filters, Tyvek®-type coveralls with hood, latex outer gloves, and overboots (see Figures 6-3 and 6-4). When an aerosolized unknown biological material is suspected, fully encapsulated PPE with a self-contained breathing apparatus is recommended. When the biological material is no longer being disseminated or aerosolized, lesser forms of PPE may be adequate. For letters, packages, or powder deposits suspected of containing biological materials, a full-face piece respirator with a P100 filter or a powered air purifying respirator with high-efficiency particulate air filter may be used. Potentially contaminated equipment requires decontamination. Responders should always observe blood-borne pathogen universal precautions as the first line of defense when treating patients. Responders should seek medical attention immediately if, after responding to

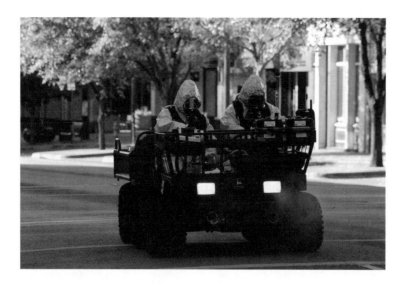

FIGURE 6-3 Responders from a National Guard Civil Support Team enter the hot zone during a training exercise. Note Level B personal protective equipment worn while conducting operations in a hazardous environment. (Image courtesy of Department of Defense, DefenseLINK.)

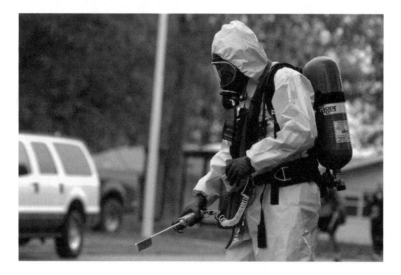

FIGURE 6-4 U.S. Air Force Master Sgt. Ken Jacobson, an Air National Guardsman assigned to the 42nd Civil Support Team, North Carolina National Guard, Charlotte, dons Level B personal protective equipment and operates in a mock hot zone to perform chemical and biological readings. (Image Courtesy of Department of Defense, DefenseLINK.)

an incident, they develop flulike or other unusual symptoms. Response personnel who suspect that they have been contaminated should seek medical attention immediately.

Isolation

Challenges in the response phase include securing the site, identifying and treating victims, decontamination of personnel, and neutralization of the agent. Assuming that the scene of the original release is known or suspected, the site and downwind hazard area must be secured. Entry into this area is restricted and zones must be established to protect

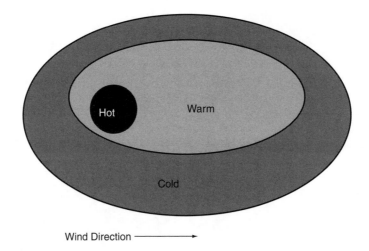

Wind Direction ———————➤

FIGURE 6-5 Here, a hypothetical release of a biological material has occurred. The incident commander establishes a Hot zone around the site of the release. The radius of this zone depends on a number of factors and can be estimated with the *Emergency Response Guidebook* (U.S. Department of Transportation, 2004) or a software program. Outside the Hot zone, the incident commander establishes a Warm zone, where decontamination operations and processing of evidence may take place. Finally, a Cold zone is established outside the Warm zone. Although this is a safe area, the operation uses this area to conduct administrative functions and keep the public from crossing into the hazardous area.

personnel and assist the incident commander in conducting operations that are consistent with an incident action plan and commensurate with the training and actions of response personnel at the levels previously described. The incident commander needs to move quickly to *isolate* the area by establishing hot, warm, and cold zones (see Figure 6-5).

The intentional release of a biological agent would make the site a crime scene. First responders need to be sensitive to protecting the crime scene and preserving physical evidence. Physical evidence has the potential to play a critical role in the overall investigation and resolution of the criminal act.

There are two universal considerations for crime scenes. The first universal consideration, often referred to as the *golden rule*, states that responders should leave any suspect object undisturbed, unless it is necessary for the performance of duties and is done in concurrence with law enforcement. The second universal consideration is that an incident should involve the fewest number of personnel possible. Protecting the populace may involve keeping some victims in the hot zone and preventing them from leaving the area before required medical evaluation and decontamination has taken place, while, at the same time, keeping people outside the hot zone from entering.

□ □ □ ▬▬▬▬▬▬▬▬▬▬▬▬▬▬▬▬▬▬▬▬▬▬▬▬▬▬▬▬▬▬▬▬▬▬▬▬▬

Critical Thinking

Consider the use of isolation and protection zones outlined in the *Emergency Response Guidebook* (ERG; U.S. Department of Transportation, 2004) in relation to a biological agent release. Are the distances specified in the guidebook practical for use by an incident commander? What environmental conditions could affect those distances?

▬▬▬▬▬▬▬▬▬▬▬▬▬▬▬▬▬▬▬▬▬▬▬▬▬▬▬▬▬▬▬▬▬▬▬▬▬ □ □ □

Standard operating procedures for WMD evidence management should be closely coordinated with the local FBI field office, evidence response team, supervisory special agent, or assistant special agent-in-charge. Establish a multiagency coordinating group for planning and coordinating crime scene evidence preservation and collection protocols.

Decontamination covers a broad scope of activities. Self-decontamination involves a responder contaminated with a hazardous substance; the responder should remove his or her clothing, decontaminate with the appropriate material, and then cover himself or herself before seeking medical evaluation.

Notification

Responders who suspect that a biological attack has taken place must follow local protocols to notify emergency services and emergency support personnel. Command authorities must be included in the chain of command and notifications made as indicated in the local emergency plan. Communication among related medical, health, and emergency personnel is critical, especially to facilitate early treatment and prevention. Numerous technical resources are available at the federal level. Acts of bioterrorism are considered WMD incidents. Accordingly, the site becomes a federal crime scene; hence, the FBI has legal jurisdiction over the incident, and the Department of Homeland Security appoints a principal federal official to take command of response and recovery efforts.

Responders need to become familiar with local and state resources and know the people that represent these agencies before an incident occurs. Response agency leads, especially at the state level, must establish ties with officials from the U.S. Public Health Service or the Centers for Disease Control. Incident commanders need to know how to contact the Federal Bureau of Investigation's WMD coordinator and determine when National Guard civil support teams will assist in processing and collecting samples from the hot zone, if applicable (Hurston, Sato, and Ryan, 2006).

Conclusion

Biological weapons are insidious. They may be deployed covertly, leaving no outward sign for days or weeks, until the first few cases begin to appear following the agent's incubation period. In this event, health-care professionals must be vigilant to note the signs and symptoms of the diseases that make Categories A, B, and C. Alternatively, there may be outward signs that a biological weapon has been deployed. As with the Amerithrax incident, the letters containing the agent came with a warning. Regardless, first responders and first receivers must be properly trained to protect themselves and contain the outbreak. The acronym RAIN provides a framework for guiding their actions. Recognition is the key to an effective response. Knowing that a problem exists precipitates a long list of actions from numerous agencies at all levels. More information about the response is found in Chapter 11. The concept RAIN was introduced here so that it may be applied to the case studies that follow.

Essential Terminology

- **First responders.** Personnel who have responsibility to initially respond to emergencies. Some examples are firefighters, HazMat team members, law enforcement officers, lifeguards, forestry personnel, ambulance attendants, and other public service personnel. In the case of hazardous materials incidents, these personnel typically respond at the site where the incident occurred.

- **First receivers.** Employees at a hospital engaged in decontamination and treatment of victims who have been contaminated by a hazardous substance(s) during an emergency incident. The incident occurs at a site other than the hospital. These employees are a subset of first responders.

- **RAIN.** An acronym that stands for recognize, avoid, isolate, and notify, which provides a framework for responders to act appropriately when faced with a life threatening situation.

- **Gold standard.** The reference method of choice, the procedure or measurement that is widely accepted as being the best available, against which new interventions should be compared. It is particularly important in studies of the accuracy of diagnostic tests.

- **Accuracy.** The relationship between test results and "gold standard" results.

- **Sensitivity.** The probability that a test will produce a true positive result when the agent is present in a sample.

- **Specificity.** The probability that a test will produce a true negative result when used on a sample that does not contain the agent.

Discussion Questions

- How are we likely to recognize the next big act of bioterrorism?
- Responders are called to a "white powder" incident at a high-rise office building. What reliable tools do they have to determine if the suspicious substance contains a biothreat agent?
- How important is it to take a "good sample"?
- What guidance is out there for biological sampling for responders to follow? Conduct an Internet search to determine if there is one method for sampling powders from nonporous surfaces.

Web Sites

Information regarding PPE for responders can be found at the web sites that follow:

Centers for Disease Control and Prevention: www.bt.cdc.gov/documentsapp/anthrax/Protective/10242001Protect.asp.

National Institute for Occupational Safety and Health: www.dhs.gov/dhspublic/index.jsp.

National Fire Protection Agency: www.nfpa.org/index.

One can get a true appreciation for the complexities associated with sampling by looking at the CDC protocol for *Bacillus anthracis*. Go to the following URL to see the extensive procedures: www.bt.cdc.gov/agent/anthrax/environmental-sampling-apr2002.asp.

References

29 Code Federal Regulations (CFR) 1910.120. Occupational Safety and Health Administration. Department of Labor. Hazardous Waste Operations and Emergency Response.

49 Code Federal Regulations (CFR) 172.101. Research and Special Programs Administration. Department of Transportation. Hazardous Materials Table.

Comprehensive Environmental Response, Compensation, and Liability Act (CERCLA, 42 U.S.C. §§9601–9675), enacted by the United States Congress on December 11, 1980.

Domestic Preparedness Program. 1999. Training Overview DPT 8.0 [CD-ROM]. Edgewood, MD: U.S. Army Soldier and Biological Chemical Command.

Douglass, C. 1993. Evaluating diagnostic tests. *Advances in Dental Research* 7:66–69.

Horton, Z. Berkowitz, and W. Kaye. 2003. Secondary contamination of ED personnel from hazardous materials events, 1995–2001. *American Journal of Emergency Medicine* 21:199–204.

Hurston, E., A. Sato, and J. R. Ryan. 2006. National Guard civil support teams: Their organization and role in domestic preparedness. *Journal of Emergency Management* 4, no. 5 (September/October):20–27.

Nunn-Lugar-Domenici Defense against Weapons of Mass Destruction Act of 1996 (Public Law 104-201).

Occupational Safety and Health Administration. 2005. *OSHA Best Practices for Hospital-Based First Receivers of Victims from Mass Casualty Incidents Involving the Release of Hazardous Substances.* Washington, DC: OSHA.

Report to Congressional Requesters. 1999. *Combating Terrorism: Opportunities to Improve Domestic Preparedness Program Focus and Efficiency.* Washington, DC: General Accounting Office.

Socher, M., and E. Leap. 2005. Training preparedness for terrorism. Chapter 33 in *Medical Response to Terrorism.* Preparedness and Clinical Practice, ed. D. Keyes, pp. 329–347. Philadelphia: Lippincott, Williams and Wilkins.

U.S. Department of Transportation. 2004. *Emergency Response Guidebook: A Guidebook for First Responders during the Initial Phase of a Dangerous Goods/Hazardous Materials Incident.* Washington, DC: U.S. Department of Transportation.

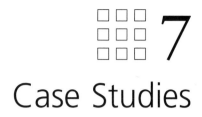

Case Studies

Every object that biology studies is a system of systems.
—François Jacob, 1974

Objectives

The study of this chapter will enable you to

1. Analyze biological events, natural, accidental, and intentional, with an eye toward understanding the challenges of detection and subsequent containment and mitigation efforts.
2. Apply the acronym RAIN in each case study explored.
3. Identify opportunities and challenges in detecting an emerging disease.
4. Compare the morbidity and mortality from natural, accidental, and intentional biological events.
5. Compare the economic and societal impact from natural, accidental, and intentional biological events.

Key Terms

Cordon sanitaire, fomite, cluster.

Introduction

The six case studies presented within this chapter should be viewed as drawing attention to weaknesses in a system of detection first, followed perhaps by issues in containment and mitigation as a result. In looking at these events from a system perspective, we should be aware that the point at which a system fails is often a weakness due to failure in other parts of the system. A *system* is defined as "a dynamic order of parts and processes standing in mutual interaction with each other" (von Bertallanfy, 1968). It is necessary, therefore, for all professionals reading this text, to examine all the parts and processes, especially the interactions among the parts.

The manner in which the case studies are presented in this chapter runs the risk of being categorized as anecdotal and, as such, dismissed by some purists. It is not practical for us to completely recreate or chronicle the accounts for the case studies presented here, for more elaborate and definitive references are easily retrieved from open sources. As such, references and web sites are provided at the end of the chapter to allow additional, in-depth exploration of the described events.

Early detection of biologic events requires an innate ability to make sense of seemingly subtle and random events, quite often lacking scientific explanation. The practice of medicine is an example of the need to combine science, experience, and instinct in the development of a plan of action. Rarely, do patients themselves progress in clinical presentation and disease etiology as the pages in a textbook might suggest. In 1973, Sacks wrote that

> We need, in addition to conventional medicine, a medicine of a far profounder sort, based on the profoundest understanding of the organism and of the life. Empirical science is the key to one form of knowledge, the generalized knowledge that gives us power over nature; the key to wisdom however, is the knowledge of particulars.

We anticipate that the reader will filter and interpret this material within the context of his or her chosen vocation. Applying some of these lessons may allow future generations, regardless of their particular vocational path, to detect early on the emergence of a biologic event and conceivably achieve improved outcomes. Herd health and well-being may take precedence over individual rights and outcomes. No doubt, this is a hard pill for some to swallow. However, improved outcomes portend a decrease in morbidity and mortality, minimization of social or economic impact, or perhaps even decreased international interest.

1. Anthrax, Sverdlovsk, USSR, 1979: Accidental Release of Weaponized Material

In April 1979, an unusual epidemic of anthrax occurred in Sverdlovsk, a city of 1.4 million people 140 km east of Moscow in the former Soviet Union (Meselson et al., 1994). Shortly after the cases emerged, Soviet officials explained that the source of the outbreak was related to the ingestion of contaminated meat. According to their report, contaminated animals and meat from an anthrax epizootic south of Sverdlovsk caused 96 cases of human anthrax (Meselson, 1988). Of these cases, 17 were cutaneous anthrax and 79 were gastrointestinal anthrax. Of the 96 cases, 64 of the gastrointestinal anthrax cases were fatal. At the time, there was great debate among officials from other nations as they tried to determine if the outbreak may have actually been due to covert Soviet bioweapons production.

The following report comes from a recently declassified Defense Intelligence Agency's *Intelligence Information Report* dated March 21, 1980:

> A fourth source reports in late April 1979, the population was awakened by a large explosion that was attributed to a jet aircraft. Four days later, seven or eight persons from the military installation were admitted to hospital number 20 in the suburbs where the military installation is located. Their symptoms were high fever (104°), blue ears and lips, choking, and difficulty breathing. They died within 6 to 7 hours, and autopsies revealed severe pulmonary edema plus symptoms of a serious toxemia. About 6 days after the illness first appeared, the source and other doctors from various hospitals were called together by the district epidemiologist. The number of fatalities had risen sharply, and the source estimated deaths by this time at 40. The epidemiologist

announced the outbreak of an anthrax epidemic and gave a lecture on the disease.
He claimed the epidemic was caused by an illegally slaughtered cow suffering
from anthrax in a town about 10 km northeast of Sverdlovsk. He said the beef
had been sold in the suburb where the fatalities were occurring. This explanation
was not accepted by the doctors in attendance because the fatalities were caused
by pulmonary anthrax as opposed to gastric or skin anthrax, which would be
more likely if anthrax-contaminated beef were eaten or handled.

As more reports emerged, U.S. intelligence reviewed satellite imagery and signal intercepts from the spring of 1979 and found corroborative signs of a serious accident. This included roadblocks and decontamination trucks around what was then known as Compound 19, a military installation in Sverdlovsk. In addition, officials learned that the Soviet defense minister had visited the city shortly after the incident. The anthrax explanation also seemed plausible, given the longstanding history of Soviet efforts to mass produce *Bacillus anthracis* into a biological weapon (Wampler and Blanton, 2001).

U.S. intelligence agency officials believed that the incident had to be due to inhalation of spores that were released from a secret bioweapons plant in the city. Victims presented with severe respiratory distress and died within a few days of the onset of symptoms (see Figure 7-1). This belief came from epidemiological data that showing that most victims lived or worked in a narrow zone extending from the bioproduction facility to the southern city limit. Furthermore, livestock downwind from the point of release died of anthrax along the same zone's extended axis. The zone paralleled the northerly wind that prevailed shortly before the outbreak (Meselson et al., 1994). Other scientists harbored doubts about the official U.S. accusation, noting that an accidental release of anthrax spores could have been in connection with a defensive biological warfare research program, which was allowed under the 1972 convention. It was later concluded that the escape of an aerosol of anthrax pathogen at the military facility caused the outbreak.

The reports of a possible anthrax outbreak in Sverdlovsk, linked to an incident at a suspected Soviet biological warfare facility, served to further deepen already worsening U.S.-Soviet relations, which were heading back toward a new Cold War in the wake of the Soviet invasion of Afghanistan. In the 1980s during the Reagan administration, Sverdlovsk would become one of the major points in the U.S. indictment of the USSR, to build the case that the Soviets were violating the ban on the use of biological weapons imposed by the 1972 Biological Warfare Convention, which both the United States and the Soviet Union had signed.

□ □ □ ▬▬▬

Critical Thinking

Could there be legitimate national security reasons for not disclosing the source of such an outbreak? If there are reasons, what are the potential ramifications for recognition, containment, and mitigation of the danger from the organism?

▬▬▬▬▬▬▬▬▬▬▬▬▬▬▬▬▬▬▬▬▬▬▬▬▬▬▬▬▬▬▬▬▬▬▬▬▬▬▬ □ □ □

The final breakthrough did not come until after the Soviet Union had ceased to exist, at the end of 1991, and Boris Yeltsin came to power as the new head of the Russian government. Yeltsin had a personal connection to the Sverdlovsk issue, as he had been

Communist Party chief in the region at the time of the anthrax outbreak, and he believed the KGB and military had lied to him about the true explanation. At a summit meeting with President George Bush in February 1992, Yeltsin told Bush that he agreed with U.S. accusations regarding Soviet violation of the 1972 biological weapons convention, that the Sverdlovsk incident was the result of an accident at a Soviet biological warfare installation, and promised to clean up this problem. In a May 27 interview, Yeltsin publicly revealed what he had told Bush in private:

> We have now circumscribed the time of common exposure to anthrax. The number of red dots we can plot on our spot map places nearly all of the victims within a narrow plume that stretches southeast from Compound 19 to the neighborhood past the ceramics factory.... we have clarified the relation of the timing of animal and human deaths and believe the exposure for both was nearly simultaneous. All the data—from interviews, documents, lists, autopsies, and wind reports—now fit, like pieces of a puzzle. What we know proves a lethal plume of anthrax came from Compound 19. (Wampler and Blanton, 2001.)

The Sverdlovsk incident represents one of the leading examples of how an unknowing population can be affected by the release of a formulated biological agents. It seems pretty clear at this point that the release was accidental. However, questions remain unanswered as to exactly how much *Bacillus anthracis* was released, how far down range did it travel, and how many people were affected by the release.

2. Salmonellosis and the Rajneesh, the Dalles, Oregon, USA, 1984: Intentional Food-Borne Outbreak

On September 9, 1984, a man was admitted to the county's only hospital, complaining of intense stomach cramps, nausea, and high fever. Two friends were also ill. All three had eaten at a local restaurant earlier that day. In the following week, 13 employees and dozens of customers of the restaurant became violently ill. Many called and threatened to sue.

Within 48 hours after the first patient presented to medical professionals, a pathologist at Mid-Columbia Medical Center had determined the cause was food poisoning from *Salmonella* bacteria. However, it was a full week before the first complaint of this food-borne outbreak was reported to the county health department. By September 21, reports of new cases had subsided; the state lab had identified the strain of *Salmonella* used. That is when the second wave struck. Two days later, every bed in the local hospital was filled with salmonella victims. Almost a third of the town's restaurants were implicated (10 in all). This was enough to basically shut down the economy of The Dalles; many of these restaurants would close forever.

On September 25, the local health department called in assistance from the CDC. By the time the first CDC officers began to arrive, the county health department had already confirmed 60 cases of *Salmonella enterica* serotype *Typhimurium* from the outbreak. They had also found the main epidemiologic connection: Most of the sick people had eaten from salad bars. By the time the CDC arrived in force, the county health department had already done the main work involved in stopping the outbreak.

Key Activities in The Dalles Outbreak

- The local public health office began immediately tracking patients through passive surveillance. For each patient, three-day food histories were completed. These interviews quickly showed that most of the ill people had eaten at a salad bar at one of the affected restaurants. Restaurants were asked to close their salad bars; all 38 restaurants in the county complied immediately.

- Colleagues were interviewing and inspecting restaurants in the county. They found nothing, though, that would indicate how 10 restaurants had created a single outbreak using the exact same pathogen.

- They found that the 10 affected restaurants used several distinct suppliers, and no supplier served more than four restaurants. In addition, the epidemiologic investigation found that various foods were risk factors at various times. The first wave of illness centered on items like potato salad; the second wave on blue cheese dressing. No major violations were found in the distributors or suppliers.

- Samples were taken from both water systems that served the area restaurants, both from the restaurants themselves and at the municipal level. These samples were negative for any form of bacteria, and all had acceptable color and chlorine levels.

Despite the suspicions of the community and the lack of any other explanation, an epidemiologic investigation failed to demonstrate that the outbreak was deliberately caused. The state did not want to be considered backward or insensitive to the Rajneeshees, and the investigation may have been influenced by such political pressure and would hold to a theory of multiple coincidental cross-contaminations throughout the county.

Critical Thinking

The Rajneeshees incident occurred in 1984. However, had this event occurred after the 2001 anthrax attacks, do you think investigators would be so quick to discount an intentional attack? Many years have passed since the 2001 attacks; do you think our vigilance has a shelf life?

In all, 751 cases of salmonellosis were confirmed from more than 1,000 patients; about 12% of the community became ill. Even though the illness struck simultaneously in 10 restaurants dispersed throughout the county, the state health department's epidemiologic investigation concluded that the outbreak was caused by unsanitary hand-washing practices at the restaurants involved. An initial criminal investigation agreed with the health department's conclusion. One year later, a representative of the Bhagwan Shree Rajneesh sect, which had a ranch in the county, announced that members of that sect had poisoned local salad bars with *Salmonella* bacteria in a test run for a plan to influence local election results in the sect's favor. A subsequent criminal investigation found that the sect had ordered the exact strain of *Salmonella* used by mail from a licensed commercial laboratory company.

When the CDC analyzed the data, things looked much different. Employees generally had symptoms at the same time as customers, and the strain of *Salmonella* encountered was not at all the same as any other area cases in recent years. The outbreak occurred in two distinct waves that flew in the face of a single exposure event. In this case, the initial state health report denied local law enforcement the probable cause they needed to open an investigation.

Even in the face of strong evidence suggesting a deliberate attack, investigators discounted this theory initially, giving several reasons why they reached this conclusion. Among the reasons were these: there was no apparent motive; no one claimed responsibility, and nothing like this had ever occurred before. These points reinforce the need to maintain a high index of suspicion and follow epidemiological clues to reach a plausible explanation of any unusual outbreak. Early involvement of law enforcement personnel may enable investigators to remain subjective in their determination and cognizant of evidentiary matters should a reasonable index of suspicion be warranted.

Had investigators used more aggressive surveillance techniques to gather more information (i.e., surveying doctor's offices for symptomatic persons), they may have received additional information for the investigation and might have produced enough evidence to change the investigator's position on whether the outbreak was accidental or intentional. Accounts from community members support the position that numerous patients did not report to the medical community and chose to stay home and treat themselves (personal communication, J. Glarum).

3. Pneumonic Plague, Surat, India, 1994: Natural Outbreak

The population of Surat, in the western state of Gujarat, boomed shortly after World War II. Surat's population grew from 237,000 to approximately 1.5 million residents. The city divided into two parts, the "old city" or city center remained the most heavily populated area, accounting for 77% of the total population. The newer settled, outer portions of the city were characterized by their universal lack of planning. Incorporating a mix of industry and lower class residences, these areas were largely devoid of proper sewage facilities and only 60% of total daily garbage produced was collected regularly (Shah, 1997). Less than half of the city had access to treated drinking water. The unhygienic conditions and poor working conditions within Surat were commonly identified by public health officials as the causes for regular epidemic outbreaks within the city of malaria, gastroenteritis, pneumonia, and diarrhea.

In September 1993, an earthquake occurred, which killed an estimated 20,000 people; and due to the poverty of the area, many of the dead were not properly buried. Floods in August 1994 created an unbelievable mix of human waste, refuse, and human and animal remains left behind. These events in addition to the poor refuse disposal and sewer services created an abundant food supply for rats and other vermin. Some reports point to a possible precursor event, which involved the die-off of rats in Mamala village to such an extent that they were "falling off rafters, dead, in great numbers" (John, 1994). By mid-September, in spite of the available epidemiological clues, 10% of the village population was ill with bubonic plague.

The Indian government initially appeared unable or unwilling to mitigate the spread of the disease created by a series of events both in and outside of the country. Poor crisis communication regarding the outbreak caused the population to take measures to keep themselves safe in the areas affected and chose to leave, potentially carrying disease with them to unaffected areas. Contact tracing was not accomplished initially, once more leading to spread of disease. Once the disease became obvious and there was little being done by the government to contain it, panic ensued and more people fled, carrying the disease. It has been estimated that 25% of the 1.5 million people fled the area.

A **cordon sanitaire**[1] may have proven useful in plague containment; however, it would have affected India's diamond-cutting and silk-production center in the area of the slums. Sealing off this area from the rest of the city would have prevented workers getting to the factory, cutting off their income, as well as slowing production. In addition, the encroachment of the holiday season with the associated visitors and large conferences with international guests drawing thousands of international tourists were planned; and tourism is one of India's major financial businesses. This is a similar situation to China's dilemma on dealing with the outbreak of SARS.

Several countries put restrictions on travelers from India, with Moscow imposing a six-day quarantine for all visitors from India and banning all travel to the country. Estimates for business losses for the city of Surat alone were over $260 million. It has been estimated that India lost over $1 billion in export earnings, and 40–60% of its anticipated tourism (Steinberg, 1995). Several million people lost income when they were unable to work, locally or internationally; many more millions suffered panic, fear, or dislocation. Thousands of squatters had their dwellings inspected and condemned. As a nation, India found its modernity, its efficiency, its health administration, and its local governance called into question. Locally, agricultural exporters saw their share prices tumble as some foreign countries not only refused Indian exports but closed their borders. The United Arab Emirates was reported to have cut off postal links with India out of fear that the plague would spread via mail.

Given the economic upheaval it is interesting to note that about 900 people fell ill with the total death toll only 56. This is the point: Fear and panic due to poor risk communication and appropriate containment measures caused the bigger problems for the financial markets and economy than the actual disease. Control of this disease outbreak would have had to include selective quarantine, contact tracing, treatment, and prophylaxis, as well as elimination of potential vectors and animal hosts.

In hindsight, investigators identified a 35-year-old man on September 12 as the first case. He had been admitted to a hospital four days earlier with respiratory symptoms and fever (Shah, 1997). Over the next week or so, through September 20, approximately 15 individuals were admitted to various hospitals, mostly to be diagnosed with and treated for malaria. Not until September 21 did the presumption of plague surface. Public health authorities were alerted, word began to spread through the medical community, and the one hospital was designated for new suspected plague admissions. Shops began closing in the most heavily affected region of the city, medical practitioners began to leave the city, and local pharmacies sold out of available tetracycline. Hospital admissions continued to grow and public health authorities were barely able to locate sufficient antibiotics to treat the ill and their care providers. Within three weeks, the case fatality rate had dropped from 80% to below 10%. Until adequate government supplies of tetracycline begin to arrive, approximately 30% of Surat's population fled, businesses closed, and public facilities (schools, swimming pools) shut down. By the end of September, adequate supplies, plans, and personnel had the epidemic under control (Shah, 1997).

---

[1] *Cordon sanitaire* is a French term that translates to "sanitary cord." It is used to denote an extreme use of quarantine where public health authorities implement large-scale quarantine measures to contain the spread of disease. In this case, a small section of the city would have been under quarantine order. As one might imagine, this would be difficult to implement and enforce.

Modern public health and medicine are capable of intervening effectively in outbreaks of bacterial diseases, such as plague, through combinations of medical screening, immunization, antibiotic treatment, and supportive care. Even in the absence of effective medical intervention, proper behavior, like contact avoidance, can profoundly alter the disease progression cycle. If any measure is overlooked or botched in its implementation, it is easy to see how containment can be slow or nonexistent.

4. Amerithrax, USA, 2001: Intentional Release of a Formulated Agent

In late September 2001, an avid outdoorsman whose pastimes were gardening and fishing left for a short vacation in North Carolina. His job as a photo editor required that most of his work time was spent reviewing photographs submitted by mail or over the Internet, so no doubt he looked forward to this trip. Soon after arriving in North Carolina, the first symptoms of illness developed; these included muscle aches, nausea, and fever. The symptoms waxed and waned for the duration of the three-day trip.

The day after he returned home, he was taken to the hospital for medical evaluation at the emergency department of a Florida medical center after he awoke from sleep with fever, emesis, and confusion. Because he was disoriented at the time of his presentation at the hospital, he was unable to provide further relevant information. Treatment with intravenous cefotaxime and vancomycin was initiated for presumed bacterial meningitis while the patient awaited a lumbar puncture (Malecki et al., 2001).

On physical examination, he was found to be lethargic and disoriented. His temperature was 39°C (102.5°F), the blood pressure was 150/80 mm Hg, the pulse was 110, and his respirations were 18. No respiratory distress was noted; his arterial hemoglobin saturation, as indicated by pulse oximetry while he was breathing ambient air, was 97%. Examination of the ear, nose, and throat detected no discharge or signs of inflammation. Chest examination revealed rhonchi without rales (Bush et al., 2001).

The initial chest radiograph was interpreted as showing basilar infiltrates and a widened mediastinum (see Figure 7-1). The results of a CT scan of the head were normal. A spinal tap was performed under fluoroscopic guidance within hours after presentation at the hospital and yielded cloudy cerebrospinal fluid.

The patient was admitted to the hospital with a diagnosis of meningitis. After a single dose of cefotaxime (a broad-spectrum cephalosporin) he was started on multiple antibiotics. A short time later, he had generalized seizures and was intubated for airway protection. The next day a new array of antibiotics was initiated, replacing those previously prescribed. He remained febrile and became unresponsive to deep stimuli. His condition progressively deteriorated, with hypotension and worsening kidney function. The patient died on October 5. Autopsy findings included hemorrhagic inflammation of lymph nodes in the chest as well as disseminated *Bacillus anthracis* in multiple organs (Bush et al., 2001).

Gram's staining of cerebrospinal fluid revealed many polymorphonuclear white cells and many large gram-positive bacilli, both singly and in chains. On the basis of the cerebrospinal fluid appearance, a diagnosis of anthrax was considered, and high-dose intravenous penicillin G was added to the antibiotic regimen. Within six hours after plating on sheep's-blood agar, the cultures of cerebrospinal fluid yielded colonies of gram-positive bacilli.

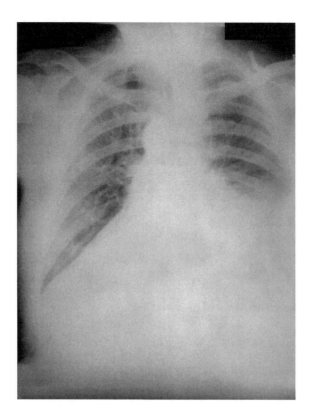

FIGURE 7-1 Typical chest X-ray from a case patient with inhalation anthrax. This aspect shows a widened mediastinum (lower separation seen on film between lobes of the lungs) and pleural effusion (opaque area below right). (Image courtesy of the Centers for Disease Control and Prevention, PHIL 1795.)

The clinical laboratory of the medical center presumptively identified the organism as *B. anthracis* within 18 hours after plating; this identification was confirmed by the Florida Department of Health laboratory on the following day. It was evident that making a diagnosis of anthrax would have serious ramifications. Although the case was reported to local public health authorities when anthrax was first suspected, final laboratory confirmation of the diagnosis was awaited before a public announcement was made.

Extensive environmental samples from the patient's home and travel destinations were negative for anthrax. Moreover, the finding of *B. anthracis* in regional and local postal centers that served the work site implicates one or more mailed letters or packages as the probable source of exposure. Coworkers report that the patient had closely examined a suspicious letter containing powder on September 19, approximately eight days before the onset of illness. This index case highlights the importance of physicians' ability to recognize potential cases in the identification and treatment of diseases associated with biologic terrorism.

☐ ☐ ☐

Critical Thinking
Based on your knowledge of inhalation anthrax, how does the clinical presentation from the index case measure up with the incubation period and final outcome?

☐ ☐ ☐

Protective suit worn by public
health personnel entering
the AMI building

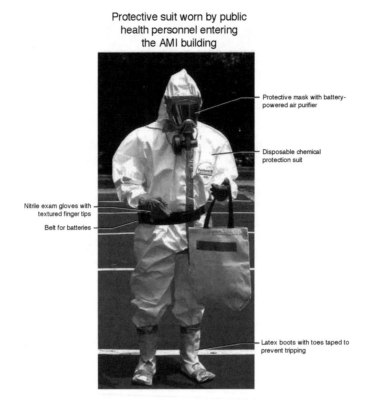

Protective mask with battery-
powered air purifier

Disposable chemical
protection suit

Nitrile exam gloves with
textured finger tips

Belt for batteries

Latex boots with toes taped to
prevent tripping

FIGURE 7-2 Federal investigators responded to the index case of inhalation anthrax in 2001 by isolating the AMI building. Despite extensive efforts to locate the source of the spores that infected the index case and one other employee, the contaminated source was never found. Interviews with AMI employees led investigators to believe that it may have been a letter.

In summary, officials believe that there were a total of five letters mailed, four of which were recovered. There were two known mailing dates, September 18 and October 9, 2001. The letter to the AMI building in Florida (see Figure 7-2), where the index case originated, was not recovered. The September 18 letters went to the offices of NBC Studios and the *New York Post* in New York City. The October 9 letters were mailed to Senators Daschle and Leahy of the U.S. Senate. The amount of formulated anthrax spores in these letters was estimated to be 1–2 grams. The letter to Senator Leahy (which was unopened at the time it was discovered) contained approximately 2 grams of highly weaponized anthrax spores.

Outbreaks of the disease were concentrated in six locations: Florida; New York (see Figure 7-3); New Jersey; Capitol Hill in Washington, D.C.; the Washington, D.C. regional area, including Maryland and Virginia; and Connecticut. The anthrax incidents caused illness in 22 people: 11 with the cutaneous (skin) form of the disease and 11 with the inhalational (respiratory) form, 5 of whom died. Demands on public health resources reached far beyond the six outbreaks of disease. Once officials realized that mail processed at contaminated postal facilities could be cross-contaminated and end up anywhere in the country, residents brought samples of suspicious powders to officials for testing and worried about the safety of their daily mail.

In dealing with this crisis, there were deficiencies in both the local public health response and the federal government's ability to manage it. Public health officials did not

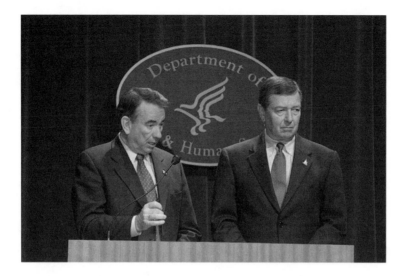

FIGURE 7-3 October 12, 2001, Health and Human Services Secretary Tommy G. Thompson and Attorney General John Ashcroft held a news conference to discuss a confirmed case of anthrax in a NBC News employee in New York City. (Image courtesy of Department of Health and Human Services, http://www.hhs.gov/news/photos/2001/.)

fully appreciate the extent of communication, coordination, and cooperation needed among responders. There were difficulties in reaching clinicians to provide them with guidance.

5. Ricin and the Amateur Bioterrorist, USA, 2004: Intentional Release

In February 2004, ricin was discovered in Senator William Frist's office in the Dirksen Office Building. After the toxin was discovered in a letter-opening machine in the senator's office, federal investigators examined some 20,000 pieces of mail, hoping to find the source of the ricin, but turned up nothing to lead them to a suspect. They were unable to determine whether the ricin had been there for hours, weeks, or even months before it was discovered by an intern in the office.

Conflicting reports on the handling of the response emerged. Some Senate employees described the hours after the toxin was found as confused and chaotic. Some employees near Dr. Frist's office went home with no medical screening after the substance was found, and others went about their activities without being advised to seek decontamination.

The authorities said the substance was first seen about 3 p.m. on Monday, when a hazardous-materials team was dispatched to Dr. Frist's offices, in the Dirksen Senate Office Building. After preliminary tests proved negative, an all-clear was given. Such an occurrence is not unusual for congressional offices, which frequently receive suspect mail that turns out to be harmless.

☐ ☐ ☐ ▬▬▬▬▬▬▬▬▬▬▬▬▬▬▬▬▬▬▬▬▬▬▬▬▬▬▬▬▬

Critical Thinking
What is the risk to overreacting and carrying out containment activities every time a suspect item is discovered at government offices?

▬▬▬▬▬▬▬▬▬▬▬▬▬▬▬▬▬▬▬▬▬▬▬▬▬▬▬▬▬ ☐ ☐ ☐

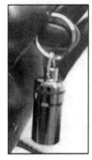

caution RICIN POISON
        Enclosed in sealed container
        Do not open without proper protection

The following is a representation of the language contained in the threat letter:

To the department of transportation: I'm a fleet owner of a tanker company.

I have easy access to castor pulp. If my demand is dismissed I'm capable of making Ricin.

My demand is simple, January 4 2004 starts the new hours of service for trucks which include a ridiculous ten hours in the sleeper berth.

Keep at eight or I will start dumping. You have been warned this is the only letter that will be sent by me.

Fallen Angel

FIGURE 7-4 Federal notice given by the U.S. Postal Service and Department of Justice concerning the 2004 ricin incident perpetrated by "Fallen Angel." The perpetrator was never arrested.

When follow-up tests detected the presence of ricin, the Capitol Police returned and began evacuating people to another area of the Dirksen building. By that time, staff members who were present said, many people had left for the day. Those who had been in the vicinity and remained in the building were directed to shower at a decontamination tent erected in a hallway between the Dirksen building and the adjacent Hart Senate Office Building. There they were interviewed by the police and allowed to go home.

Investigators have found nothing to explain how the potentially deadly powder wound up in the offices of the Senate majority leader. The investigation focused on a mysterious "Fallen Angel," who threatened to use ricin as a weapon unless new trucking regulations were rolled back. No obvious direct connection between the Frist case and the letters signed by "Fallen Angel" has been found (see Figure 7-4). Those letters were discovered in mail facilities that serve the Greenville-Spartanburg International Airport in South Carolina and the White House.

6. Norwalk Virus, Queen of the West Cruise Ship, Coastal Oregon, USA, 2002: Accidental Exposure

Like most enteric pathogens, Norwalk-like viruses (NLVs) are primarily spread by the fecal-oral route. Food-borne and waterborne NLVs are the most common of transmission. Typical food "vehicles" include salads, sliced fruits, sliced meats, wedding cake frosting—anything that gets human handling without subsequent reheating. Raw oysters are another popular choice. In contrast to bacterial pathogens, NLVs do not multiply in foods; therefore, keeping foods at the right temperature when holding or serving does not necessarily affect the pathogen once it gets into the food. It is also possible that NLVs are spread by the airborne route (Sawyer et al., 1988). It appears that aerosolized particles of NLVs are generated when infected victims vomit (or have diarrhea). In turn, these virus particles may infect people directly or settle onto surfaces that then are touched with hands and sooner or later end up in the mouth. The role of **fomites** in transmission continues to interest epidemiologists and can often defeat the best efforts of infection control practitioners in hospitals, nursing homes, and cruise ships alike.

This brings us to our final case study. In September 2002, a cruise ship known as the Queen of the West, a faux stern wheeler embarked for a week-long cruise from Portland, Oregon. The journey's route took passengers upriver as far as Hells Canyon, near Idaho, and out to Astoria at the mouth of the Columbia River, then back to Portland. With cruise rates beginning at about $2,500 per passenger, guests were treated very well. The ship had a capacity of 145 passengers and 45 crew members. Breakfast, lunch, and dinner were served on board and snacks were available at all times.

The legal jurisdiction for this epidemiological investigation was with the FDA and the Coast Guard, as the ship was a U.S. port vessel moving in interstate but not international commerce. Public health officials had been notified of a number of passengers on board with gastrointestinal distress. The ship's captain asked for assistance when it docked in Astoria. Environmental health experts were to meet the ship, and three passengers were removed to the Astoria hospital on Friday morning when the ship docked, one of whom was admitted because of dehydration.

It is interesting to note that, while local medical and public health staff recognized a **cluster** of patients with gastrointestinal distress, they may have misjudged the source of the outbreak and causative organism. Possibly, they attributed their patients' conditions due to simple food poisoning from an organism such as *Staphylococcal Enterotoxin B*, an agent that does not represent a secondary transmission source and has an incubation period of 4–10 hours postingestion. NLVs, on the other hand, may be shed by infected individuals prior to onset of symptoms and are difficult to kill, thus increasing the opportunity for secondary transmission by multiple routes including fomites. Adopting a working diagnosis of possible food poisoning rather than NLV resulted in secondary transmission to several health-care workers, who also developed symptoms.

While the patients who left the ship were being cared for at a local hospital, the local health department representatives met the ship and began organizing specimen collection, gathering information for a questionnaire, and initiating an epidemiological investigation. The ship's staff had been attempting to collect some information, following what they described as a "CDC" template. No such template was ever produced and the information the ship had collected was not easy to utilize. Instead, a questionnaire was developed and faxed to the ship and distributed to passengers on Friday night after dinner. Based on preliminary data of onset of symptoms supplied by the crew, questions were confined to meals Sunday through Wednesday, including a catered lunch that had been delivered on shore Monday. The ship got an extensive cleaning per FDA instructions in a rush to get done before the next load of passengers was to arrive Saturday afternoon.

The questionnaires were completed by 78% of the passengers. Stool specimens were collected from six passengers. The Oregon State Public Health Laboratory determined by PCR that all stool specimens were positive for Norwalk-like virus. A case definition for possible Norwalk-related illness was drafted. Passengers that experienced vomiting or three or more loose stools within a 24-hour period at any time during the cruise where considered to be suspect case patients. Unfortunately, this diagnosis came too late to prevent the exposure to the health-care workers.

No single meal or food item was identified that readily explained this outbreak. Several items and meals taken as a whole were statistically associated with illness, but they "explained" relatively few cases. Knowing that this was Norwalk, with a typical median incubation of 30–36 hours, suspicion rested on the lunch meals on the Calliope deck Sunday through Wednesday. It is interesting to note that eating lunch in the dining room on Tuesday and Wednesday seemed to exclude passengers from being case patients.

Norwalk outbreaks are very common on land and a well-known problem on cruise ships as well. Understanding the importance of vigilance in reporting and investigating in a logical manner can assist in containment efforts being accomplished in a timely manner, limiting further illness. State health officials praised the crew, officers, and management of the ship and its parent company in Seattle (America West Steamboat Company) as being extraordinarily cooperative and helpful with their investigation and zealous in their efforts to control the outbreak under guidance.

Conclusion

The six case studies presented here, in brief, should provoke the reader to delve more into the particulars of each incident. The Sverdlovsk anthrax incident illustrates the danger posed by bioweapons production. A seemingly simple accident involving the release of a small amount of formulated agent can have a dramatic effect. Imagine if the same thing occurred in the United States or Europe in the Information Age of which we are all part today. The Rajneeshee incident involving the intentional contamination of food with bacteria was the largest act of bioterrorism to occur in the United States. Acquisition of the agent, the ease of production, and the covert and simple nature of the attack emphasizes the indiscriminate and insidious nature of biological terrorism. Despite the best efforts of many people, it took more than a year and a confession of guilt from the perpetrators to convince officials that the incident was intentional.

The outbreak of pneumonic plague that took place in Surat, India, is a testimony to the importance of fast and decisive action to contain a natural outbreak of a highly contagious and deadly disease. Had this been related to an intentional act there would have been more index cases or victims initially to facilitate widespread disease. This emphasizes the importance of early detection and standard procedures for containment. The Amerithrax incident of 2001 showed us how vulnerable a nation is to a small amount of formulated biological material. Looking back on that time, the events, as they unfolded, seemed surreal. It was hard to believe that we were under attack and no one really knew for quite some time how widespread it was or when it would end. Many have criticized public officials for how they handled or mishandled the event. However, we believe that public health officials moved quickly to disseminate information and increase the awareness of the public (potential victims) and the vigilance of health-care providers (alert guardians).

Thanks to numerous evil documents circulated on the Internet, ricin production, possession, and dissemination now fits nicely into the toolbox of every amateur bioterrorist. Keeping things in perspective, ricin, in its crudest forms, is not a formidable threat, but it is deadly if delivered to the potential victim in the right way. Its production, possession, and dissemination are illegal and deserving of a rapid and formidable response. Persons that break these laws should be prosecuted to the fullest extent of the law.

Norwalk virus has hurt the cruise ship industry badly over the last 25 years. The Oregon case study briefly described here was related from first-hand experience and involvement with the event. Those involved early on in the event recognized that they had a "cluster," requested assistance immediately, and got public health officials involved to limit the spread of the contagion and determine the source. Here, quick and decisive actions led to a relatively good outcome, but this case serves to remind us that adopting a higher level of personal protective equipment in the face of a cluster may be wise.

Essential Terminology

Cluster. A grouping of health-related events that are related temporally and in proximity. Typically, when clusters are recognized, they are reported to public health departments in the local area.

Cordon sanitaire. A French term that translates to "sanitary cord." It is used to denote an extreme use of quarantine, where public health authorities implement large scale quarantine measures to contain the spread of disease. As one might imagine, this would be difficult to implement and enforce in a modern setting.

Fomite. Any inanimate object that can mechanically transmit infectious agents from one host to another.

Web Sites

The National Security Archive, volume 5, *Anthrax at Sverdlovsk. 1979.* U.S. Intelligence on the Deadliest Modern Outbreak, National Security Archive Electronic Briefing Book No. 61, ed. Robert A. Wampler and Thomas S. Blanton, November 15, 2001, available at www.gwu.edu/~nsarchiv/NSAEBB/NSAEBB61/#8#8.

Meselson, M., J. Guillemin, M. Hughes-Jones, et al. The Sverdlovsk anthrax outbreak of 1979, *Science* 266, no. 5188 (November 18, 1994): 1202–1208, available at www.anthrax.osd.mil/documents/library/Sverdlovsk.pdf.

Hoffman, R., and J. Norton. 2002. Lessons learned from a full scale bio-terrorism exercise, *Emerging Infectious Diseases* 6, no. 6 (November–December): 652–653, available at www.cdc.gov/ncidod/eid/vol6no6/pdf/hoffmann.pdf.

Mavalankar, D. 1995. Indian "plague" epidemic: Unanswered questions and key lessons, *Journal of the Royal Society of Medicine* 88, no. 10: 547–551, avail-able at www.pubmedcentral.nih.gov/picrender.fcgi?tool=pmcentrez&artid=1295353&blobtype=pdf.

Blanchard, J., Y. Haywood, B. Stein, T. Tanielian, M. Stoto, and N. Lurie. 2005. In their own words: Lessons learned from those exposed to anthrax, *American Journal of Public Health* 95, no. 3: 489–495, available at www.pubmedcentral.nih.gov/picrender.fcgi?tool=pmcentrez&artid=1449207&blobtype=pdf.

Rooney, R., E. Cramer, S. Mantha, G. Nichols, J. Bartram, J. Farber, and P. Benembarek. 2004. A review of outbreaks of foodborne disease associated with passenger ships: Evidence for risk management, *Public Health Reports* 119, no. 4: 427–434, avail-able at www.pubmedcentral.nih.gov/picrender.fcgi?tool=pmcentrez&artid=1497653&blobtype=pdf.

Discussion Questions

- Does it seem to matter if an outbreak is derived from a natural, accidental, or intentional event? In what ways are they equivocal? In what ways are they different?

Table 7-1 Refer to the Web Sites to Apply the Concept of RAIN to Each Case Study

	Anthrax, Sverdlovsk, Russia	Salmonellosis, The Dalles, Oregon	Plague, India	Anthrax, United States	Ricin, United States	Norwalk Virus, Oregon
Recognize						
Avoid						
Isolate						
Notify						

Note: In some instances, there will be insufficient details given to know how the community responded (Sverdlovsk).

- With reference to the initial response, does it matter whether an outbreak is natural, accidental, or intentional? If yes, how does it matter and to whom? If not, why not?
- Would automated biosensor programs increase, decrease, or have no effect on the vigilance of medical practitioners presented with unusual disease outbreaks?
- For each case study presented, apply the concept of RAIN to complete Table 7-1.

References

Bush, L., B. Abrams, A. Beall, and C. Johnson. 2001. Index case of fatal inhalational anthrax due to bioterrorism in the United States. *New England Journal of Medicine* 345:1607–1610.

Defense Intelligence Agency. 1980. Possible BW Accident near Sverdlovsk. *Intelligence Information Report* (March, 21).

John, T. 1994. Learning from plague in India. *Lancet* 344:972.

Malecki, J., S. Wiersma, H. Chill, et al. 2001. Update: Investigation of bioterrorism-related anthrax and interim guidelines for exposure management and antimicrobial therapy. *Morbidity and Mortality Weekly Report* 50, no. 42:909–919.

Meselson, M. 1988. The biological weapons convention and the Sverdlovsk anthrax outbreak of 1979. *Federation of American Scientists Public Interest Report* 41 (September):1.

Meselson, M., J. Guillemin, M. Hughes-Jones, et al. 1994. The Sverdlovsk anthrax outbreak of 1979. *Science* 266:1202–1208.

Sacks, O. *Awakenings*. London: Pan Books, 1973.

Sawyer, L., J. Murphy, J. Kaplan, et al. 1988. 25- to 30-nm virus particle associated with a hospital outbreak of acute gastroenteritis with evidence for airborne transmission. *American Journal of Epidemiology* 127:1261–1271.

Shah, G. 1997. *Public Health and Urban Development: The Plague in Surat*. New Delhi, India: Sage Publications Pvt. Ltd.

Steinberg, F. 1995. Indian cities after the plague—What next? *Trialog* 43:8–9.

von Bertallanfy, L. 1968. *General System Theory*. New York: Brazillier.

Wampler, R., and T. Blanton, eds. 2001. *Athrax at Sverdlovsk, 1979*, the National Security Archive, volume 5, U.S. intelligence on the deadliest modern outbreak. National Security Archive Electronic Briefing Book No. 61 available at www.gwu.edu/~nsarchiv/NSAEBB/NSAEBB61/#8#8.

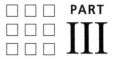

PART

III

The Threat to Agriculture

Agriculture can be defined in many ways. In very general terms, it represents the body of knowledge, science, and practice of cultivating the soil and rearing animals. Agriculture is vitally important to the development and maintenance of human society. Agricultural systems enable modern-day societies to safely and inexpensively feed their populace. Countries that have not developed a sophisticated agricultural system are unable to sustain large cities, concentrate their people, or advance their technologies.

The business of agriculture or "agribusiness" is vitally important to the economy of nations. Recent estimates from the U.S. Department of Agriculture indicate that agribusiness is responsible for more than 13% of the U.S. gross domestic product, 17% of the nation's employment, and about 20% of its exports. Therefore, agricultural products are not only essential for the survival of its people, they are paramount to a thriving economy.

Outbreaks of animal or plant diseases threaten the capacity to produce commodities essential to domestic sustenance and international trade. Outbreaks of disease have the potential for creating significant losses for the economy. Most often, we concern ourselves with foreign animal and plant diseases; however, highly contagious and serious pathogens are endemic to the United States and her allies. When it comes to food safety and agricultural security we must consider pathogens that are naturally spread and accidentally introduced. In addition, because we live in the Age of Terrorism and face the threat of asymmetric warfare, we have to be watchful for intentional acts of introducing disease agents into the agricultural sector. A directed, well-planned, intentional act could be devastating.

As we learned in Chapter 1, humans developed agriculture about 12,000 years ago. In his poignant book *Guns, Germs and Steel*, Dr. Jared Diamond discussed how agriculture enabled humans to settle in one place, efficiently sustain larger tribes, develop new tools, and gain advantage over nomadic groups and neighboring tribes. These advances, however, did not come without cost. Diamond also referred to domesticated animals as if they were "deadly gifts," because they introduced humans to new disease pathogens.

In an eloquently written article on avian influenza (Avian influenza: Virchow's reminder, *American Journal of Pathology* 168 [2006]: 6–8), Dr. Corrie Brown emphasizes that control of bird flu in the human sector will require control of the disease in the animal. To make her point she reminds us of what German physician Rudolf Virchow stated in 1855 when he defined the term *zoonoses*.

Highly pathogenic avian influenza has become the "zoonosis" of the decade and hopefully will not become the pandemic of the century. . . . On the subject of comparative medicine, Virchow stated, "Between animal and human medicine, there is no dividing line—nor should there be." Virchow is a name familiar to all pathologists because he is widely regarded as the father of modern pathology and is heralded for elucidating the cellular nature of disease, which drastically changed the course of medicine. However, it may be his emphasis on considering diseases across species lines that will be his most lasting legacy.

Regardless of how introduced, the biological threat to agriculture has the potential to rob us of our ability to feed ourselves, shake our confidence in government, undermine an economy, and pose a threat to human health. For these reasons, an entire part in this book is dedicated to the threat of biological agents to agriculture. Chapter 8 covers the threat to domesticated animals and crops and outlines the response actions and control measures used in disease containment. Chapter 9 briefly describes four case studies where foreign animal diseases have caused great harm to agribusiness.

8

Biological Threat to Agriculture

*For the life of me, I cannot understand why the terrorists have not attacked
our food supply, because it is so easy to do.*
—Tommy Thompson, Former Secretary of Health and Human Services

Objectives

The study of this chapter will enable you to

1. Discuss the importance of agriculture and food supply to the nation.
2. Describe the different ways that biological threats may harm agriculture and the food supply.
3. Define *agroterrorism*.
4. Discuss the potential effects of agroterrorism.
5. Discuss the importance of biosecurity to the agricultural sector.
6. Describe the nation's response to an outbreak of a foreign animal disease.

Key Terms

Critical infrastructure, foreign animal disease (FAD), vector, foreign animal disease diagnostician, agroterrorism, biosecurity, premises, quarantine, National Animal Health Emergency Management System (NAHEMS), ESF 11, control zones, depopulation, disinfection.

Introduction

An assessment by a panel of experts during President Clinton's administration found one of the greatest challenges for the U.S. government in the coming decade to be the effective protection of America's **critical infrastructure**. Specifically, the committee studied the security of the nation's telecommunications systems; electrical power grids; transportation systems, gas and oil delivery and storage systems; water purification and delivery mechanisms; banking and finance centers; fire, police, EMS, and disaster systems; and other government services. Specifications for the protection of America's critical infrastructure were detailed in Homeland Security Presidential Directive (HSPD) 7. Shortly after the release of HSPD 7, officials realized that America's lifeblood, agriculture, had been omitted from the list. It was not until December 2003 that agriculture and food was added to the list. The protection of our food systems and agriculture was further enhanced by HSPD 9, which "establishes a national policy to defend the agriculture and food system against terrorist attacks, major disasters, and other emergencies" (HSPD 9, January 2004).

The Critical Infrastructure Information Act of 2002 (CCI Act of 2002) provides for the protection of national infrastructure and infrastructure information sharing among federal agencies and between federal agencies and the private sector. The act creates a new framework that enables members of the private sector to voluntarily submit sensitive information regarding the nation's critical infrastructure to Homeland Security with the assurance that the information, if it satisfies the requirements of the CCI Act, will be protected from public disclosure. Some critical infrastructure systems that could obviously be affected by biological threats include water supply systems, emergency services (public safety and public health), and government operations. However, one could argue that none of these could be more seriously targeted and affected as agriculture and food systems. Agriculture and food systems are vulnerable to disease, pest, or poisonous agents that occur *naturally*, are *accidentally* introduced, or are *intentionally* delivered through an act of terrorism. Agriculture and food systems are extensive, open, interconnected, diverse, complex structures providing lucrative targets for plant and animal disease. A widespread disease outbreak, regardless of the cause, could have a dramatic effect on health and economics.

□ □ □ ▬▬▬▬▬▬▬▬▬▬▬▬▬▬▬▬▬▬▬▬▬▬▬▬▬▬▬▬▬▬▬▬▬

Critical Thinking

Originally, agriculture and food systems were not part of our nation's critical infrastructure. How could this oversight occur? Or, could you argue that they do not belong or are inconsistent with the other elements of critical infrastructure?

▬▬▬▬▬▬▬▬▬▬▬▬▬▬▬▬▬▬▬▬▬▬▬▬▬▬▬▬▬▬▬▬▬ □ □ □

The Importance of Agriculture

Today, farming employs about 1% of the U.S. workforce and accounts for less than 1% of the gross domestic product (GDP). However, its effect on the national economy is much larger, due to farming's links to a variety of industries. For instance, farmers require machinery, fertilizer, seed, feed, labor, financial services, transportation, processing, packaging, and other inputs to produce crops and livestock. Taken together, U.S. farming and its related industries accounted for 13.1% percent ($997.7 billion) of the GDP in 1996. That year, the U.S. food and fiber system employed nearly 23 million Americans, or 17% percent of the labor force (U.S. Department of Agriculture, 2006).

Today's world population exceeds 6.5 billion people (U.S. Census Bureau, 2007). Estimates suggest that the world population will reach 8 billion in 2025 and 9 billion by 2050. If these estimates are correct, that represents an amazing 50% increase in a 50-year span. The enormity of the task of feeding tomorrow's world is difficult to conceive and the challenge is aptly described by the following statement: "In the next 50 years mankind will consume twice as much food as mankind has consumed since the beginning of agriculture 10,000 years ago" (James, 2000).

□ □ □ ▬▬▬▬▬▬▬▬▬▬▬▬▬▬▬▬▬▬▬▬▬▬▬▬▬▬▬▬▬

Some Important Facts about U.S. Agriculture

- The farm sector is the largest positive contributor to the U.S. trade balance.
- The United States produces nearly 50% of the world's soybeans, over 40% of its corn, 20% of its cotton, 12% of its wheat, and over 16% of its meat.
- America has more than 2 million farms totaling over 300 million acres.
- In some states, agriculture accounts for over 10% of employment and gross state product.

▬▬▬▬▬▬▬▬▬▬▬▬▬▬▬▬▬▬▬▬▬▬▬▬▬▬▬▬▬ □ □ □

Protecting the Agricultural Sector

Agricultural products are vital to our survival and our economy. Agricultural products account for about 5% of all U.S. exports (Amber Waves, 2007). The United States has nearly 2 million farms, totaling nearly 310 million acres, where crops and animals are raised to provide the steady flow of inexpensive, high-quality, safe foods. The United States leads the world in food production. In 2005 and 2006, there was nearly $70 billion in agricultural exports per year (Amber Waves, 2007). In 2006, grains and feed generated nearly $18.4 billion in sales, soybeans generated $6.3 billion, red meat products generated $4.9 billion, and poultry generated $2.4 billion (AoTab27, USDA Web site).

Outbreaks of animal or plant diseases, regardless of the origin, could undermine the capacity to export agricultural goods, thereby generating significant losses to the economy. Most often, we concern ourselves with foreign animal and plant diseases; however, several serious pathogens are endemic to the United States. When it comes to food safety and agricultural security, we are not always worried about intentional acts. In fact, our most recent experiences with numerous naturally occurring and accidentally introduced animal diseases has had us exercising the National Animal Health Emergency Management System (NAHEMS), keeping us ever mindful that a directed, well-planned, intentional act could be devastating. Regardless of the cause of the outbreak, we must do all we can to protect the agricultural sector from the potential devastation of threat organisms.

Foreign Animal Diseases

Many **foreign animal diseases** (FAD), or serious animal diseases that *do not* exist in the United States are of great concern to U.S. animal health officials. The United States Department of Agriculture (USDA) Animal and Plant Health Inspection Service (APHIS) works with state animal health officials and veterinarians to identify, control, and eradicate these diseases (Critical Foreign Animal Disease Issues for the 21st Century, 1998). At the international level, the Office International des Epizooties/Epizootics (OIE), of the World Organization for Animal Health, is an intergovernment organization with 155 member countries responsible for animal disease information, surveillance, guidelines, and policy. The OIE tracks diseases throughout the world and provides rules for animal movement and disease control, including tests and vaccines. The OIE maintains and tracks animal diseases and outbreaks from several member countries. The World Trade

Table 8-1 OIE List A Diseases

African horse Sickness
African swine fever
Avian influenza
Bluetongue
Contagious bovine pleuropneumonia
Exotic Newcastle disease
Foot and mouth disease
Goat and sheep pox
Highly pathogenic avian influenza
Hog cholera
Lumpy skin disease
Newcastle disease
Peste des petits ruminants
Rift Valley fever
Rinderpest
Swine vesicular disease
Vesicular stomatitis

Organization recognizes the OIE as the international agency for setting animal health standards for conducting international trade. The OIE maintains a list of "transmissible diseases" (www.oie.int/eng/maladies/en_classification.htm). Until recently, this listing had been divided into List A and List B. Under the old system, List A was a compilation of diseases that "have the potential for very serious and rapid spread, irrespective of national borders; are of serious socio-economic or public health consequence; and are of major importance in the international trade of animals and animal products." List A diseases (Table 8-1) could severely damage agricultural markets, since an outbreak of one of these diseases is internationally recognized as grounds for export embargo. Under the old system, the OIE assembled a list of diseases (List B) that were considered to be of socioeconomic or public health importance within countries and significant in the international trade. List B is too long to present here. Rather, the reader is directed to the OIE web site that depicts the old listing (www.oie.int/eng/maladies/en_OldClassification.htm).

The diseases under List A (Table 8-1) are predominately viral diseases that are transmitted in three primary transmission ways. Most viruses can be transmitted through direct contact. Some can be spread through the air over great distances in aerosol form. Others, such as bluetongue virus and African swine fever virus, are spread by insect vectors.

- **Airborne transmission mode of animal diseases.** Foot and mouth disease (FMD), highly pathogenic avian influenza, and exotic Newcastle disease can spread via airborne aerosols over long distances. In 1981, three days after an outbreak of FMD in Brittany, France, single cases appeared across the English Channel on the Isle of Wight. Prevailing wind patterns corroborate the hypothesis that the virus traveled a distance of 175 miles as an airborne aerosol. Airborne diseases are extremely difficult to contain and therefore would present an enormous challenge to emergency responders in the event of an outbreak. These diseases can also be transmitted by direct contact.

- **Direct transmission mode of animal diseases.** Diseases such as rinderpest, vesicular stomatitis, hog cholera, and African swine fever can be spread by direct contact among animals, as well as by contact with contaminated objects. For example, feed troughs, water troughs, and milking machines that are used by an infected animal can transmit a virus to other animals. In addition, these viruses can travel on people's clothes, shoes, and equipment. This presents the necessity of biosecurity measures— keeping animal facilities clean and restricting human and vehicle traffic around animals.

- **Vector transmission mode of animal diseases.** Some diseases are transmitted by insect **vectors**. A tick or a mosquito acquires an agent from one animal and transmits it to another through a subsequent bite. In these cases, disease control depends on insect control.

Criteria for Inclusion on OIE Listing

As of January 2006, OIE officials combined Lists A and B into a consolidated listing that divided the diseases of concern by host (e.g., multiple species, sheep and goats, cattle, equine, swine, bees, fish, mollusks, crustaceans, and rabbits). Inclusion criteria now cover four considerations: potential for international spread, significant spread within naïve populations, zoonotic potential, and emerging diseases. Figure 8-1 explains how these criteria have been applied to compile the list.

Domestic Compliance with OIE

On the national front, the National Animal Health Monitoring System Program Unit conducts national studies on the health and health management of America's domestic livestock populations. The National Surveillance Unit (NSU) is the coordinating entity for activities related to U.S. animal health surveillance. The NSU develops and enhances animal health surveillance through evaluation, design, analysis, prioritization, and integration. The National Animal Health Reporting System (NAHRS) is a joint effort of the U.S. Animal Health Association, American Association of Veterinary Laboratory Diagnosticians, and USDA's Animal and Plant Health Inspection Service. NAHRS was designed to provide data from chief state animal health officials on the presence of confirmed World Organization for Animal Health (OIE) reportable diseases in specific commercial livestock, poultry, and aquaculture species in the United States. It is intended to be one part of a comprehensive, integrated animal-health surveillance system. NAHRS is based on the recognized presence or absence of OIE reportable diseases rather than the prevalence of disease. Within a state, data about animal disease occurrence are gathered from as many verifiable sources as possible and consolidated into a monthly report submitted to the National Surveillance Unit, where the information is verified, summarized, and compiled into a national report. The commodities currently covered are cattle, sheep, goats, equine, swine, commercial poultry, and commercial food fish.

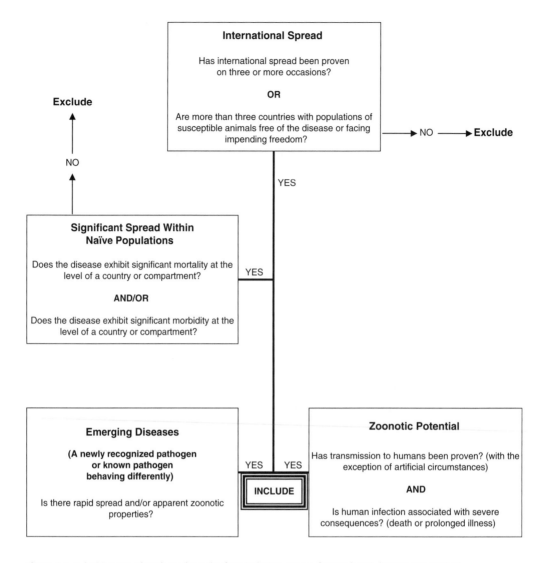

Figure 8-1 A decision tree that shows how the four inclusion criteria for OIE listed diseases are applied.

Critical Thinking

There is no doubt that foreign animal diseases are a threat to a nation's economy and food supply. What are the essential elements necessary to recognize an FAD? Apply RAIN to one such situation and discuss appropriate actions for Recognition, Avoidance, Isolation, and Notification.

One of the more immediate and severe consequences of an FAD occurrence in the United States is the effect on export markets. Other countries will ban the import of U.S. animals or animal products, as occurred following the first known case of bovine spongiform encephalopathy (BSE) in the United States, identified in Washington state. To protect the long-term health and profitability of U.S. animal agriculture, the FAD must be contained, controlled, and eradicated rapidly. Eradication efforts present short- and long-term costs to the industry and government. Accredited veterinarians are required to report all animal disease conditions whose differential diagnosis could include a foreign animal disease. A USDA-trained **foreign animal disease diagnostician** is assigned to investigate according to a standardized protocol and submits diagnostic materials to the USDA's National Veterinary Services Laboratories.

Factors that affect FAD prevention, control, management, and recovery are numerous and include free trade agreements, free trade blocks, regionalization, increased international passenger travel, intensification of animal production, the constant evolution of infectious agents, and the uncertain impact of biotechnology and bioterrorism.

Plant Pathogens and Crop Security

Plant pathogens can be devastating when they strike a large crop. Most plant pathogens are very specific for a particular plant species or group. In very few instances, the plant pathogen may produce a toxin that is harmful to humans (e.g., mycotoxins). As with livestock production, crops are often grown in highly concentrated settings over vast expanses of land. This makes them a vulnerable target for the pathogen. This is especially true for cereal grains. Rice and wheat are two crops that supply the majority of the world's daily intake of calories. Any pathogen targeting these two crops could have serious implications for the economy and nutritional status of a population.

There are numerous examples of plant diseases throughout history. For the sake of this book, we outline four important diseases that affect four different bumper crops: karnal bunt in wheat, rice blast in rice, plum pox virus in stone fruits, and soy bean rust in soy beans.

Karnal Bunt

Karnal bunt, a fungal disease of wheat, was first discovered in wheat-growing areas of India. Since then, it has been found in all major wheat-growing areas in India, Pakistan, Iraq, Afghanistan, a small area of South Africa, and Mexico. In 1996, it was found in the United States. The disease is not known to severely affect crop production, but due to international regulation of the disease, an outbreak of the disease severely affects the ability to export wheat to overseas buyers (U.S. Department of Agriculture, 2007b). The U.S. Department of Agriculture (USDA) employs an annual national survey to certify the U.S. wheat crop is free from karnal bunt. Regulations prevent the movement of contaminated seed and grain throughout the United States.

Soy Bean Rust

Asian soybean rust is a serious disease of soybeans caused by the fungus *Phakopsora pachyrhizi*. A second, similar-looking rust fungus, *P. meibomiae*, also infects soybeans but is much less virulent and occurs primarily in the Western hemisphere. It is important to differentiate between these two rust species, but this can be done reliably only using molecular techniques. Both *P. pachyrhizi* and *P. meibomiae* infect numerous leguminous plant hosts. Until recently, this disease did not occur on soybeans in the Western hemisphere, but it spread to South America in 2001. As of 2004, Asian soybean rust in the Americas is found in Argentina, Bolivia, Brazil, Paraguay, and Uruguay. In November 2004 *Phakopsora pachyrhizi* was found for the first time in Louisiana and, soon thereafter, in other southeastern U.S. states (U.S. Department of Agriculture, 2007a).

Rice Blast

Rice is one of the most important crop plants in the world, and the rice blast disease caused by the fungus, *Magnaporthe grisea*, is one of the most destructive diseases. The disease is widespread and causes severe losses. The disease is particularly destructive to upland rice crops produced without irrigation. Many rice scientists consider blast to be the most important disease of rice worldwide. This is because the disease is widely distributed in 85 countries and can be very destructive when environmental conditions are favorable. Disease occurrence and severity vary by year, location, and even within a field, depending on environmental conditions and crop management practices. Yield loss estimates from other areas of the world have ranged from 1–50%. The fungus can infect and produce lesions on most of the shoot. Rice blast has been reported in California, where it was contained to one area (Scardaci et al., 1997).

Plum Pox Virus

Plum pox is a viral disease of stone fruit trees, such as plums, peaches, and apricots. Plum pox virus (PPV) has been a devastating disease in Europe since the early 1900s. In 1992, PPV was reported for the first time in the Americas, in Chile. Plum pox virus was discovered for the first time in North America in 1999, in a peach orchard in Adams County, Pennsylvania. Shortly afterward, it was found in Ontario and Nova Scotia, Canada, in 2000. In the United States, the disease remained localized, and it was hoped that it was contained before it had a chance to spread to the other parts of the North American continent. In 2006, PPV was identified in New York and Michigan. Aphids are believed to be the primary vectors, spreading the virus from tree to tree.

Agroterrorism

Terrorist groups lack the personnel and weapons to attack in large-scale engagements against standing armies. Instead, they rely on small units to attack their civilian or military targets. The nature of guerilla warfare and insurgency has these limited terrorist groups attacking organized military forces by exploiting their weaknesses. That approach to warfare is known as *asymmetric warfare*. The Department of Defense defines *asymmetric warfare* as "unanticipated or non-traditional approaches to circumvent or undermine an adversary's strengths while exploiting his vulnerabilities through unexpected technologies or innovative means" (Ancker and Burke, 2003). The United States traditionally has little or no protection against an asymmetric threat. The term may also refer to terrorists' use of new or unexpected technology or means other than conventional weapons. The September 11, 2001, attack was unanticipated, used unconventional weapons (airplanes), took advantage of weaknesses in the American security system, and attacked innocent civilians. A weakness that may be identified by a terrorist threat includes the food and agriculture sector (Pate and Camerson, 2001).

Agricultural terrorism, or **agroterrorism,** is a term that describes *the intentional use of biological agents targeted against crop or animal agriculture.* Agroterrorism is not a new concept; it has been used throughout the ages. Centuries ago, food crops were vulnerable to attack by invaders. As people became more educated, their attention turned to perfecting the means of acquiring and increasing populations of disease-causing organisms and perfecting methods for spreading the diseases among their enemies. During the early part of World War I, the Germans mounted a biological warfare campaign in the United States while the country was still neutral. The targets were draft animals, horses, and mules purchased by Allies for use by their military forces in Europe. The Germans devised a plan to infect the animals with glanders and anthrax organisms. The first attempt failed when the organisms were found dead. Efforts were attempted again, this time in New York City and in Maryland. The Germans conducted similar operations in other countries. Military forces are not the only ones that have used agroterrorism. Some individuals or small groups have used or attempted acts of agroterrorism (Carus, 2001). Specific records of the use of biological agents against agriculture as a form of economic attack exist as early as 1915. Table 8-2 presents a chronology of known or reported biological attacks against agricultural targets.

Table 8-2 Chronology of Biological Attacks Targeting Crops and Livestock, 1915–2000

Year(s)	Location	Act
1915–1917	Argentina, Mesopotamia, Norway, Romania, United States	The German secret service mounted a covert biological campaign during World War I, using glanders and anthrax to infect draft animals, horses, and mules to be used by the Allies for the war effort in Europe. It also appears that the Germans attempted to use a wheat fungus.
1943	Isle of Wight, United Kingdom	Richard Ford, a prominent British naturalist, made the accusation that Germany dropped Colorado potato beetles on the United Kingdom during World War II, accounting for their unusual appearance in parts of the United Kingdom. According to Ford, the bombs were made of cardboard and contained 50–100 beetles.
1950	East Germany	In a Ministry of Forestry report dated June 15, 1950, the East German government accused the United States of scattering Colorado potato beetles over potato crops in May and June 1950.
1952	Kenya	The Mau Mau, a nationalist liberation movement, poisoned 33 steers at a British mission station, using what is believed to be a local toxic plant known as *African milk bush.*
1962–1997	Cuba	Cuba accused the United States of attacking Cuban crops or livestock on as many as 21 occasions. According to Raymond Zilinskas, of the few incidents for which information is available, agents include Newcastle disease (1962), African swine fever (1971, 1979–1980), sugarcane rust disease (1978), and thrips insect infestation (1997). Only in the case of the thrips did Cuba make a formal complaint. According to the Cuban account, the United States flew a crop duster operated by the State Department over Cuba and released the insects.
1982–1984	Afghanistan	Ken Alibek, first deputy chief of Biopreparat, alleges he was informed by a senior Soviet military officer that the Soviet Union attacked the Afghan mujaheddin with glanders on at least one occasion. According to Alibek this would have the dual effect of sickening the mujaheddin and killing their horses, their main mode of transportation.

(Continued)

Table 8-2 Chronology of Biological Attacks Targeting Crops and Livestock, 1915–2000—Cont'd

Year(s)	Location	Act
1983–1987	Sri Lanka	The Tamil militant group threatened to use biological agents against Sinhalese and crops in Sri Lanka. The communiqué threatened to introduce foreign diseases into the local tea crop and to use leaf curl to infect rubber trees.
1984	Queensland, Australia	Queensland's state premier received a letter threatening to infect wild pigs with foot-and-mouth disease, which was feared might spread to cattle and sheep, unless prison reforms were implemented within 12 weeks. Ultimately, this incident proved to be a hoax, as the perpetrator turned out to be a 37-year-old murderer serving a life sentence in a local jail.
1996	Florida, United States	A Florida university professor informed the CIA that a Florida citrus canker outbreak was the result of a Cuban biological weapons program. Although the CIA could not substantiate the claim, it did investigate the case.

Note: This list includes allegations and threats, along with confirmed incidents of deliberate use of biological agents to destroy preharvest crops or livestock, to cause economic damage.

Source: Carus, 1998.

Agroterrorism represents a particularly desirable option for terrorists seeking to wreak havoc on the American society for a number of reasons. First, these diseases exist in natural reservoirs; and proliferation of weaponized agents, or the knowledge to produce them, may have made them widely available. Second, U.S. agriculture is highly vulnerable. Normally, security at agricultural facilities is low, and the ease with which these agents spread requires a relatively simple method of inoculation. Once the disease has made its way into the animal or crop population, it could potentially spread widely as a result of the great mobility exhibited by these products as they are shuttled from one region of the country to the next for trade and processing. Third, use of biological agents against crops and livestock affords anonymity to the aggressor. A period of time would pass between the point at which the agent was introduced and the point at which the resultant disease was noticed. Essentially, the incubation period for the disease acts as a cloak of darkness allowing the perpetrator time to get away from the scene of the crime. Fourth, what makes these herds and crops so attractive to terrorists and potentially devastating is the nature of the business. These assets represent our fundamental and material wealth. This is America's "breadbasket." These crops, herds, flocks, and gatherings are kept in high density collections so that we can more easily manage them and maximize the use of space needed to culture them. That condition makes the introduction of a contagious pathogen more of a threat. Finally, an attack would cause great damage to the U.S. economy. As recent natural outbreaks of livestock diseases in Europe and Asia demonstrate, agricultural diseases have the potential to cause significant economic damage. Several studies estimate that a single case of foot and mouth disease in the United States would result in a loss of $12–20 billion (Schoenbaum and Disney, 2003).

Use of Plant Pathogens as a Weapon

The history of state use of plant pathogens over the last century indicates that attacks on agriculture using biological warfare agents are feasible. Both livestock and crops have long been considered viable targets; many countries have used, developed, or pursued the use of plant pathogens.

In 1939, the French anticrop program was directed primarily at the Germans, using potato beetles to destroy a food staple. Germans first developed their agricultural biological warfare program during World War I but further improved their capabilities with plant pathogens during World War II, experimenting with potato beetles, turnip weevils, antler moths, potato stalk rot, and potato tuber decay. In World War II, the Japanese also used fungi, bacteria, and nematodes on nearly all grain and vegetables grown in Manchuria and Siberia.

Late in World War II, the United States seriously considered using a fungus to destroy Japanese rice crops; however, the delayed impact made the attack impractical. During that time, the United States developed several anticrop and anti-animal agents, including wheat stem rust, rice blast fungus, and rinderpest. Between 1951 and 1969, the U.S. Army carried out at least 31 anticrop tests and stored rice and wheat blast fungus at Fort Detrick, Maryland, and at the Rocky Mountain Arsenal near Denver. In 1955, wheat stem rust became the first plant pathogen standardized by the Chemical Corps. More recently, during the Persian Gulf War, Iraq experimented with wheat stem rust and camel pox (Ban, 2000).

For plants, the list of agents that might be used is nearly endless, although some, such as wheat smut or rice blast, appear more harmful than others. Weather, season, and growth stage play important roles in the effectiveness of the agent employed.

□ □ □ ▬▬▬▬▬▬▬▬▬▬▬▬▬▬▬▬▬▬▬▬▬▬▬▬▬▬▬▬▬▬▬▬▬▬

Plant Pathogens in Biowarfare

Plant pathogens that have been weaponized or pursued for weaponization include

- Rice blast (*Mangaporthe grisea*).
- Wheat stem rust (*Puccinia graminis* f.sp. *triciti*).
- Wheat smut (*Fusarium graminearum*).

Additional plant pathogens that have weaponization potential include

- Wheat pathogens: wheat dwarf (*geminivirus*) and barley yellow dwarf virus (*Pseudomonas fascovaginaei*).
- Corn pathogens: barley yellow dwarf virus (*Pseudomonas fascovaginaei*), brown stripe mildew (*Sclerophthora rayssiae*), sugarcane downy mildew (*Peronosclerospora sacchari*), and java downy mildew (*P. maydis*).
- Soybean pathogens: soybean dwarf virus (*Luteovirus*) and red leaf blotch (*Pyrenochaeta glycines*).

Source: Kortepeter and Parker, 1999.

▬▬▬▬▬▬▬▬▬▬▬▬▬▬▬▬▬▬▬▬▬▬▬▬▬▬▬▬▬▬▬▬▬▬ □ □ □

In 1977, the Department of Defense released a report (U.S. Department of Defense, 1977) that discussed past efforts in the biological weapons program. The 1977 report said the BW program included testing, production, and stockpiling of anticrop agents (see Figure 8-2). Between 1951 and 1969, 31 anticrop dissemination trials were

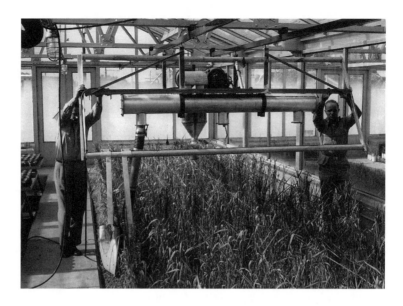

FIGURE 8-2 Circa 1955, U.S. Army workers in the Crops Division at Fort Detrick conduct testing in a greenhouse. (Photo courtesy of the U.S. Army.)

conducted at 23 locations. From 1951 to 1957, wheat stem rust spores and rye stem rust spores were produced and transshipped to Edgewood Arsenal, where they were classified, dried, and placed in storage. Between 1962 and 1969, wheat stem rust spores were produced, transshipped to Rocky Mountain Arsenal, Denver, Colorado, classified, dried, and stored. Rice blast spores were also produced during this period under contract to Charles Pfizer and Company and shipped to Fort Detrick for classification, drying, and storage. The entire anticrop stockpile was destroyed as part of the biological warfare demilitarization program completed February 1973 (Covert, 2000).

The Vast Potential of Agroterrorism

Agroterrorism could be as devastating as any other form of terrorism. An act of agroterrorism could (1) disrupt or cripple the economy of a nation; (2) destroy the livelihood of many people; (3) put the food supply at risk, perhaps for a long time; (4) spread quickly before being detected, thereby reaching difficult-to-control levels; (5) cause high mortality and morbidity in the target population; and (6) cost billions to contain, clean up, and disinfect infected premises. Simply put, an attack upon any segment of the food industry could have catastrophic effects upon the whole economy (Wilson et al., 2000).

□ □ □ ▬▬▬▬▬▬▬▬▬▬▬▬▬▬▬▬▬▬▬▬▬▬▬▬▬▬▬▬▬▬▬▬

Critical Thinking
Just how plausible is an act of agroterrorism? In your opinion, is it realistic or just someone's active imagination?

▬▬▬▬▬▬▬▬▬▬▬▬▬▬▬▬▬▬▬▬▬▬▬▬▬▬▬▬▬▬▬▬ □ □ □

The United States is vulnerable to intentional efforts to undermine its agriculture industries, either by the deliberate tampering of food during production or through the release of a biological agent, resulting in animal or plant disease. However, agricultural targets are not limited to animals or plants; they can also include transportation systems; water supplies; grain elevators or other storage facilities; producers, farmers, and farmworkers; restaurants and food handlers; grocery stores; food and agriculture research laboratories; and packing and processing facilities.

If any of these commodities were significantly impacted by a bioterrorist event, the results could be catastrophic, but the impact of a devastating attack on our food supply would not be limited to the farmer; businesses such as farm suppliers, transportation, grocery stores, restaurants, equipment distributors, and in the end, consumers all pay the price. Small towns could be wiped out, placing the supply of our food in peril, perhaps for a long time.

An attack against animals or crops is generally viewed as more benign and less offensive than if humans fell dead from a direct assault. Agricultural terrorism is not about killing animals; it is about crippling an economy. To that end, agents foreign to the U.S. livestock and poultry industries and crops would be preferred by terrorists.

Attributes of Agroterrorism Making It Attractive to a Terrorist

- **Economic impact.** Agroterrorism delivers a high-value impact.
- **Lower physical risk.** Disseminating a plant or livestock disease organism presents less physical risk to the terrorists than releasing human pathogens or using other chemical, biological, radiological, nuclear, or explosive weapons.
- **Smaller chance of outrage and backlash.** Agroterrorism is not likely to create the same kind of public reaction and backlash as using a weapon that kills people.
- **Similarity to natural outbreaks.** Use of plant or animal pathogens can create outbreaks that resemble natural outbreaks, thereby reducing the risk of early detection.
- **Lower technical barriers.** The materials needed are relatively easy to acquire. Small quantities are needed and are easier to transport to the area of intended use. Infection of a small number of animals or small groups of plants would normally be sufficient to cause an outbreak of the disease. An epidemic could be caused by dropping Newcastle disease–contaminated bird droppings into a feeding trough or foot and mouth disease by placing tongue scrapings from infected animals into the ventilation system of a large hog-production operation.

For animals, many foreign agents are readily available in nature, from low-security laboratories, even from commercial sources, that require little effort or risk to smuggle in. Most foreign animal agents pose no risk to human health, so the terrorist may feel some sense of security in handling and dispersing these pathogens. Once released, an agroterrorism event may go unnoticed for days to weeks, and by then, it may be nearly impossible to determine if the event was human-made or occurred naturally (Sutmoller et al., 2003).

Biosecurity from Field to Fork

In order to protect agriculture and the food supply, **biosecurity** must be applied from one end of the food chain to the other. Consider the entire food production scheme when you take into account the threat from biological agents. This includes pre- to postharvest, processing, packaging, and distribution. Hence, the expression *from field to fork* is applicable here. Biosecurity on the farm is a management practice designed to prevent the spread of disease. It is accomplished by maintaining a facility in such a way that there is minimal movement of biological organisms (pathogens and pests) across its borders. Biosecurity is the cheapest, most effective means of disease control available. No disease prevention program is effective without good biosecurity practices.

Identification of biosecurity hazards is a key element in preventing the introduction of disease pathogens onto a premise. Common hazards include

- People, animals, vehicles, and equipment.
- Contaminated feed or water.
- Contact with other animals.

Biosecurity has three major components: isolation, traffic control, and sanitation. This section examines some of the principles that support each component of biosecurity.

Isolation

Farmers and producers should consider their premises as an oasis and adopt a healthy attitude toward keeping the biological threat outside the fence from encroaching on their sanctuary. As the old saying goes, good fences make good neighbors. The same could be said for farms. The high-production farm should be isolated as best as possible from the outside environment. A good physical barrier with obvious markings should be in place and well maintained at all time. Figure 8-3 shows an example of a prominent border of a biosecure area.

All movement of people, animals, vehicles, and equipment on and off the property must be controlled to reduce the risk of pathogen transmission. This may include measures such as establishing a guard at entrances, locking unguarded entrances, and patrolling and repairing boundary fences. Employees have often been a source of disease introduction and should be counseled on their role in the possible mechanical transmission of disease. Strict biosecurity measures must be observed at all times.

Only authorized personnel should be allowed on the premises. Producers should know who is on the premises at all times. Producers should keep a record of all visitors and deliveries. If a disease outbreak should occur on the premises, this information could help follow-up investigations. Producers should have a single, combined entrance-exit point for their premises. This better enables the producer to control access to the premises.

Under most circumstances, housed susceptible animals are at reduced disease risk and should remain housed if possible. Producers should do whatever is practical and feasible to limit the entry of wild animals into housing facilities. Biosecurity measures should

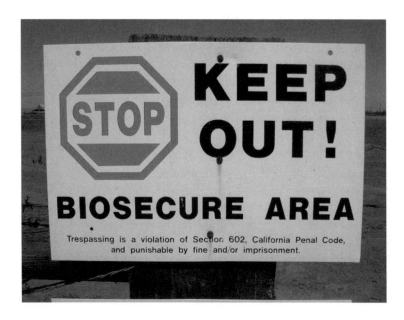

FIGURE 8-3 Biosecurity postings, like this one on a California farm, mark boundaries that are used to prevent the encroachment of animal diseases. By limiting movement into these areas, producers can restrict the flow of human and animal traffic onto and off of the premise. This simple measure is but one in a myriad of best practices that make up biosecurity program elements. (Image courtesy of California Department of Agriculture.)

be instituted at entry points of buildings. Housing facilities should also be engineered to preclude rodent infestation. Production animals should not be moved into barns or other facilities that have housed infected or potentially infected animals unless these buildings have first been thoroughly cleaned and disinfected.

If susceptible animals are penned outside, animal health officials should encourage owners to reduce the risk of pathogen transmission by implementing good biosecurity practices. In addition, owners should keep groups of animals separated by a distance sufficient to prevent pathogen transmission, not permit close or direct contact between groups of animals, and not put animals in contact with areas that have been in contact with potentially infected animals.

To the extent possible, owners should maintain flocks that are "closed" to the introduction of new animals (with population increase occurring only from flock offspring), thus decreasing the potential for transmission of disease agents from "outside" animals. All poultry should be vaccinated against common diseases.

When new animals must be introduced, they should be isolated on arrival and vaccinated to match the herd vaccination pattern. Routine disease prevention principles such as "all-in/all-out" housing also should be followed. Ideally, the premises on which animals are housed should be fenced and have a locked, gated driveway.

Feed should be purchased only from suppliers that have a high-quality assurance program in place for the safe manufacturing, storage, and delivery of their products. Special care should be taken to prevent feed and water from coming into contact with animal waste or other potentially contaminated animal products. If the owner has any reason to suspect that water has been contaminated, it should be tested before being given to animals.

Traffic Control

Limit nonessential traffic on the farm. Post signs at the entrance instructing visitors to check in at a central location, such as the farmhouse. Instruct drivers of essential vehicles, such as feed or transport trucks, to drive only where needed. Install barriers that limit vehicular traffic and address sanitation needs.

Sanitation

All vehicles entering and exiting the farm should be cleaned and disinfected. All visitors and employees, regardless of risk level, should be provided with disposable coveralls, boots, hats, and gloves for use before coming into contact with animals. They should also be required to disinfect their boots before entering biosecure areas and before exiting the premises. Disposable garments are much more economical than reusable outerwear, which must be kept in an array of sizes and which must be cleaned, disinfected, and maintained.

Mitigating Risk

The potential impact of major risk factors for the introduction of a disease can be mitigated with appropriate biosecurity actions. Producers should inspect susceptible crops and animals regularly for signs of disease. If they have any concerns, they should discuss them immediately with a veterinarian or state extension service agent.

When an outbreak is detected, the disease must be controlled, contained, and eradicated as quickly as possible to lessen the impact on industry and consumers and return the United States to a disease-free status. In doing so, selection of a control strategy will be one that

- Causes the least possible disruption to the food, farming, and tourism industries; to visitors to the countryside; and to rural communities and the wider economy.
- Minimizes the number of animals that need to be slaughtered, either to control the disease or to keep animal welfare problems to a minimum.
- Minimizes damage to the environment and protects public health.
- Minimizes the burden on taxpayers and the public at large.

Case Designations

Just as with specific human infectious diseases (refer to Chapter 2), we have a tiered diagnostic system for animal diseases. In determining designations, **premises** are evaluated by state and federal animal health officials according to the presence of one or more animals meeting the criteria for one of the following case identification terms:

- **Suspect case.** Premises containing an animal that has clinical signs consistent with a highly contagious FAD or emerging disease incident (EDI).
- **Presumptive positive case.** Premises containing an animal that has clinical signs consistent with a highly contagious FAD or EDI and additional epidemiologic information indicative of a highly contagious case.

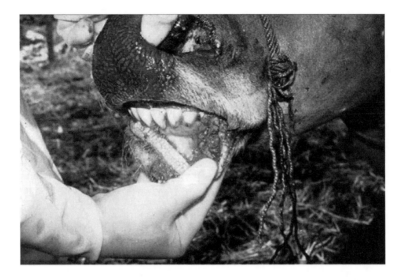

FIGURE 8-4 One of the most serious foreign animal diseases is foot-and-mouth disease. This viral disease affects cloven animals, forming lesions to their hooves and mucosal areas. Depicted here is an animal health professional revealing lesions in the mouth of an FMD-infected cow. (Image courtesy of the U.S. Department of Agriculture.)

- **Confirmed positive case.** An animal that has clinical signs consistent with a highly contagious FAD and from which the highly contagious disease agent was isolated and identified in a USDA laboratory or other laboratory designated by the Secretary of Agriculture.

For a presumptive positive of an FAD, **quarantine** of the premises, expanded surveillance and biosecurity measures will be implemented immediately. The state veterinarian, governor, or state Secretary of Agriculture is notified. The state's emergency response plan is initiated. Assistance from local responders may be necessary.

Once confirmation diagnosis of an FAD (like the foot and mouth disease shown in Figure 8-4) is obtained, further actions will be taken. A positive identification of an FAD may lead to quarantine of surrounding premises, stop movement orders in the region or state, and euthanasia. Depending on the scale of the event or the level of spread of the disease, federal agencies may become involved in the overall response. If an FAD has spread to more than one state, the U.S. Secretary of Agriculture has authority to declare federal emergencies, which provide federal resources for the situation. The National Response Framework specifies actions to be initiated. Additionally, confirmation of an FAD requires U.S. animal health officials to notify the OIE within 24 hours. If there is a report or suspicion of a possible intentional FAD outbreak or threat, the animal health authorities will notify the USDA's Office of the Inspector General, which will notify and coordinate as the situation warrants. The response process is detailed in the following section.

Animal Disease Outbreak Response

For the sake of this book, the focus of the response materials presented here is with respect to foreign animal disease outbreaks, since these may present the most challenging circumstances to response organizations. Producers and government officials will apply biocontainment measures in an animal disease outbreak. Biocontainment is the series of management practices that prevent the spread of infectious agents between animal populations on a farm or the management practices designed to prevent the infectious agent from leaving the farm.

Foreign animal diseases may be spread to susceptible species either directly or indirectly. Effective biosecurity measures are essential to the prevention of a pathogen spread via these means. During a foreign animal disease incident, biosecurity, quarantine, and stop movement procedures are used to prevent further spread of a disease and prevent unexposed animals from coming into contact with the disease agent. Properly implemented, biosecurity during an FAD outbreak is imperative, as it reduces the risk of transmission during the movement of personnel and material necessary for the extensive activities of the control and eradication campaign.

Homeland Security Presidential Directive 7 (HSPD, 2003) assigns responsibility for protecting agriculture and food (e.g., meat, poultry, and egg products) to the USDA. The Animal Plan Health Inspection Service leads the USDA efforts in exploring different methodologies for monitoring the health of the U.S. livestock and poultry populations.

APHIS reviews the animal health surveillance systems regularly to ensure the highest efficiency and capability without compromising disease-detection abilities. In addition to working with Latin American countries to design surveillance systems for that region, APHIS works with international health organizations, such as the World Organization for Animal Health (formerly known as OIE), Inter-American Institute for Cooperation on Agriculture, Food and Agriculture Organization, and others to determine trading regulations, risk analysis methods, disease surveillance, and diagnostic methods.

Veterinary Services, a department of APHIS, works with state departments of agriculture, private veterinary practitioners, and other veterinary specialty groups to design response to various threats. Veterinary Services also has created small Rapid Response Teams that can be quickly employed to investigate possible FAD outbreaks (Critical Foreign Animal Disease Issues for the 21st Century, 1998). Foreign animal disease diagnosticians and accredited veterinarians are trained to recognize exotic diseases that may enter the United States.

International Services works with U.S. agricultural trading partners to avoid importation and exportation of diseases through trade of animals and animal products, and the Resource Lab provides training resources and information. The Wildlife Research Center provides resources for studies in native, exotic species, and their interaction with humans and domestic animals.

The **National Animal Health Emergency Management System** (NAHEMS) is an integrated system for dealing with animal health incidents in the United States, such as the incursion of a foreign animal disease or a natural disaster. It encompasses the four tenets of emergency management: prevention, preparedness, response, and recovery. One cornerstone of the NAHEMS is the response guidelines series. The NAHEMS guidelines are designed for use by official response personnel in the event of a major animal health emergency. They provide information that may be integrated into the preparedness plans of other federal, state and local agencies, tribes, and additional groups involved in animal health emergency management activities.

The federal government has a National Response Framework in place to respond to any human-made or natural disaster. Local and state plans should be developed to be consistent with the National Response Framework and National Response Plan (NRP). An outbreak of a highly contagious FAD is included in the definition of disaster. USDA's APHIS is the lead agency for animal and plant emergencies for the NRP. All these activities fall under emergency support function (**ESF**) 11. As a part of ESF 11, APHIS coordinates all response efforts for incidents involving an animal disease, plant disease, or plant pests. APHIS is responsible in these instances for coordinating state, tribal, and local authorities and other federal agencies to conduct disease or pest control and eradication activities.

ESF 11 objectives for FADs are to detect, control, and eradicate a highly contagious disease as quickly as possible to return the United States to "free" status. A presumptive positive case generates immediate, appropriate local and national measures to eliminate the crisis and minimize the consequences. A confirmed positive case generates additional measures on a regional, national, and international scale.

General Considerations

Each animal disease outbreak is unique. The disease agent, animal species affected, and extent of spread affects the response and levels of control needed. Biosecurity, quarantine, isolation, and movement control procedures are an important part of an animal disease outbreak response. Responders play an important role in implementation and maintenance of these procedures. There is a basic framework that can be applied to animal disease outbreak. Inclusive of this is enhanced biosecurity, the implementation of control measures (zones and premises designations), movement restrictions, implementation of quarantine, depopulation and culling, carcass disposal, and disinfection. Each of these is discussed separately.

In an outbreak situation, all visitors should be considered high risk, especially within a control area. When an outbreak occurs, officials typically establish a control area around infected and contact premises. Information about the location and boundary of the control area should be disseminated widely and through various media outlets (television, radio, posters, publications, etc.).

As a general rule, the closer premises are to a known infected premise, the greater the hazard for exposure to the pathogen and thus the greater the necessity for implementation of rigorous biosecurity and cleaning and disinfection (C&D) measures.

If an outbreak has occurred in the United States and a premise is located outside the control area, premise owners should ensure that visitors observe biosecurity and C&D measures commensurate with the level of perceived threat. For instance, premises located immediately adjacent to the border of a control area may have stricter measures than premises located hundreds of miles away that have no livestock connections to the control area.

However, considering the multiple locations to which animals typically are moved on their way to market, premises might be vulnerable to pathogen transmission even if located a considerable distance from a control area (e.g., premises could become infected from a passing truck that has violated movement control measures).

Adequate planning for essential services, such as mortality pickups and feed delivery, should include possible separate routes and pickup sites that are not near animal rearing facilities. Additional biosecurity measures should be placed on those personnel and vehicles to minimize disease spread.

Enhanced Biosecurity

During an outbreak, enhanced biosecurity measures should be implemented at the perimeter and within the control area. Facilities such as processing plants, slaughter plants, rendering operations, feed mills, and veterinary laboratories should be considered high risk. These high-traffic facilities should have truck washing stations at entry and exit points to minimize disease spread from affected to unaffected premises in the area.

Movement Restrictions

Movement restrictions are a key component to disease containment. When movement restrictions are in place, the incident commander should institute a system of movement permits to allow movement of equipment and personnel from one premise or control zone to another. These permits should only be issued when

- No animal on the premise of origin has shown clinical signs for two or more incubation periods.
- No susceptible animals were added to the premise of origin within two or more incubation periods.
- Clinical inspection of susceptible species was conducted within 24 hours prior to movement and animals were found free of clinical signs of the disease of concern.
- Transport conveyances meet acceptable biosecurity standards.

No susceptible animal species or products posing a risk of disease transmission may leave the infected zone unless they are (1) going directly to slaughter at an approved slaughter facility established in the buffer surveillance zone, (2) going directly to a processing facility in the buffer surveillance zone, or (3) meet the criteria described on a permit. No materials posing risk of disease transmission may leave the infected zone except by permit. Nonsusceptible species are subject to normal movement control and may be allowed to move with a permit under specified conditions as prescribed by the incident commander.

Control Measures (Area, Zone, and Premises Designations)

The designation of one or more control areas and various zones is essential for effective quarantine and movement control activities. Zones most commonly used are the infected zone, buffer-surveillance zone, free zone, and surveillance zone. **Control zone** designation and size of the inclusive areas are determined by applying epidemiological methods and utilizing surveillance data gathered during the course of the outbreak. Figure 8-5 depicts the various zones in relation to a simple outbreak of vesicular disease.

- **Control area.** The control area (CA) encompasses the infected zone and a buffer-surveillance zone. The CA is established quickly to ensure rapid and effective containment of the disease. For the most serious FAD, animal health officials may declare an entire state, commonwealth, or territory a CA. As such, movement of susceptible animals are halted for a period long enough to determine the scope of the disease outbreak. Potential modes of disease transmission should be considered when determining the minimum size and shape of the CA. The incident commander

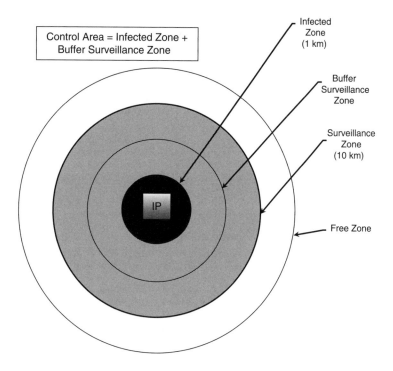

FIGURE 8-5 These are control measures that may be employed to effect containment in the event of a disease outbreak. In this simplistic example, a cow with vesicular disease was designated by an animal health official as a suspect case of FMD. The premise where the cow is located is on a farm designated IP (infected premise) in the inner-most circle. Following laboratory determination, the cow became a confirmed case of vesicular stomatitis, a highly contagious disease affecting many species of animals. To effectively contain the disease, the incident commander implements control measures around the IP to organize the workforce by task, assign responsibilities, and define actions within each of the zones. In this example, the outbreak is believed to be limited to a single premise. The incident commander establishes an infected zone of 1 kilometer, which encompasses the farm and surrounding pasture and a surveillance zone of 10 km. All at risk premises within the surveillance zone are checked by an animal health professional for the presence of the disease in susceptible animal populations. The incident commander designates a free zone for normal activities to ensue, so that production efforts outside the affected area are not hampered by the operation.

should control movement through the use of permits and maintain these restrictions until the disease is eradicated.

- **Infected zone.** The infected zone (IZ) includes the perimeter of all presumptive or confirmed positive premises and as many of the contact premises as the situation requires. The boundary of the IZ includes the borders of the confirmed infected and presumptive premises. The size and shape of the infected zone are determined by a number of factors. Terrain, weather, prevailing winds, susceptible animal populations (wild and domestic), and characteristics of the agent come into play in making this determination. Boundaries of the IZ are normally modified as surveillance and tracking results become available. Susceptible animals should not move into or through an infected zone unless they are being taken to depopulation locations inside the IZ.

- **Buffer-surveillance zone.** The buffer-surveillance zone (BSZ) immediately surrounds the IZ and is used as an area to concentrate surveillance efforts to determine the limit or spread of an FAD. No minimum size is prescribed for a BSZ. Premises within the BSZ that have clinically normal susceptible animals are known as *at-risk premises* (ARP). Surveillance on an ARP consists of a minimum of two inspections of animals per maximum incubation period of the disease under investigation. Any contact premises located outside an infected zone should be surrounded by a BSZ. The BSZ can be reduced in size as more surveillance data become available.

- **Free zone.** A free zone (FZ) is an area where the disease under consideration has been demonstrated to be absent. Requirements for disease-free (or "free") status are specified in the OIE International Animal Health Code. Within an FZ and at its borders, official veterinary control is applied for animals and animal products.

- **Surveillance zone.** Surveillance Zones (SZ) are established within, and along the border of, the free zone (FZ), separating the remainder of the FZ from the BSZ (see Figure 8-5). Surveillance efforts in the SZ focus on premises determined to be at the highest risk of infection. The suggested minimum size of the surveillance zone is 6.2 miles (10 km).

Classification of Premises

In general, in any animal disease outbreak, there are five types of premises: infected premises, suspect premises, contact premises, at-risk premises, and free premises.

- **Infected premises.** An infected premise (IP) is one where a highly contagious disease agent is presumed or confirmed to exist. The basis for this is through clinical presentation of the affected animals and laboratory results. All presumed positive premises and confirmed positive premises are classified as IPs. In addition, all other premises that meet a specific case definition are classified as IPs. For these premises, quarantine is imposed and all susceptible animals may be euthanized.

- **Suspect premises.** Suspect premises (SPs) are those that are under investigation for a report of compatible clinical signs but with no apparent epidemiological link to an IP or contact premises. These premises are under quarantine, movement restrictions, and surveillance for at least two maximum incubation periods. Surveillance consists of a minimum of three inspections of animals per incubation period of the disease under investigation. If an SP is negative after two incubation periods of surveillance, no further regular surveillance is required unless clinical signs are reported in the future. The owners of animals on an SP in an IZ may elect to euthanize and dispose of their animals, given approval of the IC.

- **Contact premises.** A contact premise (CP) is one with susceptible animals that have been exposed to animals, animal products, materials, people, or aerosol from an IP. Risk of exposure must be consistent with the transmission characteristics of the etiologic agent. The CP is quarantined and subject to disease control measures, which may include euthanasia and disposal of susceptible animals. If susceptible animals on a CP are not euthanized, they will be placed under surveillance for a period of time equal to two incubation periods. Surveillance and inspections continue until IZ or BSZ designations are removed. In the event that a CP is not located within a control area, the premises are treated as an independent IZ and surrounded by a BSZ.

- **At-risk premises.** At-risk premises are those premises in a BSZ or SZ that have susceptible animals but none of which are presenting clinically for the FAD in question. Susceptible animals from an ARP within a BSZ may be allowed to move with a permit.

- **Free premises.** Free premises (FPs) are those in the free zone, outside a surveillance zone.

Animal Quarantine Laws and Statutes

Every state has laws relating to communicable diseases among livestock and other animals and legal tools, such as quarantines and health certificate requirements, to control those diseases. Usually, the power to quarantine is given to a department of agriculture or to a livestock commission or board. The power to declare a quarantine includes the power to go onto private land and buildings to inspect for diseased animals and, if necessary, seize them. Also, if required, they are empowered, following proper procedures, to destroy diseased animals when necessary. Legal provision frequently exists for paying the owner a portion of the assessed value of the destroyed animal.

Effective quarantine and movement control are essential elements for preventing further spread of a disease agent. Movement control, in the form of a permit system, allows otherwise uninvolved entities to continue necessary movements to maintain operations. Quarantine of susceptible animals, potentially contaminated products and conveyances, and the like prevents the dissemination of the disease agent and increases the speed and likelihood of successful eradication.

Implementation of quarantines and the administration of a permit system for movement control should be described in each state's animal health emergency response plans. The USDA imposes a federal quarantine on interstate commerce from the infected state(s) and requests the infected and adjoining states (or country, if state borders are also international borders with Canada or Mexico) to provide resources to enforce the quarantine. Reimbursement formulas for this activity are set out in a cooperative agreement between the states and USDA. The federal quarantine is maintained until the disease is either eradicated or until such time as an effective control area smaller than a whole state is implemented.

Generally, state quarantines are placed on individual herds, flocks, or premises when an FAD is suspected. (i.e., under the Animal Health Protection Act of May 13, 2002, in Title 7 of the U.S. Code, Sections 8301–8317). In the absence of a declared emergency, federal quarantines are used to control interstate and international movement of diseased animals and contaminated items, whereas state quarantines are used to control intrastate movement of such animals and items.

In some instances, an extraordinary emergency may also be declared by the secretary of Agriculture, allowing federal officials to have authority to control livestock movement within a state. This can occur only after states have been notified by the secretary. Considerable disease control activity typically occurs before a federal declaration of extraordinary emergency is made.

Checkpoints and roadblocks should be located on all rural roads where they enter the control area. At checkpoints, all vehicles suspected of containing farm-related products, materials, or animals should be stopped. Although it may be impractical to establish checkpoints on interstate highways, checkpoints should be established at entrances and exits of major highways within the control area. Checkpoints should be staffed 24 hours per day and maintained for 30 days after the last infected animal is euthanized or until the situation indicates the checkpoints are no longer needed. Roadblocks may be established where human resources are limited.

Movement Control

Movement control refers to activities regulating the movement of people, animals, animal products, vehicles, and equipment based on certain criteria (determined by the disease agent suspected or confirmed). Movement control also involves record keeping of person, vehicle, or animal movement. These control measures should be established within 12 hours of a presumptive positive or confirmed positive report. The affected premises are defined as having at least one animal that is classified as having a presumptive positive or confirmed positive case of the disease in question.

Practices related to the control of movement of people, animals, vehicles, and equipment are critical to the maintenance of biosecurity during a disease outbreak or other animal emergency. Examples of practices involving movement controls include maintaining a closed herd or flock, identifying animals, keeping accurate records, and protecting animals from contact with wildlife. Movement of people (including owners, family members, employees, and visitors) is also considered a major biosecurity risk. All routine movement for services such as feed and manure removal as well as equipment on and off the premises should include biosecurity measures. Manure trucks should be covered and routes passing other susceptible species should be minimized or avoided.

Depopulation and Culling

Euthanasia of animals must be performed as rapidly and humanely as possible. Considerations must be given to owners, caretakers, and their families during this process. It is the responsibility of the responders to ensure that, when performing euthanasia on an animal, it is done with the highest degree of respect and emphasis on making the death as painless and stress free as possible. If an FAD is confirmed, depopulation (or culling) is likely to be ordered by the state veterinarian's office. **Depopulation** (culling) protocols include plans for the infected premises, contact-exposed premises, and contiguous premises. Proper destruction of all exposed cadavers, litter, and animal products is required.

Carcass Disposal

Many significant considerations pertain to animal carcass disposal, including agency response, decontamination, environmental issues, and public relations. Each concern, if inadequately addressed by decision makers before, during, or after a carcass disposal event, can yield long-term consequences (Carcass Disposal Working Group for APHIS, 2004).

Carcass disposal activities can result in detrimental effects on the environment. Factors affecting the impact on the environment include the disposal approach, type and number of carcasses, site-specific properties of the location, and weather.

A situation resulting in a large number of animal deaths causes significant public concern; disposal of carcasses on a large scale likely causes public dismay and apprehension. In fostering a positive public perception, decision makers must have access to public information professionals and make every effort to treat communication with the public as a top priority. Animal carcasses may be buried in a trench or at a landfill. Obviously, environmental considerations are associated with these two methods. In addition, removal of infected carcasses to a landfill site may violate the movement orders in place to limit the geographic spread of disease.

Animal carcasses may be incinerated as a method of disposal. Technological applications toward incineration methods have advanced a good deal in the past several years. Some reasons leading to this advancement include an increased awareness of public health, growing concerns about the environment, and economic considerations. There are three broad incineration methods: open-air burning, fixed-facility incineration, and air-curtain incineration.

Carcass composting is a natural process that utilizes oxygen in the decomposition of tissue. Under the initial phase of composting, the temperature of the compost pile increases, the organic materials break down, soft tissue decomposes, and bones soften. In the second phase, the remaining materials break down fully, and the compost turns to a dark brown or black soil. Carcass-composting systems require a variety of materials, including carbon sources (living organisms that emit more carbon dioxide than they absorb), amendments (bulking agents), and biofilter layers (layers of carbon sources or bulking materials that enhance microbial activity with proper moisture, pH, nutrients, and temperature).

Although site selection protocols may vary from state to state, a variety of site characteristics should be considered. A compost site should be constructed in a well-drained area that is at least 3 feet above the high water table level, 300 feet from sensitive water resources (streams, ponds, well, etc.), and on a slope of 1–3% to allow proper drainage and prevent pooling of fluids. Sites should be constructed downwind of nearby residences to minimize odors or dust. The site should have all-weather access to composting materials and minimal interference with other operations and traffic (Carcass Disposal Working Group for APHIS, 2004).

Disinfection

Cleaning and **disinfection** of the premises on which animals are euthanized and disposed is required. Cleaning and disinfecting are essential to contain the spread of a disease agent and are an integral part of the eradication plan. Care needs to be taken to reduce the generation and dispersal of infective dust and aerosols. This is essential to contain the spread of airborne pathogens and is an integral part of eradication. Animal facilities must be cleaned free of manure all the way down to bare concrete. A high-pressure sprayer is used to clean equipment and surfaces. A residual disinfectant is used in cleaning operations. If items cannot be adequately cleaned and disinfected, they should be disposed of by burning, burial, or other appropriate means (Carcass Disposal Working Group for APHIS, 2004).

Involvement of Local Responders

Traditional first responder and animal health practitioners may be needed in large numbers to effect disease containment, eradication, and quarantine enforcement. In zoonotic disease outbreaks, personal protective equipment (PPE) must be provided to responders. The successful use of PPE and other equipment in an animal health emergency is extremely important to the health and well-being of responders. The need for PPE and related supplies is determined by animal and human health authorities. The type of PPE required to protect responders could present additional logistic challenges to response efforts. In addition, some responders may require respirator fit testing and proficiency training to allow them to effectively wear and use their equipment.

The expertise of local responders may be essential for effective and timely containment of an FAD. Roles and responsibilities that responders may be called upon to assist with include

- Establishing quarantine perimeters for infected animal populations.
- Movement control (of animals, people, equipment, and products).
- Contact tracing of animals to identify potential exposures.
- Tracing of visitors to a producer's facility for the past 7–10 days.
- Cleaning and decontamination of equipment, vehicles, and personnel.

Food Safety

Biosecurity from field to fork implies that security measures must be in place at every link in the food chain. Food-borne pathogens received only a mention in Chapter 4. Post harvest food products and substances must be protected from microbial contamination. Notably, several bacteria have been placed in the U.S. Department of Health and Human Services Category B.

□ □ □ ▬▬▬▬▬▬▬▬▬▬▬▬▬▬▬▬▬▬▬▬▬▬▬▬▬▬▬▬▬▬▬▬▬

Category B Food-Borne Agents and Diseases

- *Clostridium botulinum* (botulism).
- *Salmonella* species (salmonellosis).
- *Escherichia coli* (strain O157:H7).
- *Salmonella typhi* (typhoid fever).
- *Shigella dysenteriae* Type 1 (shigellosis).
- *Vibrio cholerae* (cholera).

▬▬▬▬▬▬▬▬▬▬▬▬▬▬▬▬▬▬▬▬▬▬▬▬▬▬▬▬▬▬▬ □ □ □

The Food and Drug Administration is responsible for protecting the public health by assuring the safety, efficacy, and security of our nation's food supply (see the Mission Statement in U.S. Food and Drug Administration, 2007). The FDA is in partnership with the USDA, EPA, and CDC to accomplish this mission. This comprehensive and complex network of programs, initiatives, and testing laboratories is extensive. Readers interested in more details of these programs are directed to the FDA Food Protection Plan (U.S. Food and Drug Administration, 2007) and the National Food Safety Program Web site.

□ □ □ ▬▬▬▬▬▬▬▬▬▬▬▬▬▬▬▬▬▬▬▬▬▬▬▬▬▬

Food Protection Plan

Americans enjoy unprecedented choice and convenience in filling the cupboard today, but we also face new challenges to ensuring that our food is safe. This Food Protection Plan will implement a strategy of prevention, intervention and response to build safety into every step of the food supply chain.
—Michael O. Leavitt, Secretary of Health and Human Services

▬▬▬▬▬▬▬▬▬▬▬▬▬▬▬▬▬▬▬▬▬▬▬▬▬▬ □ □ □

Introduction of any of these agents into the processing, packaging, or distribution aspects of food production or preparation can and often does lead to serious outbreaks. Recall that the first and largest act of bioterrorism perpetrated in the United States was food-borne (Rajneesh cult, Salmonellosis, 1993). Each year in the United States, tens of thousands of Americans experience illness due to contaminated food. The Centers for Disease Control and Prevention maintains surveillance and database summary reports for food-borne illnesses. One such service is the Foodborne Diseases Active Surveillance Network, or FoodNet, which produces summaries of information collected through active surveillance of nine food-borne pathogens. In addition, the electronic Foodborne Outbreak Reporting System (eFORS) collects information on food-borne outbreaks that are reported each year from all 50 states and some large cities and territories. Food-borne outbreak reports are published on the Internet annually, and periodic food-borne outbreak surveillance summaries are published in the *Morbidity and Mortality Weekly Report*.

Food-borne outbreaks are reported to local, state, and federal officials. The first warning of an outbreak comes after the initial incubation and onset of symptoms in case patients. Significant or unusual outbreaks are posted to the CDC's Health Alert Network and to the news wires for mass media distribution.

Conclusion

Agriculture and food systems are the lifeblood of our nation and economy and one of the most important elements of critical infrastructure. In addition, agriculture and food systems are most vulnerable to threats from biological agents. These agents often produce devastating results when outbreaks of animal or crop disease are introduced naturally or accidentally. The malicious and intentional introduction of a crop or animal disease agent is known as *agroterrorism*. Agroterrorism has potential to undermine the economy of a nation and cause animal health professionals and government officials at all levels to muster an enormous response effort to contain the disease. Biosecurity in an agricultural setting can be described as a number of best practices aimed at reducing the threat of biological agents to the farm, animal production facility, or food processing and distribution center. Quarantine and stop movement procedures are used to prevent further spread of a disease. Involvement of the state and federal agencies is coordinated and in compliance with the National Incidence Management System and the National Response Framework. Various levels of containment are designated, based on the risk of disease. In some instances, traditional first responders may be needed to effect quarantine, movement restrictions, disinfection and carcass disposal activities.

Essential Terminology

- **Agroterrorism** (sometimes referred to as *agricultural terrorism*). The deliberate introduction of a chemical or disease agent, either against livestock or crops or into the food chain, for the purpose of undermining stability or generating fear. Agriculture is considered by many to be the perfect target for agroterrorism, because the agriculture industry is unmatched in revenue and scope.
- **Biosafety.** Efforts to prevent the transmission of biologic agents to workers or halt the spread of agents to the environment. It may include such measures as policies, procedures, personal protective safety, and elements of a facility's design. The Center for Disease Control and Prevention rates the transmission risk of agents through a classification system.
- **Biosecurity.** Generally defined as efforts to prevent the acquisition and intentional misuse of biological agents. For the purpose of this book, the definition also includes efforts to prevent the unintentional misuse or spread of pests, diseases, and agents.
- **Critical infrastructure.** A term used in the U.S. National Strategy for Homeland Security, issued in July 2002; it is defined as those "systems and assets, whether physical or virtual, so vital to the United States that the incapacity or destruction of such systems and assets would have a debilitation impact on security, national economic security, national public health or safety, or any combination of those matters."
- **Vector.** A carrier and transmission agent of a plant disease.

Discussion Questions

- How would you describe a specific form of terrorism against agriculture, often referred to as *agroterrorism*?
- Why might a terrorist "prefer" biological agents against an enemy's agricultural sector to other weapons of mass destruction and critical infrastructure?
- How does agroterrorism relate to plant biosecurity management?
- Discuss the roles of various response disciplines within each of the zones.

Web Sites

Extension Disaster Emergency Network (EDEN), available at www.agctr.lsu.edu/eden.
Guide for Security Practices in Transporting Agricultural and Food Commodities, available at www.usda.gov/homelandsecurity/aftcsecurguidfinal19.pdf.

National Association of State Departments of Agriculture, available at www.nasda.org/ NASDA.

University of Arkansas Cooperative Extension Service; Farm and Home Biosecurity Introduction, available at www.uaex.edu/biosecurity/default.asp.

American Phytopathological Society, available at www.apsnet.org.

FoodNet, available at www.cdc.gov/foodnet/reports.htm.

FDA Food Protection Plan, available at www.fda.gov/oc/initiatives/advance/food.html.

National Food Safety Programs: www.foodsafety.gov/~dms/fs-toc.html.

Farm & Ranch Biosecurity, available at www.farmandranchbiosecurity.com.

Animal and Plant Health Inspection Service (APHIS), available at www.aphis.usda.gov.

National Animal Health Laboratory Network, available at www.csrees.usda.gov/nea/ ag_biosecurity/in_focus/apb_if_healthlab.html.

National Plant Board, available at www.aphis.usda.gov/npb.

National Plant Diagnostic Network, available at www.npdn.org/DesktopDefault.aspx.

U.S. Department of Agriculture, available at www.usda.gov.

U.S. Department of Agriculture; Homeland Security, available at www.usda.gov/ homelandsecurity/links.html.

References

Amber Waves. 2007. United States Department of Agriculture, Economic Research Service, available at www.ers.usda.gov/AmberWaves/September07.

Ancker, C., and M. Burke. 2003. Doctrine for asymmetric warfare. *Military Review* (July–August): 18–26.

Ban, J. 2000. Agricultural biological warfare: An overview. *The Arena*, available at www.mipt.org/ pdf/agrobiowarfareoverview.pdf.

Bovine Spongiform Encephalopathy. 1998. In: *The Gray Book: Foreign Animal Disease*, 6th ed., by U.S. Animal Health Association, Committee on Foreign Animal Disease. Richmond, VA: Pat Campbell & Associates and Carter Printing Company.

Carcass Disposal Working Group for APHIS. 2004. *Carcass Disposal: A Comprehensive Review*. Manhattan, KS: National Agriculture Biosecurity Center.

Carus, W. 2001. *Bioterrorism and Biocrimes. The Illicit Use of Biological Agents since 1900*, rev. ed. August 1998. Washington, DC: Center for Counter-proliferation Research National Defense University.

Covert, N. 2000. Cutting Edge: A History of Fort Detrick, Maryland. The Headquarters, 4th ed., available at www.detrick.army.mil/cutting_edge/index.cfm?chapter=titlepage.

Critical Foreign Animal Disease Issues for the 21st Century. 1998. In: *The Gray Book: Foreign Animal Diseases*. Richmond, VA: Pat Campbell & Associates and Carter Printing Company.

Crop Biosecurity: Are We Prepared? American Phytopathological Society (2003).

Foot-and-Mouth Disease. 1998. In: *The Gray Book: Foreign Animal Diseases*, 6th ed., by U.S. Animal Health Association, Committee on Foreign Animal Disease. Richmond, VA: Pat Campbell & Associates and Carter Printing Company, available at www.vet.uga.edu/vpp/gray_book/pdf/FMD.htm.

Homeland Security Presidential Directive (HSPD) 7. 2003. Critical Infrastructure Identification, Prioritization, and Protection.

Homeland Security Presidential Directive (HSPD) 9. 2004. Defense of United States Agriculture and Food.

James, C. 2000. *Global Status of Commercialized Transgenic Crops: 1999*. ISAAA Briefs no. 17. Ithaca, NY: International Service for the Acquisition of Agri-biotech Applications.

Kortepeter, M., and G. Parker. 1999. Potential biological weapons threats. *Emerging Infectious Diseases* 5:523–527.

Pate, J., and G. Camerson. 2001. *Covert Biological Weapons Attacks against Agricultural Targets: Assessing the Impact against U.S. Agriculture*. BCSI Discussion Paper 2001-9. Cambridge, MA: John F. Kennedy School of Government, Harvard University.

Scardaci, S., R. Webster, C. Greer, J. Hill, J. Williams, R. Mutters, D. Brandon, K. McKenzie, and J. Oster. 1997. *Rice Blast: A New Disease. California*. Agronomy Fact Sheet Series 1997–2. Davis: Department of Agronomy and Range Science, University of California.

Schoenbaum, M., and W. Disney. 2003. Modeling alternative mitigation strategies for a hypothetical outbreak of foot-and-mouth disease in the United States. *Preventive Veterinary Medicine* 58:25–52.

Sutmoller, P., S. Barteling, R. Olascoaga, and K. Sumption. 2003. Control and eradication of foot and mouth disease. *Virus Research* 91:101–144.

U.S. Census Bureau. 2007. Population Clock, available at www.census.gov/main/www/popclock. html.

U.S. Department of Agriculture. 2006. Pre-Harvest Security Guidelines and Checklist.

U.S. Department of Agriculture. 2007a. APHIS. Soy Bean Rust Web site, available at www.aphis. usda.gov/plant_health/plant_pest_info/soybean_rust/index.shtml.

U.S. Department of Agriculture. 2007b. *Karnal Bunt: A Fungal Disease of Wheat*. Animal and Plant Health Inspection Service (USDA-APHIS), available at www.invasive.org/publications/ aphis/karnal.pdf.

U.S. Department of Defense. 1977. *Biological Testing Involving Human Subjects by the Department of Defense, 1977: Hearings before the Subcommittee on Health and Scientific Research of the Committee on Human Resources*. Washington, DC: U.S Government Printing Office.

U.S. Food and Drug Administration. 2007. *Food Protection Plan*, available at www.fda.gov/oc/ initiatives/advance/food.html.

Wilson Terrance, M., et al., 2000. Agroterrorism, biological crimes, and biological warfare targeting animal agriculture. In: *Emerging Diseases of Animals*, eds. C. Brown and C. Bolin, pp. 23–57. Washington, DC: ASM Press.

9

Recent Animal Disease Outbreaks and Lessons Learned

In nature we never see anything isolated, but everything in connection with something else which is before it, beside it, under it and over it.
—Johann Wolfgang von Goethe

Objectives

The study of this chapter will enable you to

1. Discuss foot and mouth disease and its potential devastation to the beef industry.
2. Discuss avian influenza and its potential devastation to the poultry industry.
3. Discuss classic swine fever and its potential devastation to the pork industry.
4. Discuss bovine spongiform encephalopathy and its potential devastation to the beef industry and implications for human health.
5. Discuss specific case studies of animal disease outbreaks.

Key Terms

Foot and mouth disease, picornavirus, avian influenza, influenza virus, H5N1, classical swine fever, bovine spongiform encephalopathy, mad cow disease, downer cows.

Introduction

Imagine a setting where a foreign animal disease is introduced into the United States. In response to this introduction, animal health authorities would immediately implement actions to stop the movement of affected animals and products, increase surveillance, extend quarantines, and elevate biosecurity measures. Local and state emergency management and law enforcement would be notified and may be involved in initial security and investigation. The Secretary of Agriculture, after consultation with the governors of the affected states, would declare an agricultural emergency and request a disaster declaration from the president. If terrorism is suspected, the Department of Homeland Security may declare the event an incident of national significance, a term that may become obsolete under the new national response framework. Depending on the scope of the response, state emergency operations centers (EOCs) will be partially or fully activated. USDA Animal and Plant Health Inspection Service regional and national EOCs will activate (U.S. Department of Agriculture, 2002).

Under the Homeland Security Presidential Directive 5, federal departments and agencies must follow the National Incident Management System (NIMS) in their domestic emergency management. NIMS is designed to provide a consistent nationwide approach to federal, state, and local governments to work together to prepare for, respond to, and recover from domestic incidents. At the center of NIMS is the Incident Command System (ICS), a structural management system designed to unite multiple responding agencies, including those from different jurisdictions, under a unified command structure when an incident occurs.

Following NIMS, an ICS would be initiated for the state and federal animal health officials and partner agencies to respond to an FAD. With more than one state involved, several incident command posts would be set up, with an area command for overall control. Animal health professionals would be heavily burdened with surveillance activities during the response to an outbreak and through the recovery period. The main objective of the response effort is to limit the spread of transmission and to "stamp out" the FAD (U.S. Department of Agriculture, 2003a). The ICS provides guidance and assistance to help enforce the quarantines, movement controls, and surveillance that are necessary to prevent the spread of the FAD. The ICS works closely with law enforcement to investigate and preserve the quarantined areas and the chain of custody of samples sent to the laboratories.

Surveillance and quarantined zones would be established in a specified radius of the infected premises. Any farms and ranches that may have received animals within the preceding 30 days from any of the infected premises or adjoining the infected premises would be quarantined and investigated. All livestock farms and ranches with susceptible species would be investigated to identify if they had been exposed to or infected with the FAD. At least two visits would be made to all identified farms and ranches to inspect and test for the FAD. Quarantines would remain in place until no new cases were identified and enough time had passed for the disease to occur and be identified in any additional animals. State and federal wildlife agencies would assess risk of wildlife transmission of the FAD and initiate control plans. State and federal agencies would develop and implement permit protocols for movement of nontarget species and animal and crop products from controlled areas (U.S. Department of Agriculture, 2002, 2003a).

To ensure the eradication of the FAD, the incident commander would provide resources needed for the appraisal of animals designated to be euthanized, euthanasia of the infected and exposed animals using humane methods, disposal of carcasses, and decontamination of the areas exposed to the FAD. Sampling and monitoring of the decontaminated areas would be implemented to confirm whether the areas were successfully decontaminated. Under the ICS, a legislative and public affairs official from APHIS along with a state public affairs official would provide media briefings on the disease investigation and biosecurity measures needed to contain and eradicate the disease.

Whenever found within a developed nation, foreign animal diseases have severe international trade implications for that nation's agricultural industry. To reestablish an internationally recognized free status, the country undergoing the outbreak must prove through active surveillance that it has been free from that FAD for 12 months and demonstrate that effective surveillance systems and regulatory measures are in place to prevent reintroduction.

The setting and actions in response to an FAD outbreak just detailed and in Chapter 8 present a rather idealistic view of how things are supposed to unfold and terminate. However, that is not always the way it plays out in reality. This chapter introduces the reader to four serious foreign animal diseases: foot-and-mouth disease, highly pathogenic avian influenza, classic swine fever, and bovine spongiform encephalopathy (BSE or mad cow disease). Further, the chapter discusses the *highlights* of real-world case studies for each of the four FADs. Bear in mind that it would not be practical to restate all the details for each event discussed here. Rather, the introduction of these examples should prompt the reader to look further at the details of each situation and gather the lessons learned so that they may be applied for future outbreaks. As such, suggested readings for each event are provided at the end of the chapter. Most readings come from government agencies that summarize the events and provide lessons learned.

Foot-and-Mouth Disease

Foot-and-mouth disease is a serious, highly infectious disease caused by a **picornavirus**, which is an RNA virus in the genus Apthovirus (American Veterinary Medical Association, 2007). There are seven serotypes of the FMD virus (O, A, C, SAT (South African territory) 1, SAT2, SAT3, and ASIA1). Each serotype of FMD is antigenically distinct from the other six serotypes. Foot-and-mouth disease manifests in cloven-hooved ruminants, which include sheep, cattle, swine, goats, deer, and water buffalo (American Veterinary Medical Association, 2007). Humans are not affected by the FMD virus. The FMD virus is temperature sensitive and rapidly inactivated at elevated temperatures (above 56°F). When it comes to survivability, the virus has a fairly narrow window for pH; the optimal range is 7.2–7.6. However, some pretty convincing data suggest that this virus is quite hardy in a natural setting, especially when conditions are cool and moist (Bartley, Donnelly, and Anderson, 2002). Table 9-1 lists settings and FMD virus viability.

Foot-and-mouth disease is particularly devastating to livestock. Clinically, FMD is characterized by fever ($\geq 41°C$) and the development of vesicles (blisters) on the tongue, in the mouth, the lips, nostrils, the hooves, and the teats of infected animals (see Figure 9-1). The vesicles quickly rupture to form a raw and painful surface. Vesicles cause the animal to salivate profusely and become lame (House and Mebus, 1998). Infected animals tend to lose weight and produce less milk. Pregnant animals may abort. Young animals may

Table 9-1 Practical Examples of FMD Virus Survival under Temperate Conditions

Conditions	Viability
Dry feces	14 days
Urine	39 days
Ground, summer	3 days
Ground, winter	28 days

Note: Foot and mouth disease virus can survive for long periods of time in dark, moist conditions but is rapidly inactivated by a combination of desiccation, pH, and temperature.

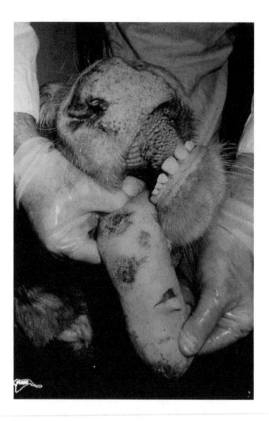

FIGURE 9-1 Foot-and-mouth disease lesions are shown in this cow from a USDA archive photo used to train animal health professionals so that they might recognize suspect cases of FMD. Note that vesicular disease in livestock can be due to a number of causes and infectious agents. (Image courtesy of USDA APHIS.)

succumb to FMD due to heart damage. Clinical signs vary in severity and the disease is often mild or not apparent in sheep (Hughes et al., 2002).

The FMD virus enters the host through the mouth, nose, or breaks in the skin. Following viral replication, virus particles may be found in saliva, milk, semen, and even the breath of the animal two days before vesicles develop. Normally, the incubation period for FMD virus infection in cattle and pigs is two to five days. The incubation period for sheep and goats appears to be longer. In fact, the incubation period may extend up to 14 days, which depends highly on the strain of FMD virus, the dose the animal receives, and the susceptibility of the individual animal (Lubroth, 2002).

The disease is extremely contagious. Inhalation and ingestion of the virus are routes of infection (Bartley et al., 2002). The virus is spread primarily from animal to animal; although other mechanisms, such as contaminated feed and fomites, are possible. Foot and mouth disease virus may also be spread by contaminated inanimate objects and people moving between infected and uninfected animals. Outbreaks are often initiated by the transport of infected animals to markets and the introduction of infected animals to a susceptible herd (Callis and McKercher, 1997). Airborne transmission of FMD virus has been documented; cattle may be more susceptible to this route of infection (Sellers, Herniman, and Gumm, 1977). Naturally, dispersion of airborne virus particles can be dramatically influenced by weather conditions.

□ □ □ ▬▬▬▬▬▬▬▬▬▬▬▬▬▬▬▬▬▬▬▬▬▬▬▬▬▬▬▬▬▬

Critical Thinking

Based on the characteristics of FMD virus, what makes it so potentially devastating to meat and milk production?

▬▬▬▬▬▬▬▬▬▬▬▬▬▬▬▬▬▬▬▬▬▬▬▬▬▬▬▬▬▬   □ □ □

Since 1921, the FMD virus has been isolated and typed from over 40 human cases (Bauer, 1997). The cases occurred in Africa, Europe, and South America. Type O predominated, followed by C, and rarely A. Infection in humans is rare and the disease is relatively mild; therefore, FMD is not considered a public health issue.

The first recorded observations of FMD occurred in Italy in 1514 (American Veterinary Medical Association, 2007). Today, the FMD virus is fairly widespread in its global distribution. The seven serotypes of FMD virus have different distribution patterns (UN Food and Agriculture Organization, 2007). Collectively, the FMD virus is found in parts of Africa, Asia, South America, and Europe. In these regions of the world, FMD is a persistent problem, since it is known to infect cloven-hooved wildlife reservoirs, which makes it extremely difficult to stamp out. Currently, 59 countries in the world are considered to be FMD free (OIE, 2007). There have been nine outbreaks of FMD in the United States, all of which occurred from 1905 to 1929. The United States has been FMD free since 1929 (American Veterinary Medical Association, 2007).

The World Organization for Animal Health (OIE) classifies foot-and-mouth disease as a List A disease requiring 24-hour notification of its first occurrence in an FMD-free country or zone or reoccurrence after a previously eradicated outbreak. In addition, the OIE considers FMD the most economically devastating livestock disease in the world. The introduction of FMD presents a worst-case scenario for livestock producers and animal health officials, due to the potential for many species to be infected, rapid spread of the contagion, and difficulty in controlling the outbreaks. Immediate notification is necessary because of its rapid spread and substantial impact on the international trade of animals and animal products.

High costs are associated with the eradication or control of FMD. Direct costs due to an outbreak of FMD include depopulating infected herds, disinfecting premises, imposition of quarantine, and enhanced surveillance. These costs are exacerbated by indirect, long-term losses brought on by the imposition of trade restrictions and subsequent higher prices paid for meat products affected by the outbreak due to interruption of the food supply. Countries that are free from FMD go to great lengths to maintain their disease-free status. Many countries that have the disease invest large sums in eradication campaigns. One estimate suggests that, if FMD became established within the United States, it would cost the nation over $27 billion in trade losses each year (Paarlberg, Lee, and Seitzinger, 2002).

In 2001, an outbreak of FMD in the United Kingdom resulted in the slaughter of more than 8 million animals and an estimated economic loss of 20 billion dollars (Davies, 2002). That event horrified the nation and nearly brought the government to its knees. The 2001 outbreak of FMD is the subject of the first case study in this chapter.

Avian Influenza

Avian influenza is an infectious disease of birds caused by type A strains of the influenza virus (Beard, 1998). All sixteen hemagglutinin subtypes of type A **influenza virus** can cause an outbreak of avian influenza. Depending on the severity of outbreak and strain of virus, avian influenza is classified as either low pathogenic avian influenza (LPAI) or highly pathogenic avian influenza (HPAI). Only hemagglutinin subtypes 5 and 7 are known to cause HPAI (Beard, 1998). Once introduced, this disease can move rapidly through a flock of domestic poultry and a flock of wild fowl. Since it is easily and rapidly spread from one bird to another, HPAI can have devastating effects, resulting in high mortality over a short period of time. Confined animal feeding operations, much like those found in the poultry industry, intensify the effects of an avian influenza outbreak due to the concentrated population of birds and uniform age of the flock.

Avian influenza was first identified in Italy in 1878. The first cases of HPAI reported in the United States were in 1924 and 1929 (American Veterinary Medical Association, 2006c). Quarantine, depopulation, cleaning, and disinfection were used to eradicate HPAI from the United States. Milder disease in poultry and wild birds caused by type A influenza virus was recognized in the middle of the 20th century; today these avian influenza viruses are termed *LPAI*. In the 1970s, surveillance for exotic Newcastle disease virus showed that migratory waterfowl were asymptomatic carriers of avian influenza. Since then, wild waterfowl (especially ducks and geese) and other aquatic birds have been shown to be reservoirs of all strains of type A influenza viruses (Stallknecht et al., 1990). Avian influenza viruses have also caused outbreaks of respiratory disease in mink, seals, and whales (Beard, 1998).

□ □ □ ▬▬▬▬▬▬▬▬▬▬▬▬▬▬▬▬▬▬▬▬▬▬▬▬▬▬▬▬▬▬▬▬▬▬▬▬▬▬

Critical Thinking

The natural reservoir for type A influenza virus is migratory water fowl. Consider that many migratory birds become infected with the virus and shed millions of virions into the aquatic environment where they live and come to rest as they migrate (Stallknecht et al., 1990). The dynamics of transmission between migratory bird populations and domestic poultry are a hot topic of debate, especially with the spread of the HPAI Asian strain of **H5N1**. Visit the WHO website to examine the patterns, if any, of spread of H5N1 from Asia into Africa and Europe. What can be done to limit the spread of a deadly HPAI strain when the dynamics of transmission are so complex?

▬▬▬▬▬▬▬▬▬▬▬▬▬▬▬▬▬▬▬▬▬▬▬▬▬▬▬▬▬▬▬▬▬▬▬▬▬▬ □ □ □

As mentioned previously, highly pathogenic avian influenza is caused only by type A influenza virus. The genetic features and severity of disease in poultry determines whether the virus is classified as low pathogenic or high pathogenic. LPAI includes viruses in all hemagglutinin subtypes (H1–H16). On the other hand, HPAI have traditionally been either H5 or H7 subtypes. H5 and H7 LPAI viruses exist and are of concern because they can mutate into HPAI strains (Beard, 1998). See Figure 9-2.

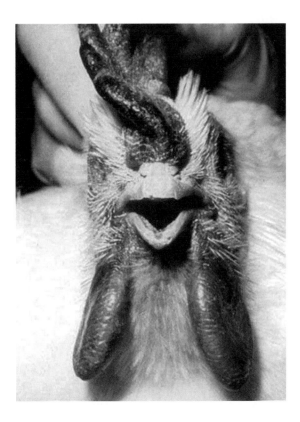

Figure 9-2 Chicken confirmed to be infected with H5N1 type A influenza virus responsible for slaughter of nearly 200 million birds worldwide since 1997. Highly pathogenic avian influenza is caused by H5 and H7 subtypes of influenza type A virus. This highly contagious disease often results in 100% mortality when it strikes a poultry operation. The H5N1 virus has been the center of attention in recent outbreaks of "bird flu" that have decimated the poultry industry in parts of Southeast Asia. (Image courtesy of USDA APHIS.)

Avian influenza can occur anywhere in the world. Migratory waterfowl are widely considered the reservoirs of avian influenza virus (Voyles, 2002). Feces and respiratory secretions contain large amounts of virus, which can infect a new host through the conjunctiva or respiratory tract. Avian influenza virus can spread by aerosol when birds are in close proximity and might be transmitted through shared drinking water (Stallknecht et al., 1990). The virus appears to be present in eggs laid by infected hens, but they are unlikely to survive and hatch. Fomites (contact with an infected object) and infected birds can transmit the disease between flocks. Domesticated birds may become infected with avian influenza virus through direct contact with infected waterfowl, other infected poultry, through contact with surfaces (such as dirt or cages), or materials (such as water or feed) that have been contaminated with the virus (Capua and Marangon, 2006).

In one outbreak in Pennsylvania, garbage flies may have spread the virus. Airborne dissemination may be possible as well as movement of infected poultry. In experimental studies avian influenza viruses can be excreted in the feces and maintained in the environment and can reemerge after a significantly stressful event. Once a flock is infected, it should be considered a potential source of virus for life. In addition, the live bird market systems that are found throughout the developing world has contributed to the westward spread of H5N1 out of Asia and into Europe.

Classical Swine Fever

Classical swine fever (CSF) is also known as *swine fever* and *hog cholera*. The etiologic agent of CSF is a Pestivirus, a positive-sense, single-stranded RNA virus from the family Flaviviridae. Flaviviruses were previously covered in Chapters 3 and 5 of this book since West Nile virus and Japanese encephalitis virus are also members of the family Flaviviridae (American Veterinary Medical Association, 2006a).

Wild boars and domestic pigs are the only natural reservoirs of CSF. Humans are not infected or affected by the CSF virus. The World Organization for Animal Health (OIE) has placed CSF on List A. Classical swine fever is endemic in parts of Africa, Asia, Europe, and Central and South America. The disease was found briefly in the United States until 1962, but the country has been CSF free since then. Classical swine fever is a reportable disease to the OIE and USDA. State or federal animal health officials should be notified immediately when CSF is suspected.

CSF occurs in acute and chronic forms. Acute CSF presents in swine as high fever, inappetence, and severe depression. In addition, acutely infected pigs present with purple discoloration of the skin, diarrhea, vomiting, coughing, hind limb weakness, and ocular discharge (Edwards, 1998). Pregnant sows infected with CSF virus often abort. Infected piglets frequently develop neurologic signs, including tremors and convulsions. There is no treatment for CSF. The case fatality rate of the acute form of CSF is 95–100% in susceptible populations. Death usually occurs in 10–15 days (Edwards, 1998).

Classical swine fever virus is spread from infected domestic pigs to susceptible pigs by direct and indirect contact. Ingestion and inhalation of the CSF virus are the most common routes of infection (Dewulf et al., 2000). Classical swine fever virus transmission also occurs via transfer of infected blood or semen. Infected animals shed the virus in saliva, feces, urine, blood, and nasal secretions. Mechanical transmission of the virus is possible with contaminated equipment, vehicles, clothing, and footwear (fomites) following outbreaks (Kleiboeker, 2002). Blood-sucking insects and birds may act as mechanical vectors of the CSF virus; although, they do not amplify it. Consumption of uncooked, infected pork scraps has resulted in outbreaks of CSF. The CSF virus can survive in these infected pork products for many months. Transplacental infection with strains of low virulence can produce chronically infected piglets, which can then be sources of infection for outbreaks. The incubation period of CSF ranges from 2–14 days. Once a pig recovers from CSF, it is capable of shedding the virus for long periods (American Veterinary Medical Association, 2006a). Therefore, recovered animals and apparently healthy but infected pigs are important sources of virus for outbreaks.

Bovine Spongiform Encephalopathy

Bovine spongiform encephalopathy (BSE), also known as **mad cow disease**, is a serious, long-term disease affecting bovines. Mad cow disease was first identified in the United Kingdom in 1986 (Brown et al., 2001). The etiologic agent of BSE is a prion (DeArmond and Prusiner, 1995). As with most other prion diseases (scrapie, Creutzfeldt-Jakob disease, chronic wasting disease), this fatal disease affects the central nervous system. In 1998, authorities in the United Kingdom instituted bans on feeding ruminants food that contained by-products of carcasses of other ruminants (American Veterinary

Table 9-2 Summary of Confirmed and Probable Cases of Variant Creutzfeldt-Jakob Disease Reported to the National CJD Surveillance Unit in the United Kingdom

Deaths from definite vCJD (confirmed)	114
Deaths from probable vCJD (confirmation pending)	1
Deaths from probable vCJD (without confirmation)	47
Number of definite/probable vCJD cases still alive	4
Total number of definite or probable vCJD cases (dead and alive)	166

Note: Figures shown are current as of November 5, 2007.

Source: www.gnn.gov.uk/Content/Detail.asp?ReleaseID=319104&NewsAreaID=2.

Medical Association, 2006b). The epidemic of BSE in cattle peaked (>37,000 new cases per year) in 1992. In 2004, the number of new cases reported in the United Kingdom was 343 and, through August 2005, was 121. New cases of BSE and variant Creutzfeldt-Jakob disease (the human form of the disease) have dropped off dramatically since 2005 (DEFRA web site, 2007). Table 9-2 provides a summary of human cases of variant Creutzfeldt-Jakob disease reported in the United Kingdom.

Cattle are the primary hosts for BSE. Other *bovid* infected include bison, kudu, gemsbok, oryx, and eland. Domestic cats on BSE-affected premises have been affected, as have some domestic cats in urban households. BSE has been experimentally transmitted to cattle, pigs, sheep, goats, mice, mink, marmosets, and macaque monkeys (Prusiner, 1998).

BSE has a long incubation period in cattle, ranging from 2–8 years. Experts generally refer to an average incubation period of five years. The most important mode of transmission of BSE between cattle is via the oral route. However, it is not an efficient transmission route. The roles of genetic predisposition and vertical transmission (mother to offspring) in the epidemiology of the disease are not well defined. However, it seems apparent that some limited transmission does occur from cows to their calves (American Veterinary Medical Association, 2006b).

Worldwide, there have been more than 170,000 cases in animals since the disease was first diagnosed in Great Britain. Over 95% of those cases have occurred in the United Kingdom (Smith and Bradley, 2003). BSE has also been confirmed in native-born cattle in Belgium, France, Ireland, Luxembourg, the Netherlands, Northern Ireland, Portugal, and Switzerland (Matthews, Vandeveer, and Gustafson, 2006). Active surveillance of cattle herds and an animal identification program have been ongoing to identify foci of infection. This, coupled with biosecurity best practices, is reducing the incidence of BSE worldwide.

Implications for Human Health

Variant Creutzfeldt-Jakob disease (vCJD) in humans was first described in 1996 in the United Kingdom (Armstrong et al., 2003). It has different clinical and pathologic characteristics from classic Creutzfeldt-Jakob disease. Typical clinical signs are associated with the terminal destruction of central nervous system tissue, which varies somewhat with each case. Signs and symptoms of vCJD are pronounced psychiatric and behavioral symptoms, accompanied by painful dysesthesias (false feelings) and delayed neurologic signs (Beisel and Morens, 2004). The median age of death for vCJD case patients is 28 years with a median duration of illness of 14 months (Bacchetti, 2003).

Epidemiologic evidence suggests the outbreak of BSE in cattle in the United Kingdom and Europe is associated with the emergence of a new variant form of Creutzfeldt-Jakob disease in humans (Croes and van Duijn, 2003). Currently, strong scientific evidence finds that the agent responsible for the outbreak of BSE in cows is the same agent responsible for the outbreak of vCJD in humans (Goldberg, 2007). Epidemiologic studies at the time suggested that the source of disease was supplements in cattle feed prepared from carcasses of cattle (meat and bone meal). Changes in the process of preparing meat and bone meal introduced during 1981 and 1982 may have been a risk factor (Hueston and Bryant, 2005). Theories about the sudden appearance of the disease in cattle include the following:

- Spontaneous occurrence and subsequent amplification when infected carcasses entered the cattle feed chain.
- Entry through the cattle feed chain from carcasses of sheep with scrapie.

High-risk tissues of cattle with or exposed to BSE include those from or contiguous with the central nervous system as well as from the distal ileum and bone marrow (Goldberg, 2007). Conventional thought is that the prion protein enters via the gut (after eating infectious material), is amplified in the local lymphoreticular tissue (tissue of the immune system) of the gut then, depending on the species of animal, might move to the spleen and possibly bone marrow, where further amplification occurs. Finally, the prion moves to the central nervous system, where there is massive terminal replication, which destroys brain tissue and leads to the observed clinical signs. Prions are thought to be spread within the bodies of affected animals through the nerves, blood, or by a combination of the two (Prusiner, 1998). If transmission through the blood is a method, then, obviously, medical use of blood and blood products (serum proteins) would constitute a source of iatrogenic infections.

Despite all this convincing evidence, the risk for vCJD is low, even after consumption of BSE-contaminated meat (Goldberg, 2007). The presence of BSE in cattle within a country creates health concerns among consumers and economic hardship because of trade restrictions. This occurred several times in the past few years in the United States and Canada. We examine this more closely in the next section.

Case Studies

Foot-and-Mouth Disease, United Kingdom, 2001

On February 19, 2001, animal health officials realized that FMD was present in several pigs at a slaughterhouse in Essex, Great Britain (U.K. Department for Environment, Food and Rural Affairs, 2002). Two days later, the Ministry of Agriculture, Fisheries and Food confirmed the presence of FMD in these pigs and in cattle on a neighboring farm near Heddon-on-the-Wall, Northumberland. From this location, officials believe that the virus spread via air current to cattle and sheep on a neighboring farm at Ponteland (~10 km). Alarmingly, the age of the lesions plus the incubation time of virus indicated that infection of the *index* case likely took place about two weeks before discovery of the disease, on or about February 5, 2001. This lag in detection enabled infected sheep from the Ponteland farm to be transported to two markets in Cumberland near the Scottish border. Here, direct and indirect contact of the animals led to widespread distribution of the disease to most of Cumbria. Subsequently, a dealer took truckloads of infected sheep to Devon, with rapid resale to Hereford, Northampton, and Wiltshire. Most of this movement had occurred by the time the disease was confirmed in Essex; therefore, the spread of the disease was, at the time, unknown (U.K. Department for Environment, Food and Rural Affairs, 2002).

By March 8, 2001, newly discovered cases reached 104, with a wide geographic distribution. By March 20, a total of 338 new cases were identified. By March 29, 1,726 cases were identified. The speed of dissemination and transmission is why early detection is a high priority for animal health officials. New cases of FMD were confirmed every day until September that year (U.K. Department for Environment, Food and Rural Affairs, 2002).

During this outbreak, the government adopted a rigorous stamping out policy. This involved the slaughter of all animals on infected premises and all those regarded as dangerous contacts. Since sheep may be asymptomatic or subclinical, animal health officials believed that the disease could have been spreading undetected through sheep. Accordingly, the state veterinary service imposed a preemptive cull of all sheep within a 3-km radius of an IP (U.K. Department for Environment, Food and Rural Affairs, 2002). This cull was later extended to pigs. In addition, the government relied on controversial FMD modeling programs, which led them to the decision to slaughter all animals on premises that were contiguous to IPs.

Because of the decisions to slaughter sheep and pigs in a 3-km radius and on contiguous premises, no one knows how many slaughtered animals were actually infected. Although a high proportion of the animals on infected premises were tested for disease, few samples were collected for testing from the large number of contiguous premises. The purpose in killing them was, it appears, less to cull infected stock rather than create a firebreak around the outbreaks of disease.

British ministers dealing with the FMD outbreak and orchestrating containment efforts faced a dilemma. They received scientific advice on vaccination that seemed conflicting. Some experts that were involved in vaccine research promoted their use. While others felt that the outbreak could be effectively contained only with stringent stamping out measures. Looking back to OIE rules in place in 2001, FMD-free status could be restored three months after the outbreak only if vaccination was not used to control it. However, if FMD vaccination of the herd was employed, FMD-free status could be achieved after a period of 12 months. This led to the view that, to get back into export markets as quickly as possible, vaccinated animals would have to be subsequently slaughtered. In addition, rapid diagnostic tests and those that could differentiate between FMD-virus-infected and -vaccinated animals had not been developed or approved. Hence, if they could not rapidly identify the problem nor differentiate between a vaccinated or infected animal they were precluded from utilizing measures that employ these techniques. When all was said and done, nearly 10,000 premises were affected and more than 8 million animals destroyed.

☐ ☐ ☐ ▬▬▬▬▬▬▬▬▬▬▬▬▬▬▬▬▬▬▬▬▬▬▬▬▬▬▬▬▬▬▬▬▬▬▬▬

Final Tally from the 2001 FMD Outbreak in the United Kingdom

No. premises where animals destroyed	9,996
Animals slaughtered or culled in epidemic control measures	4,080,001
Killed in animal welfare disposal schemes	2,573,317
Piglets, calves, and lambs killed (estimated)	2,000,000
Total of animals killed	8,653,318

Source: U.K. Department for Environment, Food and Rural Affairs, 2002.

▬▬▬▬▬▬▬▬▬▬▬▬▬▬▬▬▬▬▬▬▬▬▬▬▬▬▬▬▬▬▬▬▬▬▬▬ ☐ ☐ ☐

This classic case study of an outbreak of a foreign animal disease emphasizes many points on the breadth, depth, and scope of the problem. As stated earlier, FMD is a fast-moving contagion with devastating consequences. That, coupled with a slow-moving response, led to an all too predictable outcome. Prime Minister Tony Blair faced great adversity in his 10 years in office. The FMD outbreak was one of his nation's most challenging problems in the past 40 years. Amazingly, it caused the delay of a general election; something that had not occurred since World War II. Following the resolution of the crisis, Blair announced a reorganization of several government departments. This move by Blair was largely due to the perceived failure of the Ministry of Agriculture, Fisheries and Food to respond to the FMD outbreak quickly and effectively. The ministry was merged with elements of the Department of the Environment, Transport and the Regions to form the current department, Department for Environment, Food and Rural Affairs (DEFRA). Public reaction to the draconian measures needed for containment plus the long-term disruption felt by the cattle industry nearly brought the regime to its knees. The total loss to the economy was estimated at $20 billion. Many farmers lost their entire herds and, with it, their livelihood. Tourism was one of the industries most affected by the response to FMD in rural areas. An unforeseen outcome of the outbreak was a significant number of suicides (estimated at 85) associated with the depopulation and carcass disposal efforts. This fact emphasizes the importance of psychological first aid that should be incorporated into response and recovery operations. Animal health professionals, government officials, and animal owners are dramatically affected by the difficulty of slaughtering so many animals.

Highly Pathogenic Avian Influenza, 1983–2007

Economic losses from avian influenza vary depending on the strain of virus, species of bird infected, number of farms involved, use of control methods, and speed of implementation of control or eradication strategies. Direct losses include depopulation and disposal costs, high morbidity and mortality losses, quarantine and surveillance costs, and indemnities paid for elimination of birds. Avian influenza outbreaks have caused significant economic losses. A 1983 outbreak of HPAI (H5N2) in the northeastern United States resulted in losses of nearly $65 million, the destruction of more than 17 million birds, and a 30% increase in egg prices. During a 1999 outbreak of HPAI (H7N1) in Italy, the government paid farmers more than $100 million in compensation for 18 million birds; total indirect losses were estimated at $500 million.

Although HPAI strains of type A influenza virus do not typically infect humans, the first instance of direct bird-to-human spread of influenza A (H5N1) virus was documented during an outbreak of avian influenza among poultry in Hong Kong in 1997. The virus caused severe respiratory illness in 18 people, of whom 6 died (Horimoto and Kawaoka, 2001). Since that time, more than 300 cases of H5N1 infection in humans have been confirmed. The resultant 1997 outbreak of HPAI (H5N1) in the Hong Kong live poultry market cost $13 million for depopulation efforts and indemnities for the 1.4 million birds that were slaughtered. In 2001, there was a recurrence of H5N1 in Hong Kong, which cost $3.8 million to control; a total of 1.2 million birds were destroyed.

During August–October 2004, sporadic human cases of avian influenza A (H5N1) were reported in Vietnam and Thailand. In February 2005, human cases of H5N1 infection from Cambodia were reported. In July of the same year, human cases of H5N1 were reported from Indonesia. Since then, Indonesia has continued to report human cases and small outbreaks in birds. Currently, Indonesia has the most number of human cases of H5N1 infection and associated deaths (World Health Organization, 2007).

During the spring and summer 2002, an outbreak of LPAI H7N2 virus infected 210 flocks of chickens and turkeys in Virginia, West Virginia, and North Carolina, causing the destruction of nearly 5 million birds. Although no epidemiologic link was established, the virus was related to the LPAI H7N2 virus circulating in the live bird market system since 1994 (Senne, 2007). An avian influenza task force, composed of industry, state, and federal personnel, was utilized in the control program. Task force commanders emphasized the use of good safety and biosecurity practices. Carcass disposal options, which included burial in sanitary landfills, incineration, and composting, proved to be problematic and caused delays in depopulation of infected premises. Surveillance activities focused on once-a-week testing of dead birds from all premises, biweekly testing of all breeder flocks, and premovement testing. Additional surveillance carried out in backyard flocks and local waterfowl did not detect the H7 virus or specific antibodies to the virus. The outbreak emphasized the need to establish effective biosecurity barriers between the live bird market system and commercial poultry. A total of 197 flocks, representing approximately 20% of the 1,000 area commercial poultry farms, were infected with the H7N2 virus. Approximately 4.7 million birds, or 8.4% of the estimated 56 million birds at risk, were destroyed to control the outbreak. Turkeys accounted for 78% of the positive farms and included 28 turkey breeder flocks and 125 commercial meat-turkey flocks. Twenty-nine chicken broiler breeder flocks, 13 chicken broiler flocks, and 2 of the 3 chicken egg-layer flocks were also infected. In addition to the infected flocks in Virginia, one flock in West Virginia was infected with the H7N2 virus (Akey, 2003). The poultry industries in Virginia and West Virginia are contiguous, and it is suspected the disease was introduced into West Virginia from Virginia. Although the USDA approved the use of an H7N2 vaccine, it was not used in this outbreak because its use was controversial in the industry.

As just stated, the source of infection for the index flock was never established. However, the H7N2 strain responsible for this outbreak was shown to be genetically identical to the strain that had previously caused outbreaks in Pennsylvania and the strain that has been found in the live bird market system in the northeast United States since 1994. Federal compensation payments totaling $52.65 million were paid to growers and owners for the birds that were destroyed and for cost of bird disposal. The payments were made based on 75% of the appraised market value of the birds. An additional $13.5 million was spent on operational expenses for the outbreak task force. However, figures upward of $149 million have been used to reflect the total negative impact of the outbreak on the poultry industry and allied industries (Akey, 2003).

In 2003, the European Union reported an outbreak of H7N7, which resulted in the destruction of over 33 million birds: 30 million birds in the Netherlands (one quarter of the country's poultry stock), 2.7 million in Belgium, and 400,000 in Germany. The total costs of this outbreak are unknown (Stegeman et al., 2004).

To date, all outbreaks of HPAI in domestic poultry have been caused by H5 or H7 influenza A subtypes. Until 1999, HPAI was considered relatively rare, with only 17 outbreaks reported worldwide between 1959 and 1998; however, since 1999, the number of outbreaks occurring globally has increased significantly (Capua and Marangon, 2006). Major outbreaks of avian influenza are highlighted in Table 9-3.

Classical Swine Fever

Throughout history, swine production in many countries has suffered from outbreaks of CSF. This acute, viral disease was first recognized in the 1860s. In the United Kingdom, the disease went unchecked until 1878, when legislation for its control was introduced (U.K. Department for Environment, Food and Rural Affairs, 2007). The disease persisted for many years until it was finally eradicated from Great Britain in 1966. Much the same can be said for the status of this disease in the United States, where it was eliminated in 1963. Since that time, there were sporadic outbreaks in the United Kingdom in 1971 and 1986 (Moennig, 2000). See Figure 9-3.

However, a more serious outbreak affecting 16 farms in the United Kingdom occurred in August 2000. A total of 74,793 pigs, including those on contact farms, were slaughtered to eradicate the disease. The cause of this outbreak was never firmly established but was most likely due to pigs consuming contaminated imported pork products (U.K. Department for Environment, Food and Rural Affairs, 2007).

Mad Cow Disease (Bovine Spongiform Encephalopathy)

On December 23, 2003, officials from the USDA and Food and Drug Administration (FDA) were alerted to the first case of BSE in the United States (U.S. Department of Agriculture, 2003b). The affected cow was a dairy cow born in Canada and imported into Washington state. The cow had been slaughtered two weeks earlier and the meat and by-products from the animal traveled the normal slaughtering path: The edible parts went to meat processors for making into hamburgers and steaks, while the inedible parts went to renderers to grind into meal for animal feed and fat for soap and other products. The brain went to a USDA laboratory in Ames, Iowa, for BSE testing. Once informed that the tissue from the cow had tested positive, the FDA took immediate action, mobilizing teams of investigators in the agency's Seattle district. The FDA, along with the USDA, had to ensure recovery and destruction of as many parts of the infected cow as possible (Matthews et al., 2006). Naturally, this report generated a great deal of media attention and caused numerous nations to impose a ban on the importation of U.S. beef until the origin and extent of the outbreak could be determined. The USDA worked tirelessly to retrieve the contaminated products and determined that the cow had been brought into the United States from Canada, most likely from Alberta, where another BSE-positive cow had been found earlier that year

Table 9-3 Major Outbreaks of Avian Influenza in Domestic Poultry in the Past 25 Years

Year	Subtype	Location	Impact	Notes
1983	H5	Pennsylvania	Caused severe clinical disease and high mortality rates in chickens, turkeys, and guinea fowl; 17 million birds culled	A serologically identical but apparently mild virus had been circulating in poultry in the area for 6 months; no human cases were identified
1994–2003	H5N2	Mexico	Nearly a billion birds were affected	An LPAI virus mutated to an HPAI virus and caused an outbreak in 1994–1995; the H5N2 strain has continued to circulate in Mexico since then; no human cases have been identified
1995–2003	H7N3	Pakistan	About 3.2 million birds died from avian influenza during the initial outbreak in 1995	A vaccination campaign apparently ended the outbreak; no human cases were identified
1997	H5N1	Hong Kong	Virus isolated from chickens; avian mortality rates were high; 1.5 million birds culled in three days.	18 human cases with 6 deaths recognized; prior to this outbreak, H5N1 was not known to infect humans
2003	H7N7	The Netherlands	30 million birds out of 100 million birds were killed; 255 flocks were infected	Over 80 human cases reported and one veterinarian died; most of the human cases involved conjunctivitis
2003–2007 (ongoing)	H5N1	Asia, Europe, Africa	By far the most severe outbreak of avian influenza ever recognized; an estimated 220 million birds have died or been culled	More than 330 human cases recognized, with more than half of them fatal, in Azerbaijan, Cambodia, China, Djibouti, Egypt, Indonesia, Iraq, Lao People's Democratic Republic, Nigeria, Thailand, Turkey, and Vietnam
2004	H7N3	British Columbia	Over 19 million birds culled	Two human cases recognized; both patients had conjunctivitis
2005	H7	North Korea	About 200,000 birds culled as of April 2005	No human cases identified

Source: Center for Infectious Disease Research and Policy, available at www.cidrap.umn.edu/cidrap/content/biosecurity/ag-biosec/anim-disease/aflu.html#_Key_Outbreaks_of.

(U.S. Department of Agriculture, 2004). Eventually, this managed to quell fears of the public and beef producers and allowed for a gradual restoration of beef exportation.

In August 2005, the second BSE infected cow in the United States was found in the state of Texas (U.S. Department of Agriculture, 2005). Unlike the Washington cow, this

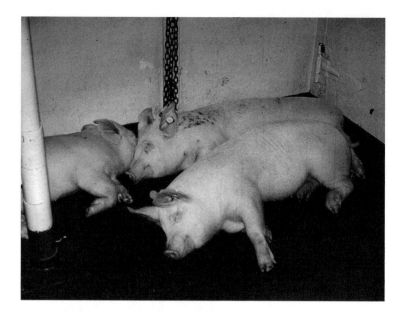

FIGURE 9-3 Pigs acutely affected with classical swine fever. These animals experience inappetence, severe depression, high fever, purple discoloration of the skin, diarrhea, vomiting, coughing, hind limb weakness, and ocular discharge. (Image courtesy of Plum Island Animal Disease Center, USDA, Agricultural and Research Service, and Department of Homeland Security.)

one was born in the United States prior to the 1997 feed ban. Despite a thorough investigation, no other positive animals could be located. The origin of infection was never determined; although animal health officials theorize that this cow probably was infected from contaminated feed.

In February 2006, the third BSE infected cow in the United States was found in the state of Alabama. In this instance, a cattle producer contacted his herd veterinarian to report that he had a downer cow. The veterinarian took the appropriate samples and notified the state veterinarian's office. A few days later, the sample was taken to the Georgia Veterinary Medical Diagnostic Laboratory. The laboratory tested the sample and got an inconclusive result based on a standard screening test. This prompted officials to issue a national press release and send the sample on for definitive testing. Several days later, the National Veterinary Services Laboratory in Ames, Iowa, completed definitive testing on the tissues and confirmed the second native case of BSE in the United States. A press release was issued on the same day, announcing the findings. Despite a thorough investigation of two farms that were known to contain the index cow and numerous others that might have supplied the index cow to the farms where the index case was known to have resided, the investigators were unable to locate the herd of origin (U.S. Department of Agriculture, 2006).

Protecting the Food Chain from BSE

All **downer cows** (live cows unable to walk) presented for slaughter are now banned from the human food chain. Any cattle suspected of having BSE (adults with neurological conditions) are held and not disposed of until results of BSE tests are confirmed. Specified risk material is prohibited from the human food chain (e.g., skull, brain, trigeminal ganglia, eyes, vertebral column, spinal cord, and dorsal root ganglia of cattle over 30 months of age). Additionally, the distal ileum and tonsils from cattle of any age are prohibited. Process quality control testing has been expanded to detect dorsal root ganglia and skull, as well as spinal cord tissue in processed-meat products. The use of air-injection stunning of cattle at slaughter has been prohibited to reduce the potential of contaminating carcasses with brain tissue.

The best way to protect cattle and humans from BSE in a given geographic location is to prevent exposure of susceptible populations to the agent. The United States is taking measures to prevent the introduction and or limit the spread of BSE (Food Safety and Inspection Service, 2004). The following measures are in effect:

- Banning importation of cattle from BSE-affected countries.
- Banning use of bovine-origin products.
- A comprehensive exam of all animals showing central nervous system signs.
- Specific label instructions that beef and dairy producers must follow when mixing feed, keeping records of all actions.
- A national animal identification system to be implemented at an accelerated rate.

Additional precautions include prohibition by the Food and Drug Administration of the use of most mammalian protein in ruminant feeds (except tallow, blood meal, and gelatin). This rule affects less than 200 rendering plants in the United States and requires a system to prevent commingling of by-products at abattoirs, as well as approved labeling and record keeping. The presence of BSE in developed countries has been an explosive issue. The threat or proclamation that it had been introduced would be enough to create a degree of disruption, economically or emotionally.

The Future of Animal Diseases

What does the future hold for animal diseases? Sociologists predict that, as the world population increases over the next 20 years, more people will reside in urban settings (from 43–60%). Sociologists also predict that there will continue to be a shift from poverty. This coupled with the Westernization of Asia suggests greater demand for protein and food from animal sources. With these trends, there is also likely to be greater reliance on confined animal feeding operations, much like what has occurred throughout North America and Europe. Therefore, acts of terrorism targeting the agricultural community could be more devastating to economies and have far greater consequences for human health. This is particularly important if the disease agent involved affects both animals and humans. Furthermore, natural and accidental outbreaks involving zoonoses may be more devastating. Regardless of the source, protecting our agricultural assets from zoonoses and FAD will be essential to our quality of life.

Conclusion

Reliance on beef, poultry, and pork has become a mainstay of Western civilization. An outbreak of FMD could cripple these industries. Classical swine fever is potentially devastating to the pork industry. Animal disease outbreaks may occur for a number of reasons. The origin of the outbreak could be natural, accidental, or intentional. Foreign animal diseases are particularly serious problems since recognition of those diseases may not be as acute among animal health practitioners and there is unlikely to be any herd immunity in the susceptible population of animals.

The 2001 foot-and-mouth disease outbreak in the United Kingdom provides evidence of the devastating effects of widespread FAD introductions. When finally brought under control, nearly 8 million cattle had been slaughtered with an estimated cost of $20 billion. More telling were the societal effects. A national election was postponed, the ministry of agriculture was completely restructured, and British meat exports were severely restricted.

Poultry is taking a heavy hit from HPAI due to H5N1 infection. The disease has now spread to more than 60 countries in a 10-year period since it first emerged in Hong Kong. Furthermore, the confirmed cases of H5N1 in humans has produced a case fatality rate of more than 60%, indicating that the problem still poses a threat and may potentially spark an influenza pandemic should the strain become more adapted to humans.

Mad cow disease threatens the beef industry and has serious implications for human health. This cryptic and debilitating disease affects cattle and human hosts in much the same way, with a long incubation period and no treatment. Officials in the United Kingdom have been battling the presence of BSE in their nation since 1997. Three small incidences in the United States with BSE mobilized the government on many levels to identify the problem and investigate the origin. Had the problem been widespread, the beef industry in the United States would have been affected for many years to come.

Essential Terminology

- **Avian influenza.** Also called *fowl plague*, *avian flu*, and *bird flu*. A highly contagious viral disease caused by influenza A virus with up to 100% mortality in domestic fowl. It is subclassified into highly pathogenic avian influenza (HPAI) and low pathogenic avian influenza (LPAI). HPAI is caused by virus subtypes H5 and H7. All types of birds are susceptible to the virus but outbreaks occur most often in chickens and turkeys.

- **Bovine spongiform encephalopathy (BSE).** Also referred to as *mad cow disease*, a fatal disease of cattle that affects the central nervous system, causing staggering and agitation. BSE is caused by a prion, which is an infectious protein particle.

- **Classical swine fever (CSF).** Also referred to as *hog cholera*. CSF is a highly contagious viral disease of swine that occurs in an acute, subacute, chronic, or persistent form. In the acute form, the disease is characterized by high fever, severe depression, multiple superficial and internal hemorrhages, and high morbidity and mortality.

- **Downer cow.** A live cow that cannot walk. This state can be caused by disease or injury. In nearly all cases it is considered by most farmers to be both humane and cost effective to slaughter the animal when it becomes a downer, rather than keep it alive and unhealthy.

- **Foot-and-mouth disease.** A highly contagious viral infection primarily of cloven-hoofed domestic animals (cattle, pigs, sheep, goats, and water buffalo) and cloven-hoofed wild animals. The disease is characterized by fever and vesicles, with subsequent erosions in the mouth, nasal passages, muzzle, feet, or teats.

Discussion Questions

- Why is it likely that future human civilizations will become ever more dependent on inexpensively produced animal protein?
- Compare and contrast the four foreign animal diseases discussed in this chapter with relation to
  - What agent caused each outbreak?
  - How quickly did the problem spread?
- How might the concept RAIN apply to these outbreaks? Construct a table similar to the one in Chapter 7.
- What were the implications for human health in each of the outbreak situations?
- What would be the affects to the economy should an outbreak like one of these occur locally? Also, determine the role of local responders.

Suggested Reading

2001 FMD United Kingdom Outbreak Summary of Findings, a comprehensive web page with numerous links to reports and fact sheets, available at www.defra.gov.uk/animalh/diseases/fmd/2001/index.htm.

U.S. Department of Agriculture, Foreign Agriculture Service, BSE Page (contains numerous reports), available at www.fas.usda.gov/dlp/BSE/bse.html#U.S.%20Reports/Reference%20Documents.

Public Health Considerations in the Application of Measures to Contain and Control Highly World Health Organization, Regional Office for the Western Pacific, Manila Philippines, April 26, 2004, Pathogenic Avian Influenza (HPAI) Outbreaks in Poultry, available at www.wpro.who.int/NR/rdonlyres/23C21802-A0BE-42B9-825F-18977C05EE58/0/Advice30042004.pdf.

Web Sites

USDA APHIS, available at www.aphis.usda.gov.

U.K. Department for Environment, Food and Rural Affairs (DEFRA) , available at www.defra.gov.uk.

Food and Agriculture Organization of the United Nations, available at www.fao.org.

The Gray Book: Foreign Animal Diseases, available at www.vet.uga.edu/vpp/gray_book02.

World Organization for Animal Health (OIE), available at www.oie.int/eng/en_index.htm.

World Health Organization. Geographical spread of H5N1 avian influenza in birds, available at www.who.int/csr/don/2005_08_18/en/print.html.

References

Akey, B. L. 2003. Low-pathogenicity H7N2 avian influenza outbreak in Virgnia during 2002. *Avian Diseases* 47:1099–1103.

Armstrong, R., N. Cairns, J. Ironside, et al. 2003. Does the neuropathology of human patients with variant Creutzfeldt-Jakob disease reflect hematogenous spread of the disease? *Neuroscience Letters* 348:37–40.

American Veterinary Medical Association. 2006a. Classical swine fever. *AVMA Backgrounder* (December 10), available at www.avma.org/reference/backgrounders/classical_swine_bgnd.asp.

American Veterinary Medical Association. 2006b. Bovine spongiform encephalopathy. *AVMA Backgrounder* (March 27), available at www.avma.org/reference/backgrounders/bse_bgnd.asp.

American Veterinary Medical Association. 2006c. Avian influenza. *AVMA Backgrounder* (September 6), available at www.avma.org/reference/backgrounders/avinf_bgnd.asp.

American Veterinary Medical Association. 2007. Foot and mouth disease. *AVMA Backgrounder* (February 14), available at www.avma.org/reference/backgrounders/fmd_bgnd.asp.

Bacchetti, P. 2003. Age and variant Creutzfeldt-Jakob disease. *Emerging Infectious Diseases* 9, no. 12 (December):1611–1612.

Bartley, L., C. Donnelly, and R. Anderson. 2002. Review of foot-and-mouth disease virus survival in animal excretions and on fomites. *Veterinary Record* 151:667–669.

Bauer, K. 1997. Foot-and-mouth disease as a zoonosis. *Annual Review Microbiology* 22:201–244.

Beard, C. 1998. Avian influenza (fowl plague). In: *The Gray Book: Foreign Animal Diseases*, 6th ed., by U.S. Animal Health Association, Committee on Foreign Animal Disease. Richmond, VA: Pat Campbell & Associates and Carter Printing Company.

Beisel, C., and D. Morens. 2004. Variant Creutzfeldt-Jakob disease (vCJD) and the acquired and transmissible spongiform encephalopathies. *Clinical Infectious Diseases* 38, no. 5 (March 1): 697–704.

Brown, P., R. G. Will, R. Bradley, et al. 2001. Bovine spongiform encephalopathy and variant Creutzfeldt-Jakob disease: Background, evolution, and current concerns. *Emerging Infectious Diseases* 7, no. 1 (January–February): 6–16.

Callis, J., and P. McKercher. 1977. Dissemination of foot-and-mouth disease virus through animal products. In: *Proceedings of the 11th International Meeting on Foot-and-Mouth Disease and Zoonosis Control*. Washington, DC: Pan American Health Organization.

Capua, I., and S. Marangon. 2006. Control of avian influenza in poultry. *Emerging Infectious Diseases* 12:1319–1324.

Croes, E., and C. van Duijn. 2003. Variant Creutzfeldt-Jakob disease. *European Journal of Epidemiology* 18:473–477.

Davies, G. 2002. The foot and mouth disease (FMD) epidemic in the United Kingdom 2001. *Comprehensive Immunology of Microbiological Infectious Diseases* 25, nos. 5–6:331–343.

DeArmond, S. J., and S. B. Prusiner. 1995. Etiology and pathogenesis of prion diseases. *American Journal of Pathology* 146, no. 4:785–811.

Dewulf, J., H. Laevens, F. Koenen, et al. 2000. Airborne transmission of classical swine fever under experimental conditions. *Veterinary Record* 147, no. 26 (December): 735–738.

Edwards, S. 1998. Hog cholera. In: *A Merck Veterinary Manual*, 8th ed., ed. S. Aeillo.Whitehouse Station, NJ: Merck & Company.

Food Safety and Inspection Service. 2004. USDA issues new regulations to address BSE, effective January 12, 2004, available at www.fsis.usda.gov/oa/news/2004/bseregs.htm.

Goldberg, A. L. 2007. On prions, proteasomes, and mad cows. *New England Journal of Medicine* 357, no. 11 (September 13):1150–1152.

Horimoto, T., and Y. Kawaoka. 2001. Pandemic threat posed by avian influenza A viruses. *Clinical Microbiological Review* 14:129–149.

House, J., and C. A. Mebus. 1998. Foot-and-mouth disease. In: *The Gray Book: Foreign Animal Diseases*, 6th ed., by U.S. Animal Health Association, Committee on Foreign Animal Disease. Richmond, VA: Pat Campbell & Associates and Carter Printing Company.

Hueston, W., and C. Bryant. 2005. Understanding BSE and related diseases. *Food Technology* 59, no. 7 (July):46–51.

Hughes, G. J., V. Mioulet, R. P. Kitching, et al. 2002. Foot-and-mouth disease virus infection of sheep: Implications for diagnosis and control. *Veterinary Record* 150, no. 23 (June 8):724–727.

Kleiboeker, S. 2002. Swine fever: Classical swine fever and African swine fever. *Veterinary Clinics of North America: Food Animal Practice* 18:431–451.

Lubroth, J. 2002. Foot and mouth disease: A review for the practitioner. *Veterinary Clinics of North America: Food Animal Practice* 18, no. 3:475–499.

Matthews, K. H., M. Vandeveer, and R. A. Gustafson. 2006. *An Economic Chronology of Bovine Spongiform Encephalopathy in North America*. From USDA Economic Research Service, June.

Moennig, V. 2000. Introduction to classical swine fever: Virus, disease and control policy. *Veterinary Microbiology* 73:93–102.

OIE (World Organization for Animal Health). 2007. *List of FMD Free Countries*, available at www.oie.int/eng/info/en_fmd.htm?eld6#Liste.

Paarlberg, P. L., J. G. Lee, and A. H. Seitzinger. 2002. Potential revenue impact of an outbreak of foot-and-mouth disease in the United States. *Journal of the American Veterinary Medical Association* 220, no. 7 (April 1):988–992.

Prusiner, S. 1998. Prions. *Proceedings of the National Academy of Science* 95:13363–13383.

Sellers, R., K. Herniman, and I. Gumm. 1977. The airborne dispersal of foot-and-mouth disease virus from vaccinated and recovered pigs, cattle and sheep after exposure to infection. *Research in the Veterinary Sciences* 23:70–75.

Senne, D. 2007. Avian influenza in North and South America, 2002–2005. *Avian Diseases* 51:167–173.

Smith, P., and R. Bradley. 2003. Bovine spongiform encephalopathy (BSE) and its epidemiology. *British Medical Bulletin* 66:185–198.

Stallknecht, D. E., S. M. Shane, M. T. Kearney, et al. 1990. Persistence of avian influenza viruses in water. *Avian Diseases* 34, no. 2 (April–June):406–411.

Stegeman, A., A. Bouma, A. R. W. Elbers, et al. 2004. Avian influenza A virus (H7N7) epidemic in the Netherlands in 2003: Course of the epidemic and effectiveness of control measures. *Journal of Infectious Diseases* 190 (December 15):2088–2095.

U.K. Department for Environment, Food and Rural Affairs. 2002. Official Report (June 2002): Origin of the UK Foot and Mouth Disease Epidemic in 2001, available at www.defra.gov.uk/animalh/diseases/fmd/pdf/fmdorigins1.pdf.

U.K. Department for Environment, Food and Rural Affairs. 2007/ FMD United Kingdom DEFRA Outbreak Report: Independent Review of the Safety of UK Facilities Handling Foot and Mouth Disease Virus, available at www.defra.gov.uk/FootandMouth/investigations/pdf/spratt_final.pdf.

UN Food and Agriculture Organization. 2007. FMD Overview, available at www.foa.org/ag/aga/agah/empres/gemp/avis/a010-fmd/index.html.

U.S. Department of Agriculture. 2002. National Emergency Management Association. *Model Emergency Support Function for Production Agriculture, Animal and Animal Industry*. Washington, DC: Government Printing Office.

U.S. Department of Agriculture. 2003a. Animal and Plant Health Inspection Service, Veterinary Services Unit, *Response Strategies: Highly Contagious Diseases*. Washington, DC: Government Printing Office.

U.S. Department of Agriculture. 2003b. USDA Makes Preliminary Diagnosis of BSE. Press Release No. 0432.03, available at www.usda.gov/wps/portal/!ut/p/_s.7_0_A/7_0_1OB/.cmd/ad/.ar/sa.retrievecontent/.c/6_2_1UH/.ce/7_2_5JM/.p/5_2_4TQ/.d/8/_th/J_2_9D/_s.7_0_A/7_0_1OB?PC_7_2_5JM_contentid=2003/12/0432. html&PC_7_2_5JM_navtype=RT&PC_7_2_5JM_parent nav= LATEST_RELEASES&P.

United States Department of Agriculture. 2004. BSE chronology, available at www.usda.gov/wps/portal/!ut/p/_s.7_0_A/7_0_1OB/.cmd/ad/.ar/sa.retrievecontent/.c/6_2_1UH/.ce/7_2_5JM/.p/5_2_4TQ/.d/2/_th/J_2_9D/_s.7_0_A/7_0_1OB?PC_7_2_5JM_contentid=bse_chrono.xml#7_2_5JM.

U.S. Department of Agriculture. 2005. Investigation results of Texas cow that tested positive for bovine spongiform encephalopathy (BSE). Press Release No. 0336.05, available at www.usda.gov/wps/portal/!ut/p/_s.7_0_A/7_0_1OB?contentidonly=true&contentid=2005/08/0336.xml.

U.S. Department of Agriculture. 2006. Animal and Plant Health Inspection Service. Alabama BSE investigation, final report, 2006, available at www.aphis.usda.gov/newsroom/hot_issues/bse/content/printable_version/EPI_Final.pdf.

Voyles, B. A. 2002. Orthomyxoviruses. In: *The Biology of Viruses*, 2d ed., p. 147. New York: McGraw-Hill.

World Health Organization. 2007. Cumulative confirmed human cases of H5N1 avian influenza, available at www.who.int/csr/disease/avian_influenza/country/en.

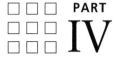

PART

IV

Initiatives, Issues, Assets, and Programs

Presently, one of the most frightening scenarios is a biological agent attack on unprotected civilians, resulting in great death and illness. Of all possible weapons of mass destruction, biological weapons are probably the most feared by government officials. This is likely due to their assessment that their communities are woefully unprepared to deal with them. The potential destructiveness of a biological attack can come in many forms and would be very difficult to detect and control. The unleashing of biological agents against an unprotected civilian population portends the ultimate medical disaster, with the capacity to completely overwhelm a community's health care system. Patients and the worried nonpatients would report to health-care facilities in unprecedented numbers. Demand for intensive and critical care would likely exceed available medical resources. Accurately defining the threat of biological weapons and determining appropriate responses to them are critical if we are to prevent the potentially devastating effects of bioterrorism. Awareness, our first challenge, centers on Recognizing that an act of bioterrorism has already happened. Response functions must included Avoidance, Isolation, and Notification procedures. In a very simplistic fashion, RAIN allows responders to approach the problem safely and protect the public they serve. However, the problems go far beyond this, and higher-level functions will be necessary to proactively detect the release of a biological agent and apply the appropriate resources in an efficient and effective manner to contain the outbreak. Clearly, local governments cannot muster the resources to respond and recover from a large-scale outbreak. National programs and strategies are needed to make these strides.

Part I of this book laid a foundation of knowledge on the threat of biological agents, the history of biowarfare, and the evolution of biodefense. *Biodefense* refers to short-term, local, usually military measures to restore security from biological threats to a given group of persons in a given area. In civilian terminology, *biodefense* may be considered a robust biohazard response. It is technically possible to apply biodefense measures to protect animals or plants, but this would not be economical. Over the years, biodefense measures have transcended into biosecurity programs. Biosecurity is the protection of people, animals, agriculture, and ecological systems against disease and other biological threats. Part II detailed the current threat to human health as related to us by Health and Human Services Categories A, B, and C. Part III explained the importance of agriculture and the threat from natural, accidental, and intentionally introduced disease to crops and animals. In this part, we cover initiatives, issues, assets, and programs that address the threat of biological agents through biosecurity. Each of these parts could have been a tome; the subject matter of each chapter a book in itself.

Chapter 10 explores some of the legal aspects of biosecurity. At the international level, there are agreements and treaties to consider. At the national level, there has been recent legislation worth note and a series of presidential directives that now guide biosecurity and biodefense programs. Chapter 11 examines numerous considerations for preparedness and response to an act of bioterrorism at the state and local levels.

Chapter 12 delves into federal government initiatives and programs that are related to enhancing biosecurity in the United States. The focus of Chapter 12 is strictly on biosecurity. Details for modern-day biodefense systems are shrouded sufficiently in secrecy; therefore, this book does not examine some recent developments within the U.S. Department of Defense or its allies. What is available in the public domain on these systems would merely present a very sketchy picture of what they were designed to do, what they are capable of, and what their limitations might be. Chapter 13 concerns the principle of consequence management and autonomous detection systems. As such, the United States Postal Service has installed the biohazard detection system. This system and the program that has been built around it represent a model biosecurity system. To appreciate this, great detail concerning the system's requirements, specifications, and validation scheme have been detailed there. Finally, Chapter 14 discusses future trends in biosecurity and directions being taken for biodefense research.

10

Legal Aspects of Biosecurity

When bad men combine, the good must associate; else they will fall one by one, an unpitied sacrifice in a contemptible struggle.
—Edmund Burke

Objectives

The study of this chapter will enable you to

1. Discuss the definitions of *terrorism* and *weapons of mass destruction* and their relation to the illicit use of biological agents.
2. List all legislative and administrative documents that address the legal aspects of the unlawful use of biological agents.
3. Discuss the prohibited uses of biological agents under United States law.
4. Discuss the prohibited uses of biological agents under international law.
5. List and briefly discuss the homeland security presidential directives that apply to biosecurity and biodefense.

Key Terms

Biological agent, biological toxin, delivery system, vector, terrorism, weapon of mass destruction, declaration, quarantine, isolation.

Introduction

Biodefense programs and initiatives have been with us since World War II. These programs were developed out of a need to counter the threat from our enemies and protect military forces and the homeland from biological attack. Biosecurity, on the other hand, is a more recent development, made up of policies and measures designed to protect the homeland, food supply, and agricultural resources from natural and accidental outbreaks and bioterrorism attacks. Many of the recent initiatives in biodefense and biosecurity came after the fall of the Soviet Union, as officials from NATO countries worried about the potential for Soviet biological weapons falling into the wrong hands. In the United States, the Clinton administration took a fairly proactive stance toward biological threat reduction. The events of 9/11 and the Amerithrax incident further solidified national resolve against weapons of mass destruction and acts of terrorism.

Politicians have felt the pressure from strong public reaction to recent acts of bioterrorism. Many articles and speeches emphasized the potential for devastating outbreaks from emerging and reemerging pathogens. Government officials had to act decisively in order to quell fears from the public and instill or renew trust in government. We can all appreciate the need to protect livestock and cash crops, which could prevent huge losses to the economy. Since the 1984 Rajneeshee incident in Oregon, lawmakers moved to enact legislation designed to define the illegality of the ill-intended use, production, dissemination, or storage of biological agents (Miller, Engelberg, and Broad, 2001).

The United States works from a federal system with two levels of government: the federal government, which exercises the powers of the U.S. Constitution; and state governments, which exercise the rights that they withheld from the federal government as sovereign states. State governments retain their basic police power. Our federal system allows for parallel tracks of the legal system on the local, state, and federal levels. The most important specific powers of the federal government are those that regulate interstate and foreign commerce, the power to provide for the national defense, and the right to tax the people and spend revenues collected for the public welfare. States and local government entities use their power to exercise their responsibility to protect the public health and safety.

Federal laws authorized by the U.S. Constitution became the "law of the land" and are binding even in the face of state laws that may be inconsistent with them. In many instances, both state and federal laws address the same issue. Statutes enact the laws that are to be followed by the executive branch and enforced by the courts at the state or federal level. In areas where there has been no legislative enactment, courts in the United States follow the legal precedents established over the years and born out of decisions related to particular controversies. Administrative agencies at both levels of government draft regulations that are legally binding and aim to apply the law to even more specific situations. At the local level, ordinances are promulgated and act as regulations within specific local municipalities. Ordinances are adopted under powers delegated from the state and establish rules applicable within the jurisdiction of the municipality that create them.

Executive orders, from either the president or a governor, are primarily regarded as directions from the head of each level of government to the officers and employees of federal and state government, respectively. As an example, the president's "declaration of emergency" is a form of executive order. Directives, such as a national security presidential directive (NSPD) or homeland security presidential directive (HSPD) are executive orders at the federal level. These directives cannot change the "law of the land," as required by the U.S. Constitution or statutes. Instead, they are intended to *direct* officers of the federal government to apply and exercise whatever discretion they may have under the rule of law in a particular fashion. These directives are important tools in creating new programs, announcing initiatives, and addressing national concerns during times of need or crisis.

□ □ □

The Law

Law is a prediction of what a court will do when faced with a particular set of facts.
—Oliver Wendell Holmes

□ □ □

This chapter seeks to identify many of the administrative aspects of biodefense and biosecurity. That is, international bodies and government at all levels have had to address the threat of biological agents, whether in a military context or civilian setting. The aim of this chapter is to discuss the most relevant treaties, laws, statutes, regulations, directives, and government directives aimed at reducing the biological threat and deal with those that use biological agents with ill intent. The chapter was not written for legal professionals. Therefore, the material is covered using plain language and in a cursory manner. In many instances, relevant text from the actual documents is used verbatim so that there is no misinterpretation on the part of the author.

In 1989, the United States was engaged on many fronts to ban the use of chemical weapons. That year, the U.S. Congress enacted the Biological Weapons Anti-Terrorism Act. It was modeled after similar legislation found in the United Kingdom, Australia, and New Zealand. Cited as the *Biological Weapons Anti-Terrorism Act of 1989*, the legislation makes it unlawful for "anyone to develop, employ, produce or stockpile any biological material that is intended to cause harm, illness, injury or death." The purpose of the Biological Weapons Anti-Terrorism Act of 1989 is to implement, within the United States, the Biological Weapons Convention (BWC). You may recall from Chapter 1 that the BWC is an international agreement, ratified by the United States Senate in 1974, and signed by more than 100 other nations, including the Soviet Union. The Biological Weapons Anti-Terrorism Act of 1989 was also detailed to protect the United States against the threat of biological terrorism. Nothing in the Biological Weapons Anti-Terrorism Act of 1989 was intended to restrain or restrict peaceful scientific research or development. Chapter 10 of the act, "Biological Weapons," is made up of four sections:

- Prohibitions with respect to biological weapons.
- Seizure, forfeiture, and destruction.
- Injunctions.
- Definitions.

For this text, the most relevant section of the Biological Weapons Anti-Terrorism Act of 1989 is *Section 175, "Prohibitions with Respect to Biological Weapons,"* which specifies that "Whoever knowingly develops, produces, stockpiles, transfers, acquires, retains, or possesses any biological agent, toxin, or delivery system for use as a weapon, or knowingly assists a foreign state or any organization to do so, or attempts, threatens, or conspires to do the same, shall be fined under this title or imprisoned for life or any term of years, or both."

It goes on to say that

Whoever knowingly possesses any biological agent, toxin, or delivery system of a type or in a quantity that, under the circumstances, is not reasonably justified by a prophylactic, protective, bona fide research, or other peaceful purpose, shall be fined under this title, imprisoned not more than 10 years, or both.

In this subsection, the terms **biological agent** and **toxin** do not encompass any biological agent or biological toxin that is in its naturally occurring environment. This means that if the biological agent or toxin "has not been cultivated, collected, or otherwise extracted from its natural source," there may be no violation of law. For purposes of this section, the term *for use as a weapon* includes the development, production, transfer, acquisition, retention, or possession of any biological agent, toxin, or **delivery system** for other than prophylactic, protective, bona fide research, or other peaceful purposes (United States Code; Title 18; Part I: Chapter 10, Section 175).

Terrorism directly threatens the foundations of government order, people, their way of life, and economic prosperity. In the modern world, populations live in densely populated urban areas, making cities conspicuous targets for terrorists WMD attacks. In accordance with United States Code (Title 18; Chapter 113B, Section 2331), **terrorism** is defined as

activities that involve an act dangerous to human life, or potential destruction of critical infrastructure or any key resource, intended to intimidate or coerce the civilian population, or influence a government, or affect a government by mass destruction, assassination, or kidnapping.

As such, acts of terrorism are a violation of the criminal laws of the United States, or any state or other subdivision of the United States in which it occurs. It goes without saying that biological agents are dangerous to life. When biological agents are used to harm or threaten another, the act will surely be classified as an act of terrorism, known as *bioterrorism*. We learned in the previous part that agriculture has been designated as critical infrastructure. Therefore, an act where someone employs a biological agent against the agricultural sector will also be considered an act of terrorism, known as *agroterrorism*.

A follow-up on Chapter 2332a, Section 921 of Title 18 of the aforementioned code defines **weapons of mass destruction** as

- "any explosive, incendiary, or poison gas, bomb, grenade, rocket having a propellant charge of more than four ounces, or missile having an explosive or incendiary charge of more than one-quarter ounce, or mine or similar device."
- "any weapon that is designed or intended to cause death or serious bodily injury through the release, dissemination, or impact of toxic or poisonous chemical or their precursors."
- "any weapon that is designed to release radiation or radioactivity at a level dangerous to human life."
- "any weapon involving a disease organism."

The last point made in that section is apropos to the threat that is the topic of this book. Indeed, what the previous two administrative documents indicate is that the illicit use of biological agents is not only unlawful; it is an act of terrorism and constitutes the use of a weapon of mass destruction. Each of these has ramifications as to how a person or persons may be investigated, charged, tried, prosecuted, and incarcerated. In addition, these terms have implications for government agencies involved in investigative and response functions. So, even the most seemingly small act that involves the unlawful use of a biological agent can bring the entire weight of the federal government down on the head of the offending party.

□ □ □ ▬▬▬▬▬▬▬▬▬▬▬▬▬▬▬▬▬▬▬▬▬▬▬▬▬▬▬▬▬▬▬▬▬▬▬▬

Critical Thinking

Consider a young gang member mashing up a small quantity of castor beans to impress his delinquent friends. Armed with a dozen castor beans and a terrorist cookbook, he generates a crude extract of ricin. He places the extract in a vial and tells his friends that he intends to use it against a rival gang. Two days later, he uses the crude extract in an attempt to poison several gang members. Is this an act of terrorism? Is this the use of a WMD? In accordance with local and state laws, what other infractions might he be charged with?

▬▬▬▬▬▬▬▬▬▬▬▬▬▬▬▬▬▬▬▬▬▬▬▬▬▬▬▬▬▬▬▬▬ □ □ □

Legislation and Presidential Directives

Select Agent Rule and Laboratory Biosecurity[1]

In June 2002, President George W. Bush signed Public Law 107-188, the *Public Health Security and Bioterrorism Preparedness and Response Act of 2002* (see Figure 10-1). The act directs the Secretary of Health and Human Services to establish and maintain a list of biological agents and toxins that have the potential to pose a severe threat to public health and safety ("select agents"). Further, the act requires all facilities and individuals in possession of those same "select agents" to register with HHS. The act created a like program at the USDA, which is being implemented through the Animal and Plant Health Inspection Service.

The Department of Health and Human Services has maintained a list of "select agents" since April 1997. The rule has since been refined and amended with the publication date of March 18, 2005 (42 CFR parts 72 and 73). The rule covers the transfer of select agents, including the registration of facilities engaging in transfers and exemptions from such registration. The intent of P.L. 107-188 was to ensure that the federal government would have visibility for all legitimate uses and inventory of biothreat organisms.

Officials from the Centers for Disease Control assembled an interagency working group to review the original list of biological agents and toxins from October 1997. From this collective wisdom, the working group proposed a revised list of agents, identified minimum quantities of toxins that would require registration, and defined genetic elements requiring regulation. Table 10-1 lists all the select agents.

In August 2002, the CDC published a *Federal Register* notice requiring all facilities in possession of select agents to notify it of their holdings. A form was sent to over

---

[1] This portion of the chapter was excerpted largely from a statement made by The Honorable John H. Marburger, Director, Office of Science and Technology Policy, before the Committee on Science U.S. House of Representatives October 10, 2002.

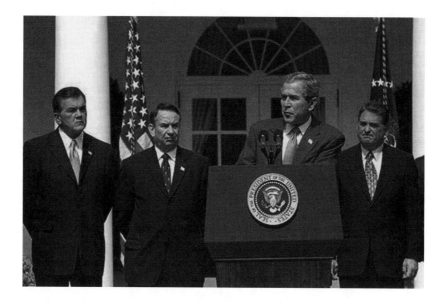

Figure 10-1 "Biological weapons are potentially the most dangerous weapons in the world," said President George W. Bush at the signing of H.R. 3448, the Public Health Security and Bioterrorism Response Act of 2002, in The Rose Garden, Wednesday, June 12. "Last fall's anthrax attacks were an incredible tragedy to a lot of people in America, and it sent a warning that we needed and have heeded. We must be better prepared to prevent, identify and respond. And this bill I'm signing today will help a lot in this essential effort." (Image courtesy of the White House. Photograph by Susan Sterner.)

Table 10-1 Department of Health and Human Services "Select Agents" and Toxins

Abrin	Cercopithecine herpesvirus 1 (Herpes B virus)
Coccidioides posadasii	Conotoxins
Crimean-Congo haemorrhagic fever virus	Diacetoxyscirpenol
Ebola viruses	Lassa fever virus
Marburg virus	Monkeypox virus
Ricin	*Rickettsia prowazekii*
Rickettsia rickettsii	Saxitoxin
Shigalike ribosome inactivating proteins	South American hemorrhagic fever viruses (Junin, Machupo, Sabia, Flexal, Guanarito)
Tetrodotoxin	Tick-borne encephalitis complex (flavi)viruses: Central European tick-borne encephalitis, Far Eastern tick-borne encephalitis (Russian spring and summer encephalitis, Kyasanur Forest disease, Omsk hemorrhagic fever)
Variola major virus (Smallpox virus) and *Variola minor* virus (Alastrim)	*Yersinia pestis*

Note: For purposes of 18 U.S.C. 175b, the list of select agents constitutes the list of select agents and toxins set forth at 42 CFR 73.3 and 73.4. Shown here are those agents specified in 73.3.

200,000 institutions for this purpose, requesting a response, even if the facilities did not possess such agents. The CDC received more than 100,000 responses to the request. Only a small proportion of those respondents declared possession of select agents.

Public Law 107-188 also requires "establishment of safeguard and security measures to prevent access for such agents and toxins for use in domestic or international terrorism or for any other criminal purpose." Therefore, the CDC working group addressed laboratory biosecurity measures, to maintain secure environments in facilities that hold and work with select agents. The fruits of that effort have been published in Appendix F of the *Biosafety in Microbiological and Biomedical Laboratories Manual* (U.S. Department of Health and Human Services, 1999), an online publication maintained by the CDC. Provisions necessary to enhance laboratory biosecurity can vary from one facility to another and depend largely on the principal function, the nature of the agents in use, the conditions for their maintenance (for example, plant or animal pathogens often require facilities different from human pathogens), and vulnerabilities or types of threats most likely to be encountered.

Another key element of P.L. 107-188 is a requirement that individuals deemed to have a legitimate need for access to select agents undergo a background check administered by the Department of Justice. This background check consists of a review of criminal, immigration, national security, and other electronic databases available to the federal government. Institutions possessing select agents are also required to have a comprehensive security plan based on threat analyses and risk assessments.

Government officials never intended that P.L. 107-188 limit the availability of biological agents and toxins for research, education, and other legitimate purposes. However, as one might surmise, the select agent rule introduced bureaucratic procedures and "red tape" into the world of scientific research. The select agent rule was not embraced by all scientists and became the incentive for some to abandon projects or destroy stocks (Cimons, 2005).

□ □ □ ▬▬▬▬▬▬▬▬▬▬▬▬▬▬▬▬▬▬▬▬▬▬▬▬▬▬

The Threat of Bioterrorism

Bioterrorism is a real threat to our country. It's a threat to every nation that loves freedom. Terrorist groups seek biological weapons; we know some rogue states already have them. . . . It's important that we confront these real threats to our country and prepare for future emergencies.
—President George W. Bush, June 12, 2002

▬▬▬▬▬▬▬▬▬▬▬▬▬▬▬▬▬▬▬▬▬▬▬▬▬ □ □ □

Presidential Directives

In the George W. Bush administration, the directives that are used to promulgate presidential decisions on national security matters are designated national security presidential directives. As discussed in NSPD 1, this new category of directives replaces both the presidential decision directives and the presidential review directives of the previous administration. Unless otherwise indicated, past directives remain in effect until they are superseded. The first directive, dated February 13, 2001, was formally approved for release by the National Security Council staff on March 13, 2001. On October 29, 2001, President Bush issued the first of a new series of homeland security presidential directives. The following is a short summary of the HSPDs that address concerns for biological agents and state initiatives in biodefense and biosecurity.

HSPD 4. National Strategy to Combat Weapons of Mass Destruction

In this directive, published in December 2002, President Bush outlined the U.S. strategy to combat WMD. The strategy contains three principal pillars: counterproliferation to combat WMD use, strengthened nonproliferation to combat WMD, and proliferation consequence management to respond to WMD use. This general document did not have much specifically to say about biological threats. In fact, it stated that

> Our approach to defend against biological threats has long been based on our approach to chemical threats, despite the fundamental differences between these weapons. The United States is developing a new approach to provide us and our friends and allies with an effective defense against biological weapons.

It did promise to advance new programs to promotion constructive and realistic measures to strengthen the Biological Weapons Convention. It also promised to strengthen the Australia Group.

HSPD 9. Defense of United States Agriculture and Food

As discussed in Chapter 8, a nation's agriculture and food systems are vulnerable to disease, regardless of whether these outbreaks are natural, accidental, or intentionally introduced. President Bush published HSPD 9 to establish a national policy to defend the agriculture and food system against terrorist attacks, major disasters, and other emergencies. The directive's intent is to protect against a successful attack on the U.S. agriculture and food system, which could have catastrophic health and economic effects. It aims to do so by

> identifying and prioritizing sector-critical infrastructure and key resources for establishing protection requirements; developing awareness and early warning capabilities to recognize threats; mitigating vulnerabilities at critical production and processing nodes; enhancing screening procedures for domestic and imported products; and enhancing response and recovery procedures.

HSPD 10. Biodefense for the 21st Century

This directive is the cornerstone of modern day biodefense and biosecurity initiatives. The components of this comprehensive national biodefense program are: threat awareness, prevention and protection, surveillance and detection, and response and recovery. National biodefense preparedness and response requires the involvement of a wide range of federal departments and agencies. Accordingly, the directive delineates responsibility and requires specific officials to optimize critical functions, such as information management and communications; research development and acquisition; creation and maintenance of needed biodefense infrastructure, including the human capital to support it; public preparedness; and strengthened bilateral, multilateral, and international cooperation. The Secretary of the Department of Homeland Security was designated as the principal federal official for domestic incident management and made responsible for coordinating domestic Federal operations to prepare for, respond to, and recover from biological weapons attacks. This HSPD detailed the following:

- A comprehensive framework for biodefense.
- The creation of the National Biodefense Analysis and Countermeasure Center.

- Increased funding for
  - New vaccines (e.g., Ebola virus).
  - Intelligence initiatives.
  - Biosurveillance.
  - Mass casualty care, to include decontamination.

□ □ □ ▬▬▬▬▬▬▬▬▬▬▬▬▬▬▬▬▬▬▬▬▬▬▬▬▬▬▬

More on the Threat of Bioterrorism

Armed with a single vial of a biological agent, small groups of fanatics, or failing states, could gain the power to threaten great nations, threaten the world peace. America, and the entire civilized world, will face this threat for decades to come. We must confront the danger with open eyes, and unbending purpose.
—President George W. Bush, February 11, 2004, included in HSPD 10

▬▬▬▬▬▬▬▬▬▬▬▬▬▬▬▬▬▬▬▬▬▬▬▬▬▬▬ □ □ □

HSPD 18. Medical Countermeasures against Weapons of Mass Destruction

This directive builds on the vision and objectives articulated in the National Strategy to Combat Weapons of Mass Destruction (HSPD 4) and Biodefense for the 21st Century (HSPD 10). In those two directives, response and recovery were identified as key components of managing the consequences of a WMD attack. Mitigating illness and preventing death are the principal goals of medical countermeasure efforts. Biological agents offer the greatest opportunity for medical mitigation, and this directive accordingly assigns priorities to countermeasure efforts. The directive recognizes that development and acquisition of effective medical countermeasures to mitigate illness, suffering, and death resulting from chemical, biological, radiological/nuclear, and explosive agents is central to consequence management efforts. Although it is not feasible to develop and stockpile medical countermeasures against every possible biological threat, the directive aimed at tackling some of the more important ones. The directive promotes the development of vaccines and drugs to prevent or mitigate adverse health effects caused by exposure to biological agents. This directive also provides for tailoring ongoing research and acquisition efforts to continue to yield new countermeasures against CBRN agents and for incorporating such new discoveries into domestic and international response and recovery planning efforts.

HSPD 21. Public Health and Medical Preparedness

This directive establishes for the United States a strategy for public health and medical preparedness. In addition, it seeks to transform national approach to protecting the health of Americans against all disasters. This strategy draws key principles from the National Strategy for Homeland Security (October 2007), HSPD 4 (December 2002), and HSPD 10 (April 2004) that can be generally applied to public health and medical preparedness. The directive outlines a strategy to accomplish the following:

- Preparedness for all potential catastrophic health events.
- Coordination across levels of government, jurisdictions, and disciplines.

- Regional approach to health preparedness.
- Engagement of the private sector, academia, and other nongovernment entities in preparedness and response efforts.
- Delineate the important roles of individuals, families, and communities.

The directive ambitiously aims to transform the nation's approach to health care in the context of a catastrophic health event in order to enable public health and medical systems to respond effectively to a broad range of incidents. Components of the directive include biosurveillance, countermeasure stockpiling and distribution, mass casualty care, community resilience, risk awareness, and education and training. Moreover, the directive outlined a framework for a functional Disaster Health System and national health security strategy. The directive specifies the creation of a task force to develop the two Disaster Health System and national health security strategy and established a deadline for an implementation plan.

Public Health and the Application of Law

In this book, a great deal of emphasis has been placed on the *R* in RAIN: recognition. After all, to do something about a problem, one has to know that it exists. Along those lines, the federal government created systems and stipulated rules and guidelines for mandatory surveillance and reporting. Specific reporting requirements vary from state to state. Depending on the state, there may be penalties for non-compliance. An example of mandatory reporting requirements is the *Model State Emergency Health Powers Act*, Article III, §301. This act stipulates that

(a) "healthcare providers 'shall' report illnesses/diseases that may be potential cause of public health emergency, including diseases listed by CDC or by Public Health Authority;"

(b) "pharmacists 'shall' report unusual pharmacy visits, prescriptions;"

(c) "within 24 hours, with detailed info about the patient and illness; and"

(d) "veterinarians, livestock owner, vet diagnostic lab director 'shall' report animal diseases that may be potential causes of public health emergency."

From this and other long-standing orders, the United States has a sophisticated reporting system for nationally notifiable infectious diseases (NNIDs). The listing covers most of the diseases caused by HHS Categories A, B, and C and many others that have significance for public health agencies. A quick review of the list, which is too long to post here, shows the comprehensive nature of the NNID surveillance system. The Web Sites section, at the end of this chapter, lists a link to the NNID listing.

In most instances, patients have a right to privacy of their medical condition and medical records. Furthermore, individuals have a right to refuse medical care, which includes treatment and prophylaxis. One of the most recent but also far-reaching legal rules governing privacy of medical records are the provisions of the Health Insurance Portability and Accountability Act of 1996 (HIPAA). Congress enacted HIPAA to ensure continuity of health insurance coverage when people changed employers. It required Congress to address how confidential medical information from one medical plan would move to another and to provide standards designed to protect the confidentiality of medical information contained in health care electronic transactions. Under HIPAA, the secretary of HHS was required to create regulations to assure confidentiality of individually identifiable health information. The rules HHS created regulate the disclosure by any public entity of any "protected health information," which is defined as information that identifies or can be used to identify an individual and relates to physical or mental health condition of, or treatment, or payment for treatment of, an individual. So, what does this have to do with an act of bioterrorism?

Clearly, an outbreak of infectious disease caused by a select agent or one in Category A, B, or C may have implications for government and public health officials. In fact, some, like smallpox, have major implications for national security and global health. That said, why should HIPAA preclude us from sharing information and stifling containment efforts when there may be time-sensitive pieces of information that should not be suppressed. For that reason, provisions of HIPAA are excluded and the information may flow when a public health emergency is declared.

Declaring a disaster or emergency is a public announcement, a statement or declaration that the government recognizes that emergency situation exists and, presumably, intends to do something about it. As such, a **declaration** is a legal determination made by an authorized official, in accordance with criteria specified by law, which has the particular effect specified in the governing law. A declaration may trigger special emergency powers, allow expenditure of emergency funds, and waive or modify normal legal requirements. In the realm of public health, a declaration is frequently optional, officials have strong powers to act without declaring "public health emergency," and "public health emergency" declarations do not normally trigger availability of significant funds. On the contrary, emergency management agency directors view declarations as critical to taking action, necessary to access emergency authorities, and required to make costs eligible for reimbursement.

□ □ □ ▬▬▬▬▬▬▬▬▬▬▬▬▬▬▬▬▬▬▬▬▬▬▬▬▬▬

Critical Thinking

At early stages of an event, consider whether a declaration is truly needed and whether it may have an adverse impact. For example, during the Amerithrax incident in Washington, D.C., the district did not declare a public health emergency. The federal government did not declare a public health emergency. The federal government did not declare a Stafford Act emergency. However, emergency resources were made available quickly from the CDC and Public Health Service. In addition, the strategic national stockpile was deployed within a few hours.

▬▬▬▬▬▬▬▬▬▬▬▬▬▬▬▬▬▬▬▬▬▬▬▬▬▬ □ □ □

Under 45 CFR §164.510(b), disclosures and uses for public health activities, a covered entity may "disclose protected health information for the public health activities and purposes" to

(i) "A public health authority that is authorized by law to collect or receive such information for the purpose of preventing or controlling disease, injury, or disability, including, but not limited to, the reporting of disease, injury, vital events such as birth or death, and the conduct of public health surveillance, public health investigations, and public health interventions;"

(ii) "A public health authority or other appropriate authority authorized by law to receive reports of child abuse or neglect;"

(iii) "A person or entity other than a governmental authority that can demonstrate or demonstrates that it is acting to comply with requirements or direction of a public health authority; or"

(iv) "A person who may have been exposed to a communicable disease or may otherwise be at risk of contracting or spreading a disease or condition and is authorized by law to be notified as necessary in the conduct of a public health intervention or investigation."

In addition, public health officials, both state and federal, may exercise principal health authorities to control communicable disease without "declaring" public health emergency, including quarantine or isolation, travel restrictions, contact tracing, and inoculations or medical examinations.

319 Emergency

A "319 Emergency" is a reference to the section of the Public Health Act authorizing a public health emergency declaration. Section 319 of Public Health Service Act is codified at 42 USC 247d. Here, the secretary of HHS may declare a public health emergency after one of the following conditions is met:

- The disease or disorder presents a public health emergency.
- A public health emergency, including significant outbreaks of infectious diseases or bioterrorist attacks otherwise exists.

The declaration enables the secretary to "take such action as may be appropriate to respond to the public health emergency," including

- Making grants.
- Providing awards for expenses.
- Entering into contracts and conducting and supporting investigations into the cause, treatment, or prevention of a disease and disorder.
- Mobilizing Pubic Health Service corps.
- Emergency approvals of medical products.
- Allow requirement waivers for Medicare, Medicaid, or other HHS programs.
- Allow waiver of any of deadlines for submission of any data or reports required under any law administered by the secretary.

State public health officials have the authority to require persons to undergo medical treatment, which is normally in the form of immunization and testing for communicable diseases, but also includes requiring persons to get definitive medical treatment. However, this authority is subject to constitution and statutory procedural protections.

States generally have authority to declare and enforce quarantine within their borders. This authority varies widely from state to state, depending on state laws. As discussed later, there is also federal isolation and quarantine authority. The Centers for Disease Control and Prevention, through its Division of Global Migration and Quarantine, also is empowered to detain, medically examine, or conditionally release persons suspected of carrying certain communicable diseases. This authority derives from section 361 of the Public Health Service Act (42 U.S.C. 264).

☐ ☐ ☐

Isolation: For People Who Are Ill

Isolation refers to the separation of persons who have a specific infectious illness from those who are healthy and the restriction of their movement to stop the spread of that illness. Isolation allows for the focused delivery of specialized health care to people who are ill, and it protects healthy people from getting sick. People in isolation may be cared for in their homes, in hospitals, or in designated healthcare facilities. Isolation is a standard procedure used in hospitals today for patients with tuberculosis and certain other infectious diseases. In most cases, isolation is voluntary; however, many levels of government (federal, state, and local) have basic authority to compel isolation of sick people to protect the public. Isolation is authorized until the person is no longer contagious.

☐ ☐ ☐

To contain the spread of a contagious illness, public health authorities rely on many strategies. Two of these strategies are isolation and quarantine. Both are common practices in public health, and both aim to control exposure to infected or potentially infected persons. Both may be undertaken voluntarily or compelled by public health authorities. The two strategies differ in that **isolation** applies to persons who are known to have an illness (see Figure 10-2) and **quarantine** applies to those who have been exposed to an illness but may or may not become ill (see Figure 10-3). As to who can invoke quarantine and isolation, that varies by state. Generally, a governor, state public health officer, city or county council, mayor, or local public health office may do so. In most states, a public health emergency declaration is not legally required, but the declaration could be useful if invoking powers for a large population. The bottom line is that one should check with a qualified attorney before powers need to be invoked.

☐ ☐ ☐

Quarantine: For People Who Have Been Exposed But Are Not Ill

Quarantine refers to the separation and restriction of movement of persons who, while not yet ill, have been exposed to an infectious agent and therefore may become infectious. Quarantine of exposed persons is a public health strategy, like isolation, that is intended to stop the spread of infectious disease. Quarantine is medically very effective in protecting the public from disease.

☐ ☐ ☐

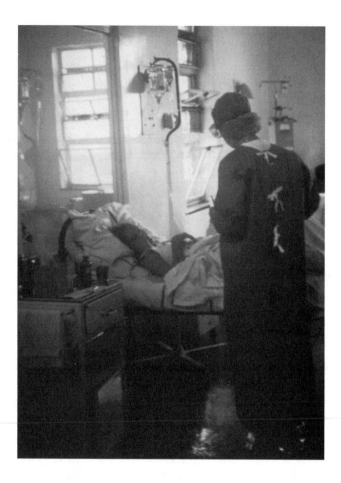

Figure 10-2 A hemorrhagic fever (Marburg virus) patient is in an isolation room in Johannesburg, South Africa. Because this virus is often spread within close contact between humans, the attending physician, like all the attendants, is fully garbed, including goggles, boots, double gloves, and gown. Droplets of body fluids or direct contact with patients, equipment, or other objects contaminated with infectious blood or tissues are highly suspect as sources of viral pathogens. (Image courtesy of Centers for Disease Control and Prevention.)

Quarantine and isolation restrict the personal liberty of individuals. Many state health laws do not spell out the procedural requirements for quarantine and isolation, while others have fairly detailed provisions. Most of these protections derived from the fact that the Constitution requires due process when depriving an individual of "liberty." The individual in question has a right to counsel. These protections may require notice and hearing requirements, showing that detention necessary to protect public health, and a reviewable final decision. If other measures are workable and protect public health, they may be required constitutionally. A court might find it unreasonable to arrest and forcibly quarantine people if a lesser restraint would be effective. It may also be important for health officials to estimate how important is 100% compliance with a quarantine order to protecting the public health. Alternatively, would a "stay at home" quarantine be effective if 80% of the population comply?

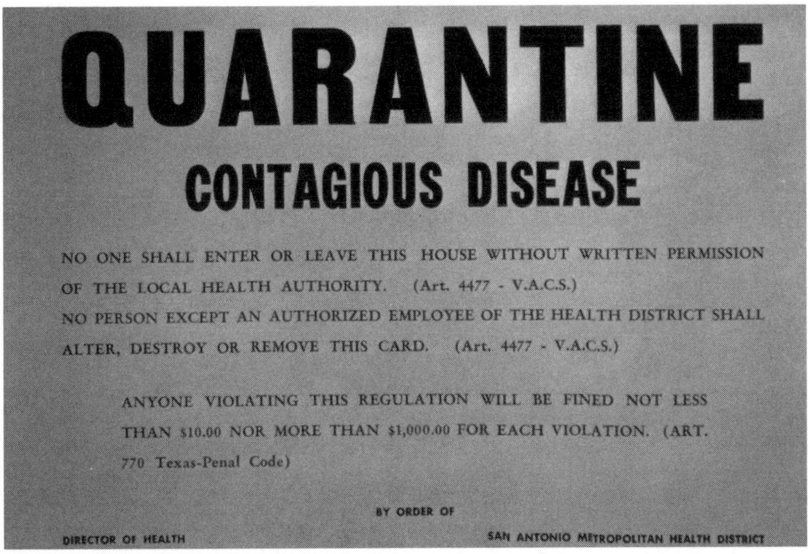

Figure 10-3 A sign informing the public that the house and its residents are under an order for quarantine. (Image courtesy of Centers for Disease Control and Prevention.)

Federal Powers: Quarantine of Travel

"A person who has a communicable disease in the communicable period

- Shall not travel from one state or possession to another . . .
- Without a permit from the health officer of the state, possession, or locality of destination, if such permit is required under the law applicable to the place of destination."

To prevent the interstate spread of disease, the federal government may restrict the movement of persons suspected of being infected with certain communicable diseases. This very old law may be a powerful tool in the hands of a qualified public health official to ensure the health and safety of the public. Only the director of the CDC can issue a permit for people within the contagious phase of certain communicable diseases (cholera, plague, smallpox, typhus, or yellow fever) to travel on board an interstate conveyance (e.g., plane, train, bus). In addition, an individual in the communicable stage of a disease may not travel from one state to another without obtaining a permit from the health officer of the destination state, assuming that such a permit is required under the law of the destination state (42 CFR §70.3). The diseases for which quarantine is authorized are listed in an executive order of the president, the most recent of which is Executive Order 13295, issued on April 1, 2005. This list now includes SARS and H5N1 influenza A virus.

Transporting Biohazardous Materials

The shipment of hazardous materials is regulated by the U.S. Department of Transportation (DOT) and the International Air Transport Association (IATA). The purpose of hazardous materials regulations is to protect the shippers, the carriers, the environment, and the recipients of each package from exposure to the contents. Failure to comply with the regulations can result in substantial fines or jail terms. The DOT defines *hazardous material* as substances that are capable of posing an unreasonable risk to health, safety, and property when transported in commerce. This includes diagnostic specimens, infectious agents, biological products, and dry ice. Such shipments must arrive at their destination in good condition and present no hazard during shipment (42 CFR, Part 72).

Individuals who ship hazardous materials are required to comply with these regulatory requirements:

- Hazardous material shipments must be properly packaged, marked, documented, and labeled.
- Individuals who offer hazardous materials for shipment must receive training.
- There are specific requirements for the packaging and labeling of biological materials. Biological materials include infectious substances (etiologic agents), diagnostic (clinical) specimens, and biological products. Proper shipping papers, Shipper's Declaration for Dangerous Goods, must be completed for shipment of infectious substances but not for biological products or diagnostic specimens. However, all three groups of materials require proper packaging. Human blood always requires "universal precautions" and may be considered a diagnostic specimen and shipped without the dangerous goods paperwork. A biohazard sticker must be present when shipping human blood, according to the OSHA Blood-Borne Pathogens standard. However, if the human blood is known to be infected with an infectious substance, it must be packaged and shipped as such and requires the dangerous goods paperwork (29 CFR, 1910.1030).

Conclusion

The administrative and legal aspects of biosecurity include international treaties (e.g., the Biological Weapons Convention), laws, statutes, regulations, and government directives aimed at reducing the threat due to the biological agents and enabling enforcers to deal with those that use them with ill intentions. These administrative measures have helped define programs and strengthen biodefense and biosecurity all over the globe. The aim of this chapter is to discuss the most relevant documents in hopes that the reader can now appreciate the authority and framework given to officials by these measures. As mentioned in the introduction, the chapter is not written for legal professionals. Rather, it is written for professionals that may have to apply the rules of law in everyday situations, especially in the public health arena. Care should be taken to consult a legal professional before utilizing any of the concepts related to public health law.

Essential Terminology

Note: The terms here are defined with the original language found in the legislative document in which they are used. The legal definitions of terms that have been used throughout this book should be applied when determining the illegality or administrative nature of whatever activity is being analyzed.

- **Biological agent.** Any microorganism (including but not limited to bacteria, viruses, fungi, rickettsiae, or protozoa), or infectious substance, or any naturally occurring, bioengineered, or synthesized component of any such microorganism or infectious substance, capable of causing
  - Death, disease, or other biological malfunction in a human, an animal, a plant, or another living organism.
  - Deterioration of food, water, equipment, supplies, or material of any kind.
  - Deleterious alteration of the environment.
- **Biological product.** A product prepared in accordance with regulations that govern vaccines, licensed biological products, and the like.
- **Biological toxin.** The toxic material or product of plants, animals, microorganisms (including but not limited to bacteria, viruses, fungi, rickettsiae, or protozoa), or infectious substances, or a recombinant or synthesized molecule, whatever their origin and method of production, and includes
  - Any poisonous substance or biological product that may be engineered as a result of biotechnology produced by a living organism
  - Any poisonous isomer or biological product, homolog, or derivative of such a substance.
- **Delivery System.** Any apparatus, equipment, device, or means of delivery specifically designed to deliver or disseminate a biological agent, toxin, or vector.
- **Diagnostic specimen.** Any human or animal material including excreta, secretions, blood, blood components, tissue, and tissue fluids being shipped for the purposes of diagnosis. Specimens that are "known or reasonably expected" to contain pathogens must be handled as infectious substances.
- **Declaration.** A legal determination made by an authorized official, in accordance with criteria specified by law, which has the particular effect specified in the governing law.
- **Etiologic agent.** A viable microorganism or its toxin that causes or may cause disease in humans or animals (DOT).
- **Infectious substances.** Substances known to contain, or reasonably expected to contain, pathogens. Pathogens are microorganisms (including bacteria, viruses, rickettsia, parasites, fungi) or recombinant microorganisms (hybrid or mutant) that are known or reasonably expected to cause disease in humans or animals (IATA).
- **Isolation.** The separation of persons who have a specific infectious illness from those who are healthy and the restriction of their movement to stop the spread of that illness.
- **Quarantine.** The separation and restriction of movement of persons who, while not yet ill, have been exposed to an infectious agent and therefore may become infectious.
- **Terrorism.** Activities that involve an act dangerous to human life or potential destruction of critical infrastructure or any key resource intended to intimidate or coerce the civilian population, or influence a government, or affect a government by mass destruction, assassination, or kidnapping.

- **Weapon of mass destruction (WMD).** A four-part definition that includes any explosive, incendiary, or poison gas, bomb, grenade, rocket having a propellant charge of more than four ounces, or missile having an explosive or incendiary charge of more than one-quarter ounce, or mine or similar device; any weapon that is designed or intended to cause death or serious bodily injury through the release, dissemination, or impact of toxic or poisonous chemical or their precursors; any weapon that is designed to release radiation or radioactivity at a level dangerous to human life; and, *any weapon involving a disease organism.*

Discussion Questions

- How may state authorities require persons to undergo medical treatment?
- With respect to quarantine and isolation, when are they authorized? Who can authorize them? What procedures need to be followed?
- What has become of the initiatives specified in HSPD 10 since it was published?
- What is the difference between isolation and quarantine?
- Can one make an argument for large-scale quarantine? When might this be applicable?

Web Sites

List of nationally notifiable infectious diseases is available at http://www.cdc.gov/EPO/DPHSI/phs/infdis.htm.

References on HIPAA

CDC/HHS Guidance on HIPAA Privacy Rule and Public Health, available at www.healthprivacy.org/usr_doc/CDC-HIPAA-PublicHealth.pdf.

Summary by the Health Privacy Project of the HIPAA Privacy Rule, available at www.healthprivacy.org/usr_doc/RegSummary02.pdf.

Preamble of HIPAA Privacy Rule: 64 Fed. Reg. 59918 (November 3, 1999) HHS Website Q & A on HIPAA Privacy Rule, available at http://www.hhs.gov/ocr/hipaa/.

CDC's Division of Global Migration and Quarantine Web Site, available at www.cdc.gov/ncidod/sars/isolationquarantine.htm.

References

Cimons, M. 2005. Rules, Regs, and Red Tape. *Howard Hughes Medical Institute Bulletin* (Winter):21–24.

International Air Transport Association. 2007. *Dangerous Goods Regulations Manual*, 48th ed. Montreal: IATA.

Miller, J., S. Engelberg, and W. Broad. 2001. *Germs: Biological Weapons and America's Secret War.* New York: Simon and Schuster.

U.S. Department of Health and Human Services. 1999. Centers for Disease Control and Prevention, Office for Health and Safety. *Biosafety in Microbiological and Biomedical Laboratories*, 4th ed., available at www.cdc.gov/OD/ohs/biosfty/bmbl4/bmbl4toc.htm.

U.S. Department of Labor. Occupational Safety and Health Administration, 29 CFR Part 1910.1030, Bloodborne Pathogens.

U.S. Department of Transportation. 49 CFR Parts 171-180 and amendments.

U.S. Public Health Service. 42 CFR Part 72, Interstate Shipment of Etiologic Agents.

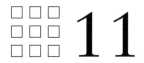

11

Response at the State and Local Level

History is a race between education and catastrophe.
—H. G. Wells

Objectives

The study of this chapter will enable you to

1. Discuss the roles and responsibilities of various key agencies in response to a biological event.
2. Discuss the need for command and coordination systems in the event of a biological attack.
3. Describe the importance of the National Incident Management System and the Incident Command System.
4. Discuss the roles of key federal agencies and officials when it comes to response to a biological event at the local level.
5. Discuss life safety issues for responders attending to the scene of a biological event.
6. Discuss considerations and describe methods for biosampling.
7. Describe outbreak containment measures employed by public health.

Key Terms

Surveillance, National Incident Management System, Incident Command System, unified command, area command, contact tracing.

Introduction

The aim of this chapter is to make the reader aware of local and state activities that affect our ability to respond effectively to natural or intentional disease outbreaks. Routine responsibility for disease prevention and outbreak investigation falls on public health agencies. Responsibility for medical management of illness caused by disease rests with the medical systems of communities. The investigational and prosecutorial aspects of

intentional acts with disease threat falls into the hands of federal law enforcement officials. Finally, responsibility for all hazards preparedness and resource allocations falls
onto the shoulders of emergency managers.

Disasters causing large numbers of casualties typically fall into the natural disaster
realm. Tornadoes, earthquakes, floods, storms, and influenza are examples that apply.
Human error or technical disasters typically do not create as many casualties. For
instance, the accidental release of 90 tons of chlorine in Graniteville, South Carolina,
and the collapse of the I35 Bridge in Minnesota are examples of technical disasters with
limited impact. Human malevolence, such as the terrorist attacks of September 11 and
the bombing of the Murrah Building, are events that may not produce casualties to extent
of natural disasters but resonate with the public into a lasting memory. Terrorist tactics are
evolving from the terrorism of the past to the new terrorism, where the targets are indiscriminate and the intent is to injure or kill as many people as possible (Martin, 2008).

Locally, emergency management officials establish programs to minimize the
adverse effects to life, property, and the environment from potential hazards based on
a jurisdiction vulnerability risk assessment. State emergency management provides the
statewide emergency management program direction, coordination, and in some cases
passage through federal funding for local emergency management programs. Response
to any event begins at the local level, unless it is based on intelligence at a higher level
and the sensitivity ("need to know") associated with such information precludes local
involvement. Unfortunately, the development of effective response strategies and operational plans is a melding of information analysis from all sources followed by implementation of joint authority. We must shift from the "need to know" manner of conducting
business, to a "need to share" philosophy. "Recommendation: Information procedures
should provide incentives for sharing, to restore a better balance between security and
shared knowledge" (9/11 Commission Report, 2004).

With respect to preparedness for an act of bioterrorism, one of the greatest challenges that community officials face is balancing preparedness and mitigation programs
for all other hazards against the low probability of a biological event. As part of the risk
assessment process, the community looks at its vulnerability to biological events, and as
the 2001 Amerithrax incident revealed, each community has some vulnerability to bioterrorism. Community planners and emergency managers need to evaluate the consequence
of such an event and ask the question, If it were to happen here, how bad might it be?
Along with this question, they must assess their organic capability to handle anticipated
consequences. That said, many community planners would determine that, even if a
biological event were to happen, the consequences would be minimal. While that assessment might prove to be true with respect to adverse effects to life, property, and the environment, it greatly underestimates the economic and societal impact of an act of
bioterrorism.

□ □ □ ▬▬▬▬▬▬▬▬▬▬▬▬▬▬▬▬▬▬▬▬▬▬▬▬▬▬▬▬▬▬▬▬

Critical Thinking

The 2001 Amerithrax incident did not create a large pool of casualties (five deaths
out of 22 total cases), which supports the argument that an intentional biological
release is a low-consequence event from a medical perspective, therefore not
requiring significant mitigation activities. On the other hand, significant resources

are now deployed to prevent and provide early detection of another similar attack. Is the main objective to minimize the medical consequences in another attack or is it an attempt to restore confidence in the government's ability to protect the American public?

This chapter is broadly subdivided into several sections. Each section covers a major area for local and state jurisdictions to consider when preparing for and responding to biological threats. The first, "Recognition," is a short discussion about the importance of surveillance and the different types of surveillance useful in recognizing that an unusual disease trend has emerged within the community. As local communities prepare for a biological event, they must develop emergency operations plans that include systems for command and coordination. Since an act of bioterrorism involves numerous agencies at all levels of government, the next section outlines NIMS, ICS, unified command, and specific agencies and officials of the federal government with which local responders must plan to work. Finally, response issues are covered, which include life safety, biosampling, and public health containment measures.

Recognition: Surveillance

The disease surveillance capacities of many state and local pubic health systems depend, in part, on the surveillance capabilities of hospitals and local primary care providers. Whether a disease outbreak occurs naturally or due to the intentional release of a harmful biological agent, much of the initial response occurs at the local level, particularly at hospitals and their emergency departments. Therefore, hospital personnel are some of the first health-care workers with the opportunity to identify an infectious disease outbreak or a bioterrorist event. The same circumstances that place these medical professionals in an optimal position to recognize the onset of an outbreak also places them at greatest risk from the disease event itself.

Infectious diseases include naturally occurring outbreaks, such as SARS, norovirus, and influenza, as well as diseases from biological agents that could be intentionally released by a terrorist, such as smallpox. An infectious disease outbreak, either naturally occurring or from an intentional release, may not be recognized for a week or more, because symptoms may not appear for several days after the initial exposure, during which time a communicable disease could be spread to those who were not initially exposed; as an example, pneumonic plague.

The initial response to an infectious disease of any type, including a bioterrorist attack, is generally a local responsibility that could involve multiple jurisdictions in a region, with states as well as the federal government providing additional support when needed or requested. Just as in a naturally occurring outbreak, exposed individuals seek out local health-care providers, such as private physicians or medical staff in hospital emergency departments or public clinics. Health-care providers should report any illness patterns or diagnostic clues that might indicate an unusual infectious disease outbreak associated with the intentional release of a biologic agent to their local health departments. Public health provides medical professionals with a list of "reportable" diseases to assist public health in recognizing clusters or unusual cases.

In order to be adequately prepared for infectious disease outbreaks in the United States, state and local public health agencies need to have several basic capabilities, either directly or have access to them through regional agreements:

- Public health departments need to have disease surveillance systems and epidemiologists to detect clusters of suspicious symptoms or diseases in order to facilitate early detection of disease and treatment of victims.
- Laboratories need to have adequate capacity and necessary staff to test clinical and environmental samples in order to identify an agent promptly so that proper treatment can be started and reduce spreading of infectious diseases.
- All organizations involved in the response must be able to communicate easily with one another as events unfold and critical information is acquired, especially in a large-scale infectious disease outbreak.

In the event of an outbreak, hospitals and their emergency departments would be on the front line, and their personnel would take on the role of *first receiver*. Because hospital emergency departments are open 24 hours a day, seven days a week, exposed individuals would likely seek treatment from the medical staff on duty. Such staff need to be able to recognize and know how to report any illness patterns or diagnostic clues that might indicate an unusual infectious disease outbreak to their local health department. Hospitals need the capacity and staff necessary to treat severely ill patients as well as implement appropriate prevention and control measures to limit the spread of infectious disease (U.S. Government Accountability Office, 2003). Every facility providing medical care should have an exposure control plan in place.

Because infected individuals might go to emergency departments for treatment, hospital personnel would likely be some of the first health-care workers with the opportunity to identify an emerging infectious disease outbreak. Therefore, the disease surveillance capacities of many state and local public health systems depend, in part, on the surveillance capabilities of hospitals. Hospitals as well as general medical providers are in many respects the "gatekeepers" for a healthy and safe public. **Surveillance** can be defined as ongoing systematic collection, collation, analysis, and interpretation of data and the dissemination of information to those who need to know for action to be taken. Effective communicable disease control relies on an effective surveillance and response system that promotes better coordination and integration of surveillance functions (WHO, 2007). Surveillance is a continuous and systematic process consisting of three primary activities:

- *Collection* of relevant data for a specified population, time period, and/or geographic area.
- Accurate *analysis* of data.
- Rapid *dissemination* of interpreted data.

The primary objective of disease surveillance is to idenitfy trends in infectious disease and determine the risk of disease transmission so that prevention and control measures can be applied to minimize the burden of illness. Surveillance data must be timely and complete to accurately reflect the occurrence and distribution of disease. The types of surveillance currently used are

- *Passive* disease surveillance refers to the receipt of reports of infections and diseases from physicians, laboratories, and other health professionals required to submit to submit reports required by public health statute.

- *Active* disease surveillance is guided by public health statute in each state and refers to the routine gathering of data in an effort to identify cases. This type of surveillance can be seasonal or initiated by a mass casualty event that has resulted in an increased number of individuals or potential cohorts presenting with similar symptoms or illnesses.

- *Syndromic surveillance* has been used for early detection of outbreaks, to follow the size, spread, and tempo of outbreaks; to monitor disease trends; and to provide reassurance that an outbreak has not occurred. Syndromic surveillance systems seek to use existing health data in real time to provide immediate analysis and feedback to those charged with the investigation and follow-up of potential outbreaks.

The fundamental objective of syndromic surveillance is to identify illness clusters early, before diagnoses are confirmed and reported to public health agencies, and to mobilize a rapid response, thereby reducing morbidity and mortality. Passive surveillance systems rely on laboratory and hospital staff, physicians, and other relevant sources to take the initiative to provide data on illnesses to the health department, where officials analyze and interpret the information as it arrives. In contrast, in an active disease surveillance system, public health officials contact sources, such as laboratories, hospitals, and physicians, to obtain information on conditions or diseases in order to identify cases. Active surveillance can provide more complete detection of disease patterns than a system that is wholly dependent on voluntary reporting. Having dedicated personnel to accomplish active surveillance is a challenge for any administrator. Public health departments are traditionally thin on staffing. Taking staff time to look for a problem that may or may not exist, at the expense of one of the many ongoing daily health department programs, is problematic.

Command and Coordination

Command and coordination are essential to effectively respond to a biological incident. Whenever an act of biological terrorism occurs, no matter how seemingly insignificant, facets of the federal government are set into motion. As such, local communities and state governments must be prepared to receive and work with elements of the federal government. Previous incidents, disasters, and catastrophic events made it clear that the nation needed a uniform approach to managing an incident. Accordingly, Homeland Security Presidential Directive Number 5 called for the **National Incident Management System** (NIMS) to manage domestic incidents by establishing a single, comprehensive national incident management system. The framework allows for a consistent command structure and clear, concise communications through common language to support interoperability between responders from the local level to the federal level. For hospitals, this framework has been extended through the Hospital Incident Command System. For public health agencies, a similar but new framework, known as the *Public Health Incident Command System*, is being adopted (Qureshi, K. Gebbie, and E. Gebbie, 2005). Regardless of the agency, small or large, the framework remains the same, although the roles and responsibilities vary based on the agencies' jurisdictional duties and statute.

□ □ □

The Incident Command System

The **Incident Command System** is a component of the National Incident Management System. Federal, state, local, and tribal governments had to be in full compliance with NIMS by September 30, 2006. The ICS is a proven modular management tool that expands and contracts as the incident warrants. ICS provides a framework for coordinated effort to ensure an effective response and the efficient safe use of resources, regardless of the size or agencies involved. The concept of ICS was developed more than 30 years ago, in the aftermath of a devastating wildfire in California. Over a 13-day period in 1970, 700 structures were destroyed and 16 lives were lost, some due to lack of coordination and poor command and control. As a result, Congress mandated that the U.S. Forest Service design a system to effectively coordinate interagency actions. As such, Firefighting Resources of California Organized for Potential Emergencies (FIRESCOPE) was established as a primary command and control system (California Office of Emergency Services, FIRESCOPE, 2004). Its organization delineated job responsibilities and organizational structure for managing day-to-day operations of all types of emergency incidents. FIRESCOPE eventually led to the Incident Command System.

□ □ □

Regardless of its application, ICS is a management system designed to enable effective and efficient domestic incident management by integrating a combination of facilities, equipment, personnel, procedures, and communications operating within a common organizational structure, designed to enable effective and efficient domestic incident management (U.S. Department of Homeland Security, 2004). The ICS is the combination of facilities, equipment, personnel, procedures, and communications operating within a common organizational structure, designed to aid in domestic incident management activities. It is used for a broad spectrum of emergencies, from small to complex incidents, both natural and human made, including acts of catastrophic terrorism. ICS is used by all levels of government: federal, state, local, and tribal. ICS is usually organized around five major functional areas: command, operations, planning, logistics, and finance and administration (U.S. Department of Homeland Security, 2004a). A sixth optional function, Intelligence, may be needed to collect and establish facts in the investigation.

The ICS organization has the capability to expand or reduce to meet the needs of the incident; but all incidents, regardless of size or complexity, will have an incident commander (IC). A basic ICS operating guideline is that the IC is responsible for on-scene management until command authority is transferred to another person, who then becomes the IC. Command primarily consists of the IC and command staff. Command staff positions are established to assign responsibility for key activities not specifically identified in the general staff functional elements. These positions may include the public information officer, safety officer, and liaison officer, in addition to various others, as required and assigned by the IC. The general staff comprises the incident management personnel who represent the major functional elements of the ICS, including the operations section chief, planning section chief, logistics section chief, and finance/administration section chief. The command staff and general staff must continually interact and share vital information and estimates of the current and future situation to develop recommended courses of action for consideration by the IC.

Unified Command

A mass casualty incident, such as a major outbreak of an infectious disease, requires a **unified command** within the ICS structure. Figure 11-1 illustrates the ICS structure. The branches and units remain the same between agencies, yet the functional roles and responsibilities vary. In a mass casualty incident, the Department of Health and Human Services is the lead coordinating agency for Emergency Support Function 8 (Health and Medical Annex of the Federal Response Plan). This responsibility remains the same at the state and local level. In a declared emergency, all information must be directed through the Emergency Operations Center, with the defined organizational structure to ensure integrated communications and an effective response. A public health liaison officer facilitates communication between the health department and medical community, including primary care providers, hospitals, home health agencies, nursing homes, foster homes, community-based health centers as well as any agency responsible for the health and medical needs of vulnerable populations. How this is coordinated may vary, depending on the size and demographics of the community, yet the organizational structure will remain the same within ICS.

Unified command is an important element in multijurisdictional or multiagency domestic incident management. It provides guidelines to enable agencies with different legal, geographic, and functional responsibilities to coordinate, plan, and interact

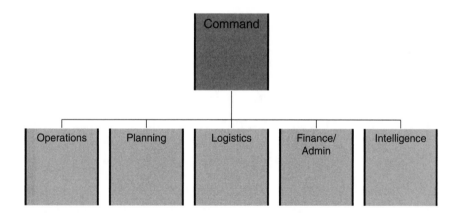

Figure 11-1 Basic National Incident Management System (NIMS) incident command structure (ICS) involving the five functions of ICS, plus an optional sixth function, known as *intelligence*. The analysis and sharing of information and intelligence are important elements of ICS. In this context, intelligence includes not only national security or other types of classified information but also other operational information, such as risk assessments, medical intelligence (i.e., surveillance), weather information, geospatial data, structural designs, toxic contaminant levels, and utilities and public works data, which may come from a variety of different sources. Information and intelligence must be appropriately analyzed and shared with personnel, designated by the IC, who have proper clearance and a *"need-to-know"* status to ensure that he or she supports decision making. In this graphic depiction, intelligence is shown as a separate function. Traditionally, information and intelligence functions are located in the planning section. However, in exceptional situations, the IC may need to assign the information and intelligence functions to other parts of the ICS organization.

effectively. As a team effort, unified command overcomes much of the inefficiency and duplication of effort that can occur when agencies from different functional and geographic jurisdictions or at different levels of government operate without a common system or organizational framework.

All agencies with jurisdictional authority or functional responsibility for any aspects of an incident participate in the unified command structure and contribute to the process of determining overall incident strategies, selecting objectives, ensuring that joint planning for tactical activities is accomplished in accordance with approved incident objectives, ensuring the integration of tactical operations, and approving, committing, and making optimum use of all assigned resources. The exact composition of the unified command structure depends on the location and the type of the incident. In some cases, **area command** is activated only if necessary, depending on the complexity of the incident and span-of-control considerations. An area command is established either to oversee the management of multiple incidents that are being handled by separate ICS organizations or to oversee the management of a very large incident that involves multiple ICS organizations. It is important to note that area command does not have operational responsibilities. For incidents under its authority, the area command

- Sets overall agency incident-related priorities.
- Allocates critical resources according to established priorities.
- Ensures that incidents are managed properly.
- Ensures effective communications.
- Ensures that incident management objectives are met and do not conflict with each other or with agency policies.
- Identifies critical resource needs and reports them to the Emergency Operations Center(s).
- Ensures that short-term emergency recovery is coordinated to assist in the transition to full recovery operations.
- Provides for personnel accountability and a safe operating environment.

Role of Federal Agencies at a WMD Incident

The response to any terrorist incident within the U.S. will entail a highly coordinated, multiagency local, state, and federal response. The following primary federal agencies will likely provide the core response as discussed in the National Response Plan (U.S. Department of Homeland Security, 2004b).

The *Secretary of the Department of Homeland Security* is the *principal federal official* for domestic incident management. The secretary is responsible for coordinating federal operations within the United States to prepare for, respond to, and recover from terrorist attacks, major disasters, and other emergencies. The *attorney general* has lead responsibility for *criminal investigations* of terrorist acts or terrorist threats by individuals or groups inside the United States or directed at U.S. institutions abroad, where such acts are within the federal criminal jurisdiction of the United States (U.S. Department of Homeland Security, Homeland Security Presidential Directive 5). The *Federal Bureau of Investigation*, under the authority of the attorney general, handles all crime scenes where a terrorist act involving a WMD has occurred.

☐ ☐ ☐ ▬▬▬▬▬▬▬▬▬▬▬▬▬▬▬▬▬▬▬▬▬▬▬▬▬

Critical Thinking

The *National Response Plan* incorporates best practices and procedures from incident management disciplines—homeland security, emergency management, law enforcement, firefighting, public works, public health, responder and recovery worker health and safety, emergency medical services, and the private sector—and integrates them into a unified structure. It forms the basis of how the federal government coordinates with state, local, and tribal governments and the private sector during incidents. Following an act of bioterrorism, assistance will come from various federal agencies under the NRP, depending on the scope of the incident. How big a footprint will federal agencies have in a community? What impact do they have on an operation even after the event has been through all incident phases? Where does the national response framework fit into all this?

▬▬▬▬▬▬▬▬▬▬▬▬▬▬▬▬▬▬▬▬▬▬▬▬▬ ☐ ☐ ☐

Department of Homeland Security

The Department of Homeland Security is the nation's lead agency in dealing with terrorism and chemical, biological, radiological/nuclear, and explosives destruction. The goals of the department are to make the nation less vulnerable to terrorism, prevent attacks, minimize the damage from attacks, and oversee recovery efforts. The DHS works closely with other federal agencies and state and local governments to coordinate disaster planning and relief efforts.

Department of Justice

The Department of Justice has the primary responsibility for preventing and investigating terrorist incidents and oversees a number of important assets, including the Critical Incident Response Group (CIRG), evidence response team, and the FBI.

The CIRG facilitates the FBI's rapid response to and the management of crisis incidents. The CIRG was established in 1994 to integrate tactical and investigative resources and expertise for critical incidents. Each of the three major areas of CIRG—Operations Support Branch, Tactical Support Branch, and the National Center for the Analysis of Violent Crime—furnishes distinctive operational assistance and training to FBI field offices as well as state and local law enforcement agencies.

The evidence response team is responsible for crime scene documentation and evidence collection. An FBI evidence response team recovered both black boxes from the aircraft that crashed into the Pentagon on September 11, 2001. An evidence response team can vary in number from 8 to 50. The FBI's evidence response teams include special agents and support personnel who specialize in organizing and collecting evidence, using a variety of technical evidence recovery techniques.

The FBI coordinates federal crisis management efforts. It is the lead federal investigative agency for CBRNE incidents through the CBRNE operations unit. There are 56 FBI field offices, 4 specialized field installations, and more than 40 foreign liaison posts. Representatives from 20 federal agencies are assigned to the Counterterrorism Center at FBI headquarters.

At the field-operational level, the FBI has approximately 60 Joint Terrorism Task Force teams based out of its field offices. The task forces are designed to maximize inter-agency cooperation and coordination among federal, state, and local law enforcement. The FBI has five rapid deployment teams that can respond to multiple incidents (two teams stationed in Washington, D.C.; one each in New York City, Miami, and Los Angeles). The FBI's hazardous materials response unit, based in Quantico, Virginia, is designed to enhance evidence-gathering capabilities in extreme environments.

The National Response Center (NRC) serves as the sole federal point of contact for reporting all oil, chemical, radiological, *biological*, and etiological discharges into the environment anywhere in the United States and its territories. The NRC gathers and compiles data concerning spills or discharges for federal on-scene coordinators and serves as the communications and operations center for the national response team. In addition to these functions, the NRC also prepares terrorist/suspicious activity reports.

Federal Emergency Management Agency

The Federal Emergency Management Agency is a department within DHS. FEMA's response division coordinates federal response efforts relating to all hazards and terrorist attacks. FEMA promotes the effective response by federal agencies at the national level and at the scene of an incident. FEMA is responsible for the Metropolitan Medical Response System (MMRS), which is utilized in the event of a CBRNE incident with mass casualties. The MMRS provides initial on-site response and safe patient transport to emergency rooms in the event of terrorist attack. It also provides medical and mental health care to victims of such attacks and can move victims to other regions should local resources be overrun. MMRS is a local resource activated by local authorities; however, its members are federally trained and funded. The team is characterized by specially trained responders, special pharmaceuticals and decontamination equipment, on-site health care, and enhanced emergency medical transportation and emergency room capabilities.

Environmental Protection Agency

The Environmental Protection Agency provides technical support to the lead federal agency, typically monitoring and assessing chemical, biological, and *radiological threats*. After the initial emergency response phase, the EPA operates the Federal Radiological Monitoring and Assessment Center. EPA's on-scene coordinators helped monitor air quality in New York following the September 11, 2001, attacks. The EPA's environmental response team supports on-scene coordinators. The response teams have portable chemical agent instruments to detect and identify agents in low- and subparts-per-million quantities. The teams can also measure alpha, beta, and gamma radiation. The environmental response teams offer 24-hour access to chemical decontamination equipment, and members have access to Levels A through C protective gear.

Department of Health and Human Services

The Department of Health and Human Services works with states to build the strongest possible network of protection and response capability for Americans faced with health and medical problems in emergencies. The Centers for Disease Control and Prevention, under the HHS, helps assess incident effects and develops strategies for public health aspects of an emergency; two key roles are disease surveillance and disease investigation. The Department of Health and Human Services, Office of Preparedness and Response, maintains responsibility for the National Disaster Medical System. This system includes disaster medical assistance teams and disaster mortuary response teams. Disaster medical assistance teams deploy to disaster sites with adequate supplies and equipment to support themselves for 72 hours, while providing medical care at a fixed or temporary medical site. Further, highly specialized medical response teams deal with specific medical conditions, such as crush injury, burns, and mental health emergencies. Disaster medical assistance teams are principally a community resource to support local, regional, and state requirements; however, they can be federalized to provide interstate aid. Also, a part of the National Disaster Medical System, the disaster mortuary response teams can be rapidly deployed to disaster sites to help identify, track, and process fatalities at a CBRNE event. Their specialty is forensics, identification of remains, and temporary holding of corpses pending outcome of the investigation.

Department of Energy

The Department of Energy responds to incidents involving nuclear or radiological materials. DOE maintains management systems that would assist in the event of a CBRNE incident. The Atmospheric Release Advisory Center uses sophisticated models to predict the consequences from atmospheric releases of nuclear, chemical, or biological hazardous material incidents, which include spills, fires, and explosions. The Atmospheric Release Advisory Center's mission is to provide public agencies real-time mapping and predictions of health and safety consequences from dispersion of radioactive, chemical, or biological materials released to the atmosphere during an accident or incident.

Response: Safety

All responders with the potential to encounter contaminated victims or exposure to contaminated material must wear the appropriate level of personal protective equipment and respiratory protection to the hazard. Responders can ensure the maximum safety of themselves and victims by following safety precautions and local protocol (29 CFR, Part 1910.120).

PPE is associated with a number of physical and psychological potential limitations, including those that follow:

- *Time to put on.* The higher the level, the more time it takes to don and doff PPE.
- *Impaired communication.* Wearing a face piece or mask may result in poor communication or speech intelligibility.
- *Impaired vision.* Face pieces may limit field of vision. Prescription eyewear cannot be worn with a self-contained breathing apparatus.
- *Heat-related issues.* Encapsulation and moisture-impermeable materials invariably lead to heat stress.
- *Increased weight.* The suit and SCBA add additional weight.

- *Encapsulation.* Gear adds to psychological trauma to both responders and patients.
- *Limited duration of use.* Wearing PPE Level B is contingent on many factors, including the total air supply, weather, work stress, and breathing.
- *Limited oxygen availability.* SCBAs can be used only for the period of time allowed by the air in the tank. Air-purifying respirators can be used only in environments in which the ambient air provides sufficient oxygen.
- *Dexterity issues.* Weight and bulkiness of the PPE may result in impaired mobility.

When wearing PPE, responders should always use the buddy system (29 CFR, Part 1910.120). All actions should be done in groups of two or more. The buddy system is used so responders can assist each other should one of them become fatigued. The approach to any potentially hazardous atmosphere, including biological hazards, must be made with a plan that includes an assessment of hazard and exposure potential, respiratory protection needs, entry conditions, exit routes, and decontamination strategies. Any plan involving a biological hazard should be based on relevant infectious disease or biological safety recommendations by the Centers for Disease Control and Prevention and other expert bodies including emergency first responders, law enforcement, and public health officials. The need for decontamination and treatment of all first responders with antibiotics or other medications should be decided in consultation with local public health authorities. Safety recommendations reiterated here come from an interim statement issued by the CDC in October 2001 following the Amerithrax incident (Centers for Disease Control, 2001). They are based on current understanding of the potential threats and existing recommendations issued for biological aerosols.

Personal Protection against Biological Agents

When using respiratory protection, the type of respirator is selected on the basis of the hazard and its airborne concentration. For a biological agent, the air concentration of infectious particles depends on the method used to release the agent. Current data suggest that the self-contained breathing apparatus, shown in Figure 11-2, that first responders currently use for entry into potentially hazardous atmospheres provides those responders with respiratory protection against biological exposures associated with a suspected act of biological terrorism (National Fire Protection Association, 2008).

Protective clothing, including gloves and booties, also may be required for the response to a suspected act of biological terrorism. Protective clothing may be needed to prevent skin exposure or contamination of other clothing. The type of protective clothing needed depends on the type of agent, concentration, and route of exposure.

The interim recommendations for personal protective equipment, including respiratory protection and protective clothing, are based on the anticipated level of exposure risk associated with different response situations, as follows:

- Responders should use a National Institute for Occupational Safety and Health (NIOSH)–approved, pressure-demand SCBA in conjunction with a Level A protective suit in responding to a suspected biological incident where any of the following information is unknown or the event is uncontrolled:
  - The type(s) of airborne agent(s).
  - The dissemination method.

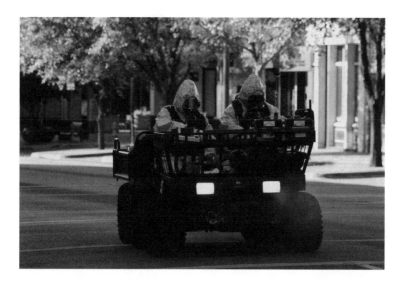

Figure 11-2 Two members of a WMD civil support team move during an exercise to establish a perimeter in a hot zone and perform reconnaissance efforts. Note that they have donned Level B personal protective equipment, which includes a splash suit and a self-contained breathing apparatus. (Photo courtesy of the U.S. Department of the Defense, Armed Forces Press Service.)

  o If dissemination via an aerosol-generating device is still occurring or it has stopped but there is no information on the duration of dissemination or what the exposure concentration might be.

- Responders may use a Level B protective suit with an exposed or enclosed NIOSH-approved pressure-demand SCBA if the situation can be defined in which the suspected biological aerosol is no longer being generated or other conditions may present a splash hazard.
- Responders may use a full face-piece respirator with a P100 filter or powered air-purifying respirator with high efficiency particulate air filters when it can be determined that an aerosol-generating device was not used to create high airborne concentration or dissemination was by a letter or package that can be easily bagged.

Care should be taken when bagging letters and packages to minimize creating a puff of air that could spread pathogens. It is best to avoid large bags and to work very slowly and carefully when placing objects in bags. Disposable hooded coveralls, gloves, and foot coverings also should be used. NIOSH recommends against wearing standard firefighter turnout gear into potentially contaminated areas when responding to reports involving biological agents.

Decontamination

Decontamination of protective equipment and clothing, shown in Figure 11-3, is an important precaution to make sure that any particles that might have settled on the outside of protective equipment are removed before taking off gear. Decontamination sequences currently used for hazardous material emergencies should be used as appropriate for the level of protection employed. Equipment can be decontaminated using soap and water, and 0.5% hypochlorite solution (one part household bleach to nine parts

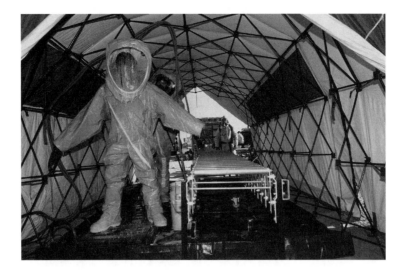

Figure 11-3 Members of the sixth WMD civil support team go through a decontamination cleanup station after inspecting a vessel for hazardous materials during an exercise in U.S. Coast Guard Station, Galveston, Texas, January 25, 2007. The sixth civil support team is using Coast Guard expertise to help train for boarding and inspecting vessels at sea. (Photo courtesy of the U.S. Department of the Defense, Armed Forces Press Service. U.S. Coast Guard photo by Petty Officer 3rd Class Adam Eggers.)

water) can be used as appropriate or if gear has any visible contamination. Note that bleach may damage some types of firefighter turnout gear (one reason why it should not be used for biological agent response actions). After taking off gear, response workers should shower using copious quantities of soap and water. In a known or suspected release, decontamination of biological materials is a four-step process. That process is detailed as follows:

1. *Wet* down the person; this allows the biological material (contamination) to adhere to clothing and skin, thus reducing the airborne hazard and the potential for ingestion and inhalation.
2. *Strip* contaminated clothing.
3. *Flush* the victim with a large amount of water, using soap if available, to remove any remaining contamination from skin and hair. Do not use bleach solutions to decontaminate skin surfaces.
4. *Cover* for protection and modesty.

Cross-contamination could occur during decontamination procedures if responders do not have appropriate PPE; therefore, the victims may perform self-decontamination. If this is the case, self-decontamination (for ambulatory victims) involves the removal of hazardous contamination from their own bodies. Victims should be advised to remove their own clothing (if contaminated) and the contaminating material in any way possible.

Response: Biosampling

Biological agents pose new challenges to both law enforcement and public health officials in their efforts to minimize the effects of a biological attack and apprehend those responsible for the attack. In the past, it was not uncommon for law enforcement and public health officials to conduct separate, independent investigations. However, a biological attack requires a high level of cooperation between these two disciplines to achieve their respective objectives of identifying the biological agent, preventing the spread of the disease, preventing public panic, and apprehending those responsible. The lack of mutual awareness and understanding, as well as the absence of established communication procedures, could hinder the effectiveness of law enforcement's and public health's separate, but often overlapping, investigations. Due to the continued likelihood of biological attacks, the effective use of all resources during a biological incident is critical to ensure an efficient and appropriate response.

When communities are faced with biocrimes, responders may be called on to collect and preserve microbial forensic evidence (Schutzer, Budowle, and Atlas, 2005). These actions are paramount to efficient and successful investigation and attribution. If evidence is not collected, degrades, or is contaminated during collection, handling, transport, or storage, the downstream characterization and attribution analyses may be compromised. Many experts believe that the inherent rigidity in a standard operating protocol for crime scene processing could be unwieldy and impractical in a bioterrorism event, which may compromise evidence collection in some cases. Therefore, consultation among the different entities involved in a response should provide best-practice options framed on established guidelines. The plan can be modified after greater scrutiny of the crime scene or as more information is obtained during the course of the investigation. If the forensic situation fits a pattern or template for which a sample collection methodology or sampling strategy already has been validated, then the sampling activities could be well defined and more focused (Budowle et al., 2006). One such scenario involving suspicious powdery substances found on hard surfaces provides the setting for routine sample collection and is the subject of this guidebook. Figure 11-4 shows a response exercise in progress.

Numerous "white powder" incidents occur each year. If a ricin or anthrax incident occurred, it would be extremely unlikely that this would be a natural event. Therefore, any incident involving biological agents should be treated as a terrorist or criminal incident until proven otherwise. This requires that the FBI be notified, which would in turn notify the Department of Homeland Security Operations Center. The Terrorism Incident Law Enforcement Annex of the NRP provides additional information on the FBI's role in pursuing the investigative response to a terrorist event.

For credible threats involving biological agents, the responding hazmat team should also notify local public health and emergency management officials through local procedures. Local public health officials should notify the CDC, which in turn will notify HHS headquarters. HHS and the National Response Center, staffed by U.S. Coast Guard personnel, should also receive notification via the HSOC.

A Protocol for Biological Agent Sample Collection

ASTM International, one of the largest voluntary standards development organizations in the world, announced the approval and availability of a new standard for collecting, packaging, and transporting visible powder samples suspected of being biological agents. ASTM (2006) Standard E2458, Standard Practices for Bulk Sample Collection and Swab Sample Collection of Visible Powders Suspected of Being Biological Agents from

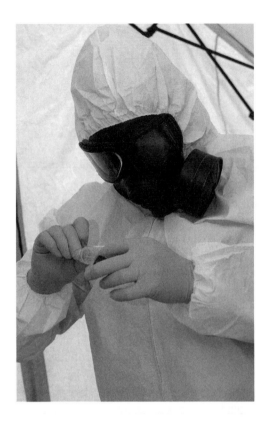

Figure 11-4 A survey team member from a WMD civil support team prepares a specimen for presumptive analysis. This was a local major accident response exercise, where a suspicious package containing unknown substances was left on a military member's desk. (Image courtesy of U.S. Department of Defense, Armed Forces Press Service.)

Nonporous (Hard) Surfaces, is the first standard to address the subject. E2458 incorporates reference guidance to comply with appropriate federal regulations regarding biosafety and biosecurity. *The standard is applicable to nonporous surfaces only.*

The development of a sample collection standard was initiated by the U.S. Department of Homeland Security in order to address the problems associated with haphazard sample collection and screening. DHS assigned the National Institute of Standards and Technology to coordinate and lead a task group whose charge was to develop a standard protocol for the collection of powders that are suspected biological agents. DHS funded Association of Analytical Communities International to organize and coordinate meetings of the task group and organize validation studies.

Formed in April 2005, the AOAC Sampling Standard Task Group consisted of experts from many different organizations, such as the FBI, the CDC, the EPA, the International Association of Fire Chiefs, health departments of U.S. states, and various segments of the U.S. Army. The resulting document was submitted to ASTM Committee E54 on Homeland Security as the basis of a full consensus standard. The stakeholders within E54 provided significant input and feedback, which resulted in hundreds of comments and three ASTM ballots of the draft standard. The final document reflects the true breadth of the homeland security effort within ASTM International. From start to finish, the standard was completed and adopted in approximately one year.

Two-Step Procedure

E2458 is a two-step procedure that is performed after an initial risk assessment is conducted and a visible powder is deemed a credible biological threat. The first step of the procedure, Method A, covers the bulk collection and packaging of the suspicious visible powders from solid nonporous (hard) surfaces. Bulk samples are collected and transported in a manner that permits public health and safety and law enforcement agencies to obtain uncompromised samples for confirmatory analysis and forensic testing. The second step, Method B, covers swab sampling of residual suspicious powders for presumptive on-site biological screening.

Sample Collection Procedure Proven to Work

A study was conducted in March 2006 to validate the reliability of the sampling procedure at the U.S. Army Dugway Proving Ground. The study demonstrated that the sampling procedure can be used by trained emergency responders in simulated emergency conditions to consistently recover samples. The study also proved that a sufficient number of *Bacillus anthracis* spores can be detected by emergency responders to make a presumptive, on-site determination, even after all bulk samples have been collected. The evaluation study was designed to determine the recovery efficacy on seven environmental surface types, which included stainless steel, food-grade painted wood, rubber, tile, concrete, finished wood, and plastic. The study involved six teams that included four National Guard civil support teams, shown in Figure 11-5, the Navy's Chemical Biological Incidence Response Force, and a hazmat team from the Florida Hazard Materials Response Unit. Team members wore Level C personal protective equipment during the entire study so that the efficacy of the sample collection procedure could be tested under as close-to-real-life conditions as could be attained.

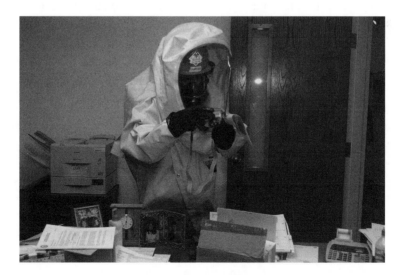

Figure 11-5 A survey team member from the 101st WMD civil support team photographs a suspicious package containing a white power. This was a local major accident response exercise, where a suspicious package containing unknown substances was left on a military member's desk. (Image courtesy of U.S. Department of Defense, Armed Forces Press Service.)

Response: Containment

Controlling the spread of a communicable disease in a community requires a multifaceted approach that includes traditional epidemiology, education of medical providers and the public, and provision of treatment and prophylaxis (Chapter 12), if available. Once an index case has been identified, contact tracing should begin. Also, specific conditions may dictate the need for more extensive control measures designed to limit contact between persons who are (or may be) contagious and others who are susceptible to infection. Isolation and quarantine are two such measures. The legal aspects of these two important elements were covered in Chapter 10. As stated, the legal authority to impose isolation and quarantine exists in most local health jurisdictions, but the success-ful implementation of either measure on a broad scale within a community requires careful planning.

Contact Tracing

On initiation of an outbreak and recognition that a problem exists, the public health officer assigns an epidemiologist to begin a disease outbreak investigation and **contact tracing**. The epidemiologist will trace contacts to determine the extent of the spread and possible secondary transmission. Once a potential contact has been identified, there are escalating methods of dealing with limiting the spread of infection by an individual. Passive monitoring is a process where the contact is asked to perform self-assessment at least twice daily and to contact authorities immediately if respiratory symptoms or fever occur. It may be useful for situations in which the risk of exposure and subsequent development of disease is low, and the risk to others if recognition of disease is delayed is also low. The benefits are that it requires minimal resources and places few constraints on individual freedoms. It does rely on self-reporting and affected persons may not be able to perform an adequate self-assessment. To help assure fulfillment of these responsi-bilities, the public health official may provide necessary supplies (thermometer, symptom log, written instructions) and staff a hotline to notify authorities about symptoms or needs.

If warranted, the next step in escalation of this process might include active monitoring by a health-care worker designee, such as a community health nurse or local emergency medical services provider. The contact is evaluated on a regular basis by phone or in person for signs and symptoms suggestive of disease. This monitoring may be called for in situations where the risk of exposure to and subsequent development of disease is moderate to high, resources permit close observation of individuals, and the risk of delayed recognition of symptoms is low to moderate. The benefit is, once again, few constraints on individual liberties, but it does require trained staffing and a system to track information and verify monitoring and appropriate actions based on findings.

Isolation and Quarantine

By definition, both isolation and quarantine restrict the movement of individuals. While voluntary isolation and quarantine are often successful, involuntary restriction may be required in some circumstances or with particular individuals, especially early in an emerging infection. Any plan for implementation of isolation or quarantine requires clear delineation of the relevant legal authorities and responsibilities. To avoid unnecessary and potentially dangerous delays and barriers, it is crucial that public health personnel, law enforcement, the judicial system, and other local authorities are familiar with these legal issues.

Isolation means separation, during the period of communicability, of a person infected with a communicable disease, in a place and under conditions to prevent direct or indirect transmission of an infectious agent to others. It may mean extremely limited contact with an ill person who is diagnosed with, or suspected of having, a communicable disease. The isolation can occur in a hospital setting in a negative airflow room for very infectious airborne diseases. Isolation usually requires health-care providers and visitors to use gowns, masks or respirators, goggles, and gloves as a means of protecting the visitors but also to protect the patient from exposure to new diseases that his or her weakened immune system may not be able to overcome.

Quarantine means restrictions, during or immediately prior to a period of communicability, of activities or travel of an otherwise healthy person who likely has been exposed to a communicable disease. The restrictions are intended to prevent disease transmission during the period of communicability in the event the person is infected. This period is commonly known as the *incubation period* of a disease. This means the person to be quarantined has been exposed to an individual with a communicable disease and may be developing the disease as well. Some diseases are not communicable until symptoms appear; other diseases may be communicable for hours or days before the person shows any signs of the disease.

Quarantine can be accomplished by a variety of means including having the person stay in his or her own home and avoid contact with others (including family members) to having the person or group of persons stay in a designated facility, to restricting travel out of an affected area. The contact remains separated from others for a specified period (generally 10–14 days postexposure), during which he or she is assessed on a regular basis for signs and symptoms of disease. Persons with fever, respiratory, or other early influenza symptoms require immediate evaluation by a trained health-care provider. Restrictions may be voluntary or legally mandated; confinement may be at home or in an appropriate facility.

Group Quarantine

Group quarantine may be considered when specific groups are at risk and is designed to reduce interactions and thereby transmission risk within the group. When focused, the intervention is applied to groups or persons identified in specific sites or buildings, most but not necessarily all of whom are at risk of exposure. It may be useful when transmission is believed to have occurred, where the links between cases are unclear at the time of evaluation, and where restrictions placed only on persons known to have been exposed is considered insufficient to prevent further transmission. It may be difficult to achieve compliance if popular buildings are closed or events cancelled. Excellent communication skills explaining the rationale, duration, support services, and replacement sites for critical activities are required. Canadian health authorities used voluntary home quarantine during the SARS outbreak and obtained good public compliance (SARS Commission, 2006).

□ □ □

Critical Thinking: Draconian Measures

At first, quarantine sounds like a prudent measure for public health officials to use during an outbreak. However, large-scale quarantine comes with many requirements and responsibilities. If a public health official is going to confine people to a location, the city or state must provide for their needs. Also, if a public health official is going to mandate them to remain under control, that mandate must be enforced. Is deadly force an acceptable method of enforcing quarantine? Does a law enforcement officer have the authority to shoot someone who is fleeing from a quarantine barrier? Would images such as these undermine a community official's authority or ability to quell fear? What about the kinder and gentler measure of social distancing programs? Can we count on the public to limit their contact with others?

□ □ □

Community Quarantine

In extreme circumstances, public heath officials may consider the use of widespread or communitywide quarantine, which is the most stringent and restrictive containment measure. Strictly speaking, *widespread community quarantine* is a misnomer, since *quarantine* refers to separation of exposed persons only and usually allows provision of services and support to affected persons. Widespread community quarantine involves asking everyone to stay home. It may involve a legally enforceable action and it restricts travel into or out of an area circumscribed by a real or virtual "sanitary barrier" or "cordon sanitaire" except to authorized persons, such as public heath or health-care workers.

Large-scale quarantine requires a wide range of services to be provided for individuals confined to one location. In the United States, payment for these services must be addressed up front. Will this cost be borne by the entity ordering the quarantine, state, or federal agencies? And will reimbursement change based on a community declaring a state of emergency or disaster? Will individuals be required to pay for food, services, and supplies they receive while in quarantine and how can they support such expenditures if they are unable to work? Will private for-profit entities be allowed to compete with government or social service providers, and how much can they charge? Who and how will repairs be handled for essential utility and communication services?

The community must be clear what local, state, and federal legislative framework allows restriction of movement of individuals for the purposes of controlling communicable diseases, and who has the authority to declare a public health emergency in the jurisdiction. In some cases, connecting the implementation of isolation or quarantine to a declaration of an emergency may be beneficial in achieving desired results and smoothing over supportive activities.

An effective and comprehensive response to a fast-moving, contagious, and potentially fatal disease with limited possibilities for prevention, treatment, or other medical intervention requires the unprecedented coordination and collaboration of a wide range of government and nongovernment parties. Government officials must provide leadership, but they cannot provide all of the services required to contain a disease and support an affected community.

Similarly, while response to a public health crisis must rely heavily on public health, medical, and scientific experts, it will also require support from law enforcement personnel, mental health providers, transportation authorities, emergency management directors, and other key service providers, who may know little about disease transmission or control measures.

Medical Surge

The approach to meeting surges in demands for care requires partnerships and rationing of care not typically seen. Systems of triage and ongoing assessment to assure that those initially assigned to lower levels of care can be transferred to higher-level care sites when indicated and vice versa. An extension of this strategy is the promotion and support of home care. Taken together, these strategies are geared to lessen the chance that emergency departments and hospitals will be inundated with patients who could be successfully managed in nonhospital or lower-level care settings, reserving hospital care for those most in need. Exactly who will provide this care, protocols that are to be followed, reimbursement for services, and protection against liability are issues to be solved locally by all preparedness partners.

Zoonotic Connection

Thinking back to the points made in Part III of this book, one cannot forget that in many instances, animal health and human health may be inextricably linked. The release of a disease agent, regardless of the intended target, may have implications for both animal and human hosts. A bioterrorist incident aimed at human populations may manifest in animals. In fact, the animals may show signs of the disease before the human targets. In this way, animals may act as a sentinel host. In addition, animals may also be infected by the release and serve to maintain the pathogen in an area. In this instance, the animals may act as a reservoir for the disease agent. What this suggests is that animal health and human health officials should have good working relationships and that surveillance data must be shared.

Conclusion

The consequences of a biological incident are potentially complex and are likely to result in a convergence of state and federal government agencies on the scene of the incident. Many agencies from the federal government will respond to a CBRNE incident, providing necessary resources. Planners within local jurisdictions need to maintain a list of the agencies, the contact numbers, and the resources available from each. State and local governments must be fully compliant with NIMS. This includes the adaptation of the ICS. Unified or area command is an essential element in domestic incident management in which multiple jurisdictions and agencies are involved. It provides guidelines to enable agencies with different legal, geographic, and functional responsibilities to coordinate, plan, and interact effectively. Unified or area command removes much of the inefficiency and duplication of effort that can occur when agencies from different functional and geographic jurisdictions or agencies at different levels of government operate without a common system or organizational framework.

Acts of bioterrorism may also result in a mass casualty incident, where there are many victims and serious implications for first responders and public health agencies. The life and safety of responders and civilians are vitally important functions. First responders and health-care personnel need to be equipped with the knowledge to handle the immediate issues of a biological attack. Public health officials will need to be familiar with containment measures that enable them to limit the spread of the disease and restore the community back to its predisaster state.

Essential Terminology

- **Area command.** An organization established to oversee the management of multiple incidents that are each being handled by an ICS organization or to oversee the management of large or multiple incidents where several incident management teams have been assigned. Area command has the responsibility to set overall strategy and priorities, allocate critical resources according to those priorities, ensure that incidents are properly managed, and ensure that objectives are met and strategies followed. Area command becomes unified area command when incidents are multijurisdictional. Area command may be established at an emergency operations center facility or at some location other than an incident command post.

- **Contact tracing.** The identification and diagnosis of persons who may have come into contact with an infected person. For sexually transmitted diseases, this is generally limited to sexual partners; but for highly virulent diseases, such as viral hemorrhagic fevers and plague, a thorough contact tracing would require information regarding casual contacts.

- **Incident Command System.** This is a systematic tool used for the command, control, and coordination of emergency response. ICS allows agencies to work together using common terminology and operating procedures to control personnel, facilities, equipment, and communications at a single incident scene. It facilitates a consistent response to any incident by employing a common organizational structure that can be expanded and contracted in a logical manner based on the level of required response.

- **National Incident Management System.** This is a system mandated by Homeland Security Presidential Directive 5 that provides a consistent nationwide approach for governments, the private sector, and nongovernmental organizations to work effectively and efficiently together to prepare for, respond to, and recover from domestic incidents, regardless of cause, size, or complexity.

- **Surveillance.** The systematic collection, analysis, interpretation, and dissemination of health data to assist in the planning, implementation, and evaluation of public health interventions and programs.

- **Unified command.** This is one of two methods of performing the command function that employs multiple ranking personnel. Unified command is used when an incident affects multiple political or legal jurisdictions or involves several responding agencies with contrasting functional responsibilities and missions.

Web Sites

DHS, The National Incident Management System, available at www.biosecuritycenter. org/content/gvmtDocs/nims.pdf.

FEMA, Introduction to the Incident Command System, available at http://training.fema. gov/EMIWeb/IS/is100.asp.

The Public Health Incident Command System, School of Public Health, University at Albany, State University of New York, available at www.ualbanycphp.org/pinata/ phics/default.cfm.

References

ASTM International. 2006. Standard Practices for Bulk Sample Collection and Swab Sample Collection of Visible Powders Suspected of Being Biological Agents from Nonporous Surfaces. Technical Report E2458-06. West Conshohocken, PA: ASTM International.

Budowle, B., S. Schutzer, J. Burans, D. Beecher, T. Cebula, R. Chakraborty, W. Cobb, J. Fletcher, M. Hale, R. Harris, M. Heitkamp, F. Keller, C. Kuske, J. LeClerc, B. Marrone, T. McKenna, S. Morse, L. Rodriguez, N. Valentine, and J. Yadev. 2006. Quality sample collection, handling, and preservation for an effective microbial forensics program. Applied and Environmental Microbiology 72, no. 10:6431–6438.

California Office of Emergency Services, FIRESCOPE. 2004. Field Operations Guide 420-1: Incident Command System Publication, available at www.firescope.org.

Centers for Disease Control and Prevention. 2001. Interim Recommendations for the Selection and Use of Protective Clothing and Respirators against Biological Agents, available at www.bt.cdc. gov/documentsapp/Anthrax/Protective/10242001Protect.asp.

Martin, G. 2008. Essentials of Terrorism: Concepts and Controversies. Thousand Oaks, CA: Sage Publications.

National Fire Protection Association. 2008. Standard 472: Standard for Professional Competence of Responders to Hazardous Materials/Weapons of Mass Destruction Incidents. Quincy, MA: NFPA.

9/11 Commission. 2004. Final Report of the National Commission on Terrorist Attacks upon the United States. New York: W. W. Norton & Company.

Qureshi, K., K. Gebbie, and E. Gebbie. 2005. Public Health Incident Command System: A Guide for the Management of Emergencies or Other Unusual Incidents within Public Health Agencies, vol. 1. Albany, NY.

SARS Commission. 2006. Final Report, vol. 2, Spring of Fear: The Story of SARS. Toronto: SARS Commission.

Schutzer, S., B. Budowle, and R. Atlas. 2005. Biocrimes, microbial forensics, and the physician. PLoS Medicine 2, no. 12:1242–1247.

U.S. Code of Federal Regulations, 29 CFR, Part 1910.120 Hazardous Waste Operations and Emergency Response, Final Rule.

U.S. Department of Homeland Security. 2003. Homeland Security Presidential Directive-5.

U.S. Department of Homeland Security. 2004a. The National Incident Management System. Washington, DC: Government Printing Office.

U.S. Department of Homeland Security. 2004b. National Response Plan. Washington, DC: Government Printing Office.

U.S. Government Accountability Office. 2003. Infectious Disease: Gaps Remain in Surveillance Capabilities of State and Local Agencies. Washington, DC: U.S. Government Accountability Office.

World Health Organization. 2007. Integrated Disease Surveillance and Response, available at www.who.int/csr/labepidemiology/projects/diseasesurv/en.

12

Biosecurity Programs and Assets

We refuse to remain idle when modern technology might be turned against us. We will rally the great promise of American science and innovation to confront the greatest danger of our time.
—President George W. Bush, at the signing of the Project BioShield Act, July 21, 2004

Objectives

The study of this chapter will enable you to

1. Relate recent initiatives in biosecurity to the four phases of emergency management.
2. Discuss the goals and objectives of the BioShield project.
3. Define the phrase *dual-use research of concern* and discuss the role of the National Scientific Advisory Board for Biosecurity.
4. Discuss how mass prophylaxis caches affect a nation's preparedness and ability to respond to a major disease outbreak.
5. Discuss the Cities Readiness Initiative.
6. Discuss the goals and objectives of the BioWatch program and how it provides early warning and detection capabilities for biothreat pathogens.
7. Discuss the goals and objectives of the BioSense program.
8. Discuss the role of the Laboratory Response Network and the function of its three tiers.
9. Describe the mission of the FBI Hazardous Materials Response Unit.
10. Describe the mission of the National Guard's WMD Civil Support Teams.

Key Terms

Preparedness, mitigation, response, recovery, overt, covert, the Australia Group, BioShield, dual use, mass prophylaxis, strategic national stockpile, BioWatch, BioSense, Laboratory Response Network, Hazardous Materials Response Unit, WMD civil support team.

Introduction

The aim of this chapter is to make the reader aware of biosecurity programs and assets that exist mostly in the United States. The construction of this chapter follows the four phases of comprehensive emergency management (**preparedness, mitigation, response, and recovery**). Biosecurity programs and assets have been developed over the last 10 years to enable the nation to establish policy, provide early warning and detection, improve readiness, and provide specialized response and recovery capabilities.

A specialist in disaster mitigation, Dennis Mileti (1999), said that we "always seem to be preparing for the last disaster." Certainly, much could be said the same for facing the threat of biological terrorism. Since the anthrax attacks of 2001, the nation has been preparing to respond to two forms of bioterrorism: covert and overt attacks. **Covert** attacks would normally be characterized as silent releases of a biological agent into a population, which later would correspond to many patients presenting to clinics and hospital emergency departments with a similar clinical syndrome. In this setting, syndromic surveillance is of paramount importance. Indeed, there may be a number of indicators for a covert act of bioterrorism. Table 12-1 lists some of the indications and characteristics of an outbreak due to bioterrorism.

An **overt** biological attack would be characterized by the release of a biological agent with corresponding notification of the release by the perpetrator. Typically, local fire, law enforcement, and emergency management would arrive on the scene within a few minutes to manage the incident. If this were an isolated incident, federal and state agencies would join local authorities within a few hours to take charge of the scene, since this falls into the realm of the use of weapons of mass destruction.

Officials from all levels of government are charged with preparing their communities for the worst possible disaster. The biological challenge, whether overt or covert, poses one of the most difficult set of circumstances for response organizations to tackle. Local community government officials know that they have limited ability to respond to the release of a biological agent, be it overt or covert. Frankly, it would be prohibitively expensive for all communities, especially small ones, to build the critical mass needed for them to effectively recognize the problem, respond, contain the outbreak, and treat the casualties. Most state governments have built a capacity for dealing with the biological challenge, but lack the resources needed to contain widespread outbreaks. For this reason, the federal government has accepted the responsibility of building critical infrastructure to recognize the threat and effectively deal with it.

Table 12-1 Characteristics of Outbreaks Indicative of Possible Bioterrorism

1. A large number of cases appearing at the same time, particularly in a discrete population.
2. Many cases of a rare disease or those that fall within HHS Category A or B.
3. More severe cases than typical for a given disease.
4. A disease related to an unusual route of exposure (anthrax and inhalation).
5. A disease that is unusual in a given place or out of season.
6. Multiple simultaneous outbreaks of the same disease or different diseases.
7. Unusual disease strains or uncommon antibiotic resistance to an organism.

□ □ □

Critical Thinking

The 2001 Amerithrax incident was both covert and overt. Covertly, anthrax spores were sent to the AMI building in Boca Raton, Florida, without obvious notification that the act had taken place. The incident led to two cases of inhalation anthrax. The letters sent to government officials and media moguls contained a note that informed the victims that they had been attacked with "anthrax." Why would the perpetrator(s) act first covertly and then overtly about a week later?

□ □ □

Mitigation: Establishing Policy and Oversight

Hazard mitigation addresses the causes of a disaster, reducing the likelihood that it will occur or limiting its impact. The focus of mitigation is to stop disasters before they happen (Lindell, Prater, and Perry, 2007). How could you stop a biological disaster before it happens? Indeed, how could you prevent a terrorist or group of belligerents from using biological agents? Laws with stiff penalties for breaking them may be a deterrent to some amateur terrorist or prankster; however, to others determined to advance their agenda, laws are of no consequence. Those concerned about the proliferation of bioweapons might enact policies for limited exchange or trade of questionable substances. Governments concerned about scientific advancements or sensitive information ending up in the public domain might assemble a group to provide guidelines and oversight. Finally, developments in disease prevention and new treatments might be fostered, so that the threat from certain biological agents might dissipate, especially if you could protect a nation from such.

Covered under the umbrella of mitigation are three examples of government attempts to mitigate disaster due to potential use of biological weapons: the Australia Group, the BioShield project, and the National Science Advisory Board for Biosecurity. The Australia Group represents one of the few international efforts aimed at providing oversight for the Biological and Toxin Weapons Convention. Project BioShield was initiated shortly after the terrorist attacks of September 11, 2001. The $5.6 billion appropriated for this project is supposed to give the United States new countermeasures to mitigate a biological attack against the American people. Finally, the National Scientific Advisory Board for Biosecurity is a panel of experts assembled by the Department of Health and Human Services to develop policy and establish guidelines to deal with scientific advances that might be exploited by would-be terrorists or adversaries of the United States.

The Australia Group

At the international level, **the Australia Group** was formed in 1985 by the government of Australia as an informal body aimed at reducing the proliferation of chemical and biological weapons. More relevant, the Australia Group has strived to support the objectives of the Biological and Toxin Weapons Convention, which has been in force since 1975. The group's main objective has been to enhance the effectiveness of national export licensing measures for specific chemical and biological agents. Following its first meeting in Brussels, it quickly established export controls, which have been modified over the years to address emerging threats and challenges. The number of countries participating in the Australia Group has grown from 15 in 1985 to more than 40. All of the participants in the Australia Group are parties to the BWC.

Evidence of the diversion of dual-use materials (discussed later) to biological weapons programs in the early 1990s led to the participants' adoption of export controls on specific biological agents. The agent control lists developed by the group have been expanded over the years to include technologies and equipment that can be used in the manufacturing or disposal of biological weapons. This comprehensive listing was subsequently used by the U.S. Department of Health and Human Services to construct Category A, B, and C lists.

Project BioShield

On July 21, 2004, President George W. Bush signed a bill to provide funding for Project **BioShield,** an effort jointly directed by the Department of Homeland Security and the Department of Health and Human Services. BioShield is intended to provide medical countermeasures to protect the American public from chemical, biological, radiological, or nuclear attacks. Project BioShield legislation was the result of a bipartisan effort in response to the catastrophic events of September 11 and the anthrax and ricin attacks directed against members of Capitol Hill and other Americans. The BioShield project has three primary goals. First, the project authorized funds to purchase and stockpile of vaccines aimed at countering specific biothreat agents. Second, the project authorized funding for increased research and development of new pharmaceuticals for the diseases caused by specific biothreat pathogens. Third, the project proposed sweeping changes in government authorization regarding medical response to a bioterror crisis and approval processes for new drugs and vaccines.

□ □ □ ▬▬▬▬▬▬▬▬▬▬▬▬▬▬▬▬▬▬▬▬▬▬▬▬▬▬▬▬▬▬▬▬▬▬

Project BioShield Summary

Project BioShield institutes a secure funding source for the purchase of critical medical countermeasures, such as vaccines, therapeutics, and diagnostics. Project BioShield authorizes $5.6 billion in funding over 10 years for the advanced development and purchase of high-priority medical countermeasures. This "special reserve fund" was provided in the fiscal year 2004 Department of Homeland Security Appropriations Act and becomes available to the Secretary of Health and Human Services for procurements following interagency and White House approval. The Office of Public Health Emergency Countermeasures) has authority for all procurement activities for Project BioShield. Acquisitions under Project BioShield are restricted to products in development that are potentially licensable within eight years from the time of contract award (Russell, 2007).

▬▬▬▬▬▬▬▬▬▬▬▬▬▬▬▬▬▬▬▬▬▬▬▬▬▬▬▬▬▬▬▬▬▬ □ □ □

Consider the preexisting state of affairs whereby a private company considers the research and development costs of producing a new drug or vaccine for a disease that is rare or not normally known to occur in the United States. After spending tens to hundreds of millions of dollars up front, what would be the likelihood that the product would sell in sufficient quantity to enable the company to show a profit? There is virtually no way for new drug makers to see a potential profit in any of these ventures unless they were able to predict when, where, and what agent would be used in the next act of bioterrorism, if any.

The Project BioShield bill gave authority to the Food and Drug Administration (FDA) to use unapproved drugs in national (public health) emergencies. The BioShield Project bill also authorizes federal officials to contract with private enterprises to purchase these medications while they are still under development. However, the final approval for purchase is contingent on clinical trials and tests that indicate the treatments are safe and efficacious. Project BioShield was intended to remove some of the uncertainties companies face in producing these drugs. Perhaps one of the most important aspects of this is the preemergence of a buyer (the federal government) for a product that will take tens of millions of dollars to research and produce. In this way, the speculative nature of any new venture is reduced, to a degree.

Although the federal government has guaranteed funding, biotechnology companies are still charged with the task of creating a safe and efficacious product. Therefore, failure to effectively produce a viable medication would be economically devastating to that company after many years of investment. This is probably why so few companies are actively engaged in BioShield and working toward these goals.

There are other concerns about BioShield from the biotechnology sector. Biotech executives complain that language in BioShield does not offer sufficient protection from product liability should a newly developed pharmaceutical have adverse effects on patients or fail to protect them against a specific pathogen.

Perhaps due to the initial shortfalls of the BioShield bill, President Bush signed into law the formation of a new regulatory division, the Biomedical Advanced Research and Development Authority (BARDA). BARDA provides another $1 billion in funding for continuation of research and development initiatives addressed under Project BioShield. Now, the government will assist with the cost of establishing domestic manufacturing facilities. It will also provide liability coverage to those companies whose products, not yet licensed with the Food and Drug Administration, will be used during biological attacks. Under these new guidelines, clear evidence of intentional misconduct must be present for a company manufacturing one of these pharmaceuticals to be sued. BARDA also provides funding for the development of experimental animal models to be used in clinical trials for testing of drugs and vaccines against diseases that are too dangerous for human subjects (i.e., VHF, smallpox, pneumonic plague).

So far, only a small fraction of the anticipated treatments and vaccines envisioned under BioShield are available. Drug companies waited months, if not years, for government agencies to decide which treatments they want and in what quantities. Unable to attract large pharmaceutical corporations to join the endeavor, the government is instead relying on small start-up companies that often have no proven track record.

A number of biosecurity and biodefense experts have expressed concerns about Project BioShield:

- Some have opined that the expedited peer review process reduces the quality of the research. Peer reviews were designed to maximize the probability that proposals with the greatest scientific advantage would get funding.

- Some suggest that the government will end up purchasing countermeasures that will eventually fail to be approved. It is a fact that most drugs and vaccines that begin the approval process fail to become approved treatments.

- Critics of such programs suggest that, because of the high product failure rate in advanced development, the government will inevitably fund products that will never be usable. In addition to removing the development risks that industry has traditionally borne, it also inserts government decision makers into the countermeasure development process, a role they argue is better suited to experts and entrepreneurs in industry. Some critics would prefer to have the government set the requirements and have industry figure out how best to meet them.

□ □ □ ▬▬▬▬▬▬▬▬▬▬▬▬▬▬▬▬▬▬▬▬▬▬▬▬▬▬▬▬▬▬▬▬▬▬▬▬▬

Officials Remain Optimistic

2007 will be a big year for BioShield: HHS has almost finished a road map for how to deal with 15 WMD threats and will soon release a new anthrax strategy and a new request for acute radiation drugs. We are nowhere near where we should be, but it's the nature of the business that developing drugs and vaccines takes years and some failures.

—Carol Linden, HHS, quoted in Marek, 2007

▬▬▬▬▬▬▬▬▬▬▬▬▬▬▬▬▬▬▬▬▬▬▬▬▬▬▬▬▬▬▬▬▬▬▬▬▬ □ □ □

Although much of what has been written so far on BioShield does not seem positive, there is some hope the project will produce effective medical countermeasures for specific biological threats. In fact, up to the time of this writing, HHS has viable acquisition programs to address four threat agents: *Bacillus anthracis*, smallpox virus, botulinum toxins, and radiological/nuclear agents. Seven contracts have been awarded: (1) recombinant protective antigen anthrax vaccine, the next-generation anthrax vaccine; (2) anthrax vaccine adsorbed, the currently licensed anthrax vaccine; (3) anthrax therapeutics (monoclonal antibody technology); (4) anthrax therapeutics (human immune globulin); (5) a pediatric formulation of potassium iodide; (6) chelating agents to treat ingestion of certain radiological particles; and (7) botulinum antitoxins. Additional acquisition contracts are expected to be awarded in the next fiscal year (Russell, 2007).

National Science Advisory Board for Biosecurity

The National Science Advisory Board for Biosecurity (NSABB) was established in 2005. The NSABB is a critical component of a set of federal initiatives to promote biosecurity in life science research. The Department of Health and Human Services created this advisory board to provide advice, guidance, and leadership regarding biological research that has the potential for misuse and could pose a biologic threat to public health or national security (NSABB web site, 2007). This is often referred to as **dual-use** *research of concern*. That is, research that can be reasonably anticipated to "provide knowledge, products, or technologies that could be directly misapplied by others to pose a threat to public health, agriculture, plants, animals, the environment, or materiel." The NSABB has proposed a series of experimental outcomes that should be given special consideration for their "dual-use" potential.

The NSABB is charged specifically with guiding the development of a system of institutional and federal research review that allows for fulfillment of important research objectives while addressing national security concern. The NSABB also developed guidelines for the identification and conduct of research that may require special attention and security surveillance. The NSABB developed professional codes of conduct for scientists and laboratory workers that can be adopted by professional organizations and institutions engaged in life science research and materials and resources to educate the research community about effective biosecurity.

The NSABB is made up of 25 voting members that have a broad range of expertise in molecular biology, microbiology, infectious diseases, biosafety, public health, veterinary medicine, plant health, national security, biodefense, law enforcement, and scientific publishing. The NSABB also includes nonvoting ex officio members from 15 federal agencies and departments. These include

- Executive Office of the President.
- Department of Health and Human Services.
- Department of Energy.
- Department of Homeland Security.
- Department of Veterans Affairs.
- Department of Defense.
- Department of the Interior.
- Environmental Protection Agency.
- Department of Agriculture.
- National Science Foundation.
- Department of Justice.
- Department of State.
- Department of Commerce.
- Intelligence community.
- National Aeronautics and Space Administration.
- Others as appropriate.

The principal aim of the NSABB is to enhance biosecurity in life sciences research. In this light, *biosecurity* refers to "processes and procedures that are designed to minimize the likelihood that biological research will be misused for the production or enhancement of biological weapons" (NSABB web site, 2007). This initiative includes implementation of the *Public Health Security and Bioterrorism Preparedness and Response Act* through the *Select Agent Program*, which were previously covered in Chapter 10. It supports the following actions, with the guidance of the NSABB:

- Developing guidelines for oversight of dual-use research and ongoing evaluation and modification of these guidelines as needed.
- Working with the scientific community, including journal editors, to ensure the development of guidelines for the publication, public presentation, and public

communication of potentially sensitive research and encouraging the adoption of these guidelines by international organizations.

- Providing guidance on the development of a code of conduct for scientists and laboratory workers.
- Developing mandatory programs for education and training in biosecurity issues for all scientists and laboratory workers at federal and federally funded institutions.

The NSABB advises all federal departments and agencies that conduct or support life science research. The board recommends specific strategies for the efficient and effective oversight of dual-use biological research, including the development of guidelines for the case-by-case review and approval by institutional biosafety committees. The NSABB takes into consideration both national security concerns and the needs of the research community. This includes strategies for fostering continued rapid progress in public health research (e.g., new diagnostics, treatments, vaccines and other prophylactic measures, and detection methods), as well as in food and agriculture research while being mindful of national security concerns.

Preparedness

Preparedness protects lives and property and facilitates rapid recovery (Lindell, Prater, and Perry, 2007). Preparedness for bioterrorism consists of plans, procedures, and resources that must be defined in advance. The components of preparedness are designed to support a timely and effective emergency response and recovery process. The threat of bioterrorism and concerns about pandemic influenza in the United States brought increased attention to the need for state and local public health authorities to provide their communities with rapid, reliable access to prophylactic medications. In fact, the federal government recently called on all states to devise comprehensive mass prophylaxis plans to ensure that civilian populations have timely access to necessary antibiotics and vaccines in the event of future outbreaks (Hupert et al., 2004).

Prophylaxis is defined as the medical care or measures provided to individuals to prevent or protect them from disease. This medical care or protective measure may be performed to entire populations or large sectors considered to be at risk. When this becomes the objective, the campaign or program may be referred to as **mass prophylaxis**. Traditionally, these measures include dispensing medications or implementing vaccination. Effective public health response to a large-scale outbreak hinges on the ability to recognize the outbreak, to mobilize supplies of needed materials to affected populations in a timely manner, and to provide ongoing medical care for affected individuals (Hupert et al., 2004).

Accordingly, there has been a major expansion of federal assets to assist local public health providers to plan and implement mass prophylaxis campaigns for bioterrorism and disease outbreak response. This expansion includes mass prophylaxis caches, the BioWatch program, the BioSense program, and the Cities Readiness Initiative. Each of these components will be considered in this section of the chapter.

Mass Prophylaxis Caches

The CDC maintains the **strategic national stockpile** (SNS) of prophylactic agents and provides technical assistance on dispensing operations to local public health and emergency management planners throughout the United States. However, the SNS and its support staff do not constitute a stand-alone, first response operation. Similarly, the National Disaster Medical System was established by HHS to provide rapid response capability for medical disasters throughout the United States, but this system is not designed to supplant comprehensive local planning and operations for mass prophylaxis campaigns either (Hupert et al., 2004).

The ready availability of drugs and vaccines may limit the response capacity to a serious outbreak. The federal government created the SNS, which is composed of a number of ready-to-deploy *push packs* containing medical supplies to treat thousands of patients affected by CDC Category A agents. In addition, predesignated pharmaceutical supply caches and production arrangements and/or vendor-managed inventory, may be used for large-scale ongoing prophylaxis or vaccination campaigns. States, some large municipalities, and a few medical facilities across the United States have developed smaller stockpiles and secure supply chains for critical antibiotics and medical material for use in an outbreak (Hupert et al., 2004).

Federal mass prophylaxis assets and resources are intended to build on the local and regional first-response infrastructure for carrying out mass prophylaxis. Every public health jurisdiction in the country has the responsibility to develop and maintain the capability to carry out first-response and federally assisted mass drug dispensing and vaccination campaigns tailored to its local population. At least four reasons underlie this rule:

Local mass prophylaxis activities need to be under way prior to the arrival of any federal assets.

Federal or state assistance will not include sufficient personnel to fully command or staff communitywide mass prophylaxis dispensing operations.

Mass prophylaxis operations are likely to remain under local control even after federal or state assets are delivered.

Dispensing and follow-up operations are likely to continue after the departure of federal or state assets (HHS and AHRQ 17-19).

Once requested, assets from the SNS are likely to arrive in less time than it takes to set up a network of fully functional dispensing or vaccination centers. Each center must have a well-defined supply route linking it to the receive, stage, and storage site for these SNS materials as well as to any local stockpiles. Most local stockpiles are predesignated for use by local first responders, hospital, and emergency management personnel to ensure that they are ready to work with the public as soon as or before federal assets arrive.

Onsite stockpile management requires the ability to ensure proper storage (e.g., coolers), inventory management, and security of supplies. If the center is dispensing drugs or vaccines under investigational new drug protocols, local staff may have to track the patients to whom those supplies are distributed. However, recent legislative proposals call for the creation of emergency use authorizations to facilitate rapid dispensing of *off-label* or investigational medicines and vaccines in the setting of mass prophylaxis (Hupert et al., 2004).

BioWatch: Early Warning and Detection

BioWatch is an early warning system for aerosolized biological agents initiated by the Department of Homeland Security. President George W. Bush announced the BioWatch program to the American public in his 2003 State of the Union Address. With early detection and medical treatment, people exposed to a biological agent have a much greater chance of recovery and the consequences of such an attack can be mitigated.

Using a network of cabinets or stations, BioWatch collectors gather samples of airborne particles into a filter system. Each day, filters are collected manually by a technician and taken to a CDC Laboratory Response Network facility for processing. The sensor filters are tested for six specific organisms: *Bacillus anthracis* (anthrax), *Brucella* species (brucellosis), *Burkholderia mallei* (glanders), *B. pseudomallei* (melioidosis), *Yersinia pestis* (plague), *Variola major* and *V. minor* (smallpox virus), and *Francisella tularensis* (tularemia). BioWatch has analyzed over a half million samples (Crawford, 2006). The time of air sample collection, transport, and sample processing introduces at least a 36-hour turnaround time from the moment when a sample is collected until the moment local officials could be notified to make appropriate responses.

□ □ □ ▬▬▬▬▬▬▬▬▬▬▬▬▬▬▬▬▬▬▬▬▬▬▬▬▬▬▬▬▬▬▬▬▬▬▬▬

BioWatch Summary

BioWatch provides early warning of a biological attack by sampling the air of high-risk cities continuously and expeditiously identifying six biothreat pathogens. The mission of BioWatch is to deploy, sustain, and maintain a continuous operational ability to detect, mitigate, respond to, and recover from a bioterrorist event. Goals of the BioWatch program are to provide early warning of a biological attack, determine the extent and type of the attack, assist in the identification of the attackers, and determine the scope of the contamination as it is related to the infected population and area (U.S. Department of Homeland Security, Office of the Inspector General, 2007, p. 2).

▬▬▬▬▬▬▬▬▬▬▬▬▬▬▬▬▬▬▬▬▬▬▬▬▬▬▬▬▬▬▬▬▬▬▬▬ □ □ □

Reportedly, in 31 cities across the United States, the exact location of the sampling monitors and the cities where they are deployed has not been made public for obvious security reasons (Shea and Lister, 2003). BioWatch is a component of the National Bio-Surveillance Integration System, which combines human health data from the CDC, agricultural diseases data from the USDA, food safety data from the USDA and HHS, and environmental monitoring from BioWatch to improve detection and response (Brodsky, 2007).

BioWatch is a joint program involving several federal agencies. The Department of Homeland Security is overly responsible for BioWatch. The CDC and EPA conduct the daily activities that make it function. The EPA is responsible for monitor deployment, site security, and accessing monitor technology (Pike, 2006). The CDC processes the samples. In addition, Los Alamos National Laboratory and Lawrence Livermore National Laboratory cooperate with EPA and CDC on the more technical aspects of the program.

Federal funding of the BioWatch Program for the fiscal year 2003 was $40 million. This represented 12% of the total budgeted money for biological countermeasures that year (Shea and Lister, 2003). In fiscal year 2005, President Bush requested that BioWatch funding be increased to $118 million to expand the program and increase research and the development efforts for improved biosensors. In 2007, Congress cut BioWatch funding by $13 million, which was originally allocated for the purchase of new sensors. In a brief issued by the Nuclear Threat Initiative, the annual estimated cost of maintenance and collection per city is $1 million, with a final program budget estimated at $85 million (Brodsky, 2007). BioWatch is not a stand-alone, autonomous detection system. It requires lots of hands to pull the pieces together. As previously mentioned, someone has to collect the filter, transport it to laboratory, extract the sample, process the material, and run the test. All this labor represents about 75% of the operational cost of the program (Cohen, 2007).

The fundamental challenge of the BioWatch system is to detect a biological attack when there is no information about where the event might take place or what meteorological conditions may exist during the event (Shea and Lister, 2003). A critical step in designing the BioWatch monitoring system was deciding where to site the air-sampling collectors. With a limited number of collectors to deploy and a multitude of potential sites, the goal was to maximize the probability that the network will detect the release of a biological agent while also maximizing the protection provided to the people of a given city. To reach this goal, the efficacy of each collector site and its contribution to the entire collector network had to be objectively evaluated using a standard set of metrics. To address this challenging problem, Los Alamos National Laboratory developed a geospatial application to provide analysts with a quantitative, decision-making tool for choosing collector sites. The BioWatch regional sensor siting tool (BioWatch tool) was developed within a commercial, off-the-shelf geographic information system. The tool uses and extends features of a commercial geographic information system package through customized menu-driven interfaces and integration with regional-scale dispersion models (Linger, 2005).

□ □ □ ▬▬▬▬▬▬▬▬▬▬▬▬▬▬▬▬▬▬▬▬▬▬▬▬▬▬▬▬▬▬▬▬▬▬▬

Critical Thinking: Tularemia, BioWatch, and the U.S. Capitol

On September 25, 2005, low levels of *Francisella tularensis* (tularemia) were detected on BioWatch filters in and around the Washington, D.C., area. These positive results came one day after a war protest took place on the Capitol Mall. Department of Homeland Security officials first suspected a problem when six sensors used in the BioWatch biological agent surveillance system collected air samples that indicated tularemia might have been present on the Mall. Subsequent testing at the CDC confirmed that there were low levels of tularemia bacteria on the Mall. However, those results were not considered entirely definitive under BioWatch standards, so DHS officials did not inform local public health officials in Washington for several days to avoid a public panic. In fact, it was not until September 30 that local health officials and the public were told to watch out for symptoms of the disease, which include chills, fever, headache, muscle aches, and pneumonia. Department of Homeland Security officials announced nearly a week later that the bacteria was naturally occurring and posed no health threat (Francis, 2006).

Two questions come to mind when reading this brief. First, why did it take federal government officials so long to notify local government agencies of a potential public health threat? After all, BioWatch is a system that stands for early warning and detection. Second, whenever we look for a problem, we will eventually find it, but we are looking for things that occur naturally. So, how do we sort out background levels of these natural pathogenic agents from something that truly poses a threat? The technologies being employed to detect these agents merely tell us of their existence, they do not necessarily tell us that they are viable. Diagnostic methods based on an organism's genetic structure do not yield results equivocal to that samples ability to infect a host.

□ □ □

The BioWatch is not without its critics. Several issues outlined in a 2007 Department of Homeland Security report, including a lack of cooperation in regard to the reporting requirements and the lack of follow-through when after-action reports were received (U.S. Department of Homeland Security, Office of the Inspector General, 2007). One of the biggest issues with BioWatch is the cost of the program. As the program moves into advanced developmental phases, it has the potential to become what it was originally intended to be, an autonomous sampling and detection system. Its function and cost will come into question if it never proves its worth in an actual attack. In the fall of 2005, an incident with BioWatch occurred in Washington, D.C. The way the incident was handled generated controversy and discussion, as explained in the section above "Tularemia, BioWatch, and the U.S. Capitol."

BioSense

BioSense is a web-based software application designed to collect nationwide public health data and disseminate that information to public health officials to increase situational awareness for a possible biological event. The BioSense system gathers real-time disease occurrence data from medical treatment facilities and compares the data to historical data to identify trends or peaks in disease occurrence. Aberrations of disease occurrence data may be the first indication of a potential biological terrorism incident (Loonsk, 2004). The CDC developed BioSense to enable early detection and localization of possible bioterror attacks or other significant outbreaks. The primary goals and objectives of BioSense are to provide the standards, infrastructure, and data acquisition for early detection; enable near real-time reporting, analytic evaluation, and implementation; and provide early event detection support for state and local public health officials (Bradley et al., 2005). Consider the multitude of diseases covered in this text that manifest initially with flulike symptoms. An episode or spike in *influenza-like illnesses* during the summer may be indicative of a biological incident (pandemic influenza, plague). This is precisely what BioSense strives to identify.

BioSense is part of the Public Health Information Network initiative, which is the CDC's "vision for advancing fully capable and interoperable information systems in the many organizations that participate in public health" (CDC, 2007a). The initiative comprises early event detection; routine public health surveillance; secure communications among public health partners; information dissemination and knowledge management, analysis, and interpretation; and public health response systems (CDC, 2007a). BioSense also serves as a platform for routine public health surveillance. The BioSense initiative formed the BioIntelligence Center, which has primary responsibility for monitoring BioSense at the federal level. The BioIntelligence Center looks for anomalies or aberrations in the data that may be indicative of a chemical or biological incident (Bradley et al., 2005). Its functions are "to conduct daily monitoring and investigation of

BioSense national data, support state and local system monitoring and data anomaly investigations, engage in communication with state and local public health officials in all relevant data anomaly investigations, and develop standard operating procedures for data evaluation" (Bradley et al., 2005). Additionally, the BioIntelligence Center has been intimately involved with the improvement and enhancement of the BioSense application, recommending changes and discovering any issues with the application (Bradley et al., 2005).

The Public Health Security and Bioterrorism Response Act of 2002 (P.L. 107-188) authorized the development and funding of the Public Health Information Network and BioSense. BioSense gets its funding through the CDC, receiving nearly $200 million since 2003 (U.S. Government Accountability Office, 2005, 2006). The implementation of the BioSense initiative was composed of various codependent developments. One component of the initiative was the development of the BioSense application itself. This involved developing software capable of receiving medical data, analyzing it for anomalies, and displaying the data and analysis to the user (Yates, 2007). The BioSense application "uses near-real time reporting of health data, performing analysis and data visualization techniques on diagnostic and pre-diagnostic electronic data sources and providing the results to state and local public health departments for use in detecting and characterizing events of potential public health importance" (Bradley et al., 2005).

Another component of the BioSense initiative is the acquisition and mechanism for continued acquisition of public health–related data. "BioSense has implemented three national data sources: Department of Defense (DOD) Military Treatment Facilities, Department of Veterans Affairs (VA) treatment facilities, and Laboratory Corporation of America (LabCorp) test orders" (Bradley et al., 2005). In 2006, the BioSense system received near real-time data from more than 30 hospitals spread out over 10 communities.

The DOD and VA provide ambulatory-care data in the form of *International Classification of Diseases*, Ninth Revision, clinical modification (ICD-9-CM) diagnosis codes and current procedural terminology medical procedure codes (Bradley et al., 2005). LabCorp, on the other hand, provides the test orders along with the reason for the tests in ICD-9-CM coding (Bradley et al., 2005). BioSense then organizes the data into 11 syndromes, which have been assigned priority by the likelihood that the syndrome is indicative of an act of bioterrorism (Sokolow et al., 2004). A multiagency groups the 11 syndromes, from highest to lowest, as follows: botulism-like, fever, gastrointestinal, hemorrhagic illness, localized cutaneous lesion, lymphadenitis, neurologic, rash, respiratory, severe illness and death, and specific infection (Bradley et al., 2005).

Many questions surfaced about the efficacy and value of BioSense. Critics ask if the right data are being collected in a timely manner to make the system useful. Specifically, where are the data being collected and what subset of the population it represents or does not represent? A second concern for the BioSense initiative is the lack of nationwide coverage. Currently, the system collects timely data only from about 30 cities in less than 20 states (Caldwell, 2006). Although the CDC hopes to expand the system, nationwide metropolitan coverage is still far from being achieved and still ignores the more rural areas of the country. Another concern for the data is the presence of duplicative or erroneous records (Bradley et al., 2005). As with any information system or database, the system is only as good as the data going into it. Duplicate records or erroneously entered data can have significantly detrimental effects on the efficacy of the system. According to one report, BioSense data were "opportunistic and noisy" (Bradley et al., 2005).

In 2005, the U.S. Government Accountability Office (GAO) reviewed the BioSense initiative along with other major public health initiatives. The GAO report on BioSense and the Public Health Information Network (PHIN) stated this in its summary: CDC's PHIN initiative includes applications at various stages of implementation; as a whole, however, it remains years away from fully achieving its planned improvement to the public health IT [information technology] infrastructure . . . "CDC and DHS are pursuing related initiatives, but there is little integration among them and until the national health IT strategy is completed, it is unknown how their integration will be addressed . . ." In addition, state and local public health agencies report that their coordination with federal initiatives is often limited (U.S. Government Accountability Office, 2005).

Also, according to the GAO report, "CDC's BioSense application . . . is available to state and local public health agencies, but according to the state and local officials with whom we spoke, it is not widely used, primarily because of the limitations of the data it currently collects" (U.S. Government Accountability Office, 2005).

Because the BioSense application gathers data from DOD and VA facilities, the geographic distribution of these facilities affects the populations covered. Areas that have small military or veteran populations and no DOD or VA facilities would be underrepresented in the system (Yates, 2007). A recent study that examined the use of the BioSense system for monitoring influenza activity also cited the need for additional data sources beyond the DOD, VA, and LabCorp. According to this report, "the addition of more data sources to BioSense . . . will be needed to increase the utility of BioSense for influenza monitoring" (Tokars et al., 2006).

The CDC has spent nearly $200 million on the BioSense project, which the GAO states may be years away from being fully operational and may be duplicative to other surveillance programs (U.S. Government Accountability Office, 2005). Additionally, the GAO reports, "syndromic surveillance systems are relatively costly to maintain compared to other types of disease surveillance and are still largely untested" (U.S. Government Accountability Office, 2005). This brings into question, whether this is the most efficient use of these funds. Some state and local officials have suggested that they would prefer to receive data from the CDC that they can use for their own analysis (U.S. Government Accountability Office, 2005).

Additionally, the GAO noted that "while HHS and other key federal agencies are organizing themselves to develop a strategy for public health surveillance and interoperability, decisions regarding development and implementation are being made now without the benefit of an accepted national health IT strategy that integrates public health surveillance-related initiatives" (U.S. Government Accountability Office, 2005). Because of this, initiatives, such as BioSense, may be developed such that they are not consistent and interoperable with other national biological and surveillance systems (U.S. Government Accountability Office, 2005).

However, one of the biggest potential problems with the BioSense program is the prevalence of false positives (Yates, 2007). According to one report, "during June–November 2004, of the approximately 160 data anomalies examined, no events involving disease outbreaks or deliberate exposure to a pathogen were detected" (Sokolow et al., 2004). Another report noted the following: "from February through May 2005, eight Sentinel Alerts were issued for [New York state] on the BioSense web site: two for Crimean-Congo hemorrhagic fever, two for cryptosporidiosis, two for typhoid fever, one pneumonic plague, and one Russian spring–summer encephalitis. Upon follow up, all eight alerts were determined to not represent cases of immediate public health significance" (Thoburn et al., 2006). The conclusions from the report were that "false alarms generated by new surveillance systems should be viewed as opportunities to test and improve communication pathways across national, state, and local levels" and that "caution should be exercised when assessing ICD-9 coded syndromic surveillance data" (Thoburn et al., 2006). It appears as though BioSense has a long way to go. In many ways, its half steps toward nationwide surveillance do little at this point to mitigate the threat from a biological attack.

Cities Readiness Initiative

The cities readiness initiative (CRI) is a recently developed program created by the Department of Health and Human Services under the CDC's Public Health Emergency Preparedness Project (Centers for Disease Control, 2004). The intent of the cities readiness initiative is to develop an increased capacity to respond to biological outbreaks and radiological incidents (Centers for Disease Control, 2007b) through the development of a strategic national stockpile and a system of disseminating the SNS in the case of an emergency, which includes increased planning and cooperation among all levels of government. The CRI is designed to allow for dissemination of medications to the affected population within 24–48 hours of the incident's onset.

The CRI sprang from an earlier emergency preparedness program that began in 1999 to enhance the strategic national stockpile and its ability to rapidly dispense antibiotics and other pharmaceuticals. The initial program worked primarily with state governments; however, the CRI program was later expanded to deal with radiological and biological threats to large metropolitan areas (Centers for Disease Control, 2006). In 2004, 21 pilot cities were included in the program. In 2005, an additional 15 cities were selected to participate. In 2006, another 36 cities were added, which brought the total to 72 cities inclusive of all 50 states and the District of Columbia (Centers for Disease Control, 2007c).

The funding for the Cities Readiness Initiative is through the CDC's Public Health Emergency Preparedness program (Centers for Disease Control, 2007c). Since 2001, the overall funding for the CDC's Public Health Emergency Preparedness project has decreased from about $900 million to $700 million (National Association of County and City Health Officials, 2007). The CDC's Public Health Emergency Preparedness project allows funding to be used for preparedness across the depth of an entire metropolitan area. For instance, the CRI grant for Philadelphia also includes funding for Wilmington, Delaware, and Camden, New Jersey (Centers for Disease Control, 2006). While the program's funding comes from the CDC, only four metropolitan areas are funded directly; New York City, Los Angeles, Chicago, and Washington, D.C. The other 68 cities receive their funds through the allocation of state funds from the CRI program. Each year, states apply for and receive CRI grants, which now go out to all 50 states (Lindell, Prater, and Perry, 2007).

There has been an interesting and creative component to the CRI program. Some CRI grant recipients have reached out to the U.S. Postal Service (USPS) and negotiated a working relationship whereby the USPS will be used in these cities to disseminate medications for mass prophylaxis campaigns (Centers for Disease Control, 2007c). The door-to-door delivery mechanism was arranged in 2005. To accomplish this, USPS employees must be trained on specific requirements for handling and storage of the pharmaceuticals (Centers for Disease Control, 2007d). The stated intent of this arrangement is to assist with a targeted response plan in reaction to the dissemination of aerosolized *Bacillus anthracis* spores within a densely populated area where such a release would rapidly affect a large percentage of the population (Centers for Disease Control, 2007d). Getting the antibiotics out in this way may be more efficacious than attempting mass prophylaxis by other means.

Response and Recovery

Emergency response begins when the event occurs (Lindell, Prater, and Perry, 2007). In some cases, early warning and detection systems may alert officials to the initiation of the event before the first index case becomes symptomatic. For the record, this early warning or occurrence has happened. During an overt attack, the perpetrator's notification or display triggers officials to mount the response. Regardless of the nature of the attack or the lag time between dissemination of the agent and awareness of the incident, a rapid assessment of the contaminated area is needed. Emergency response has three goals: protect the public, limit the damage, and minimize the extent of secondary spread. Local emergency responders dominate the response period, which is characterized by uncertainty and urgency. Response leads us to recovery. Recovery from disaster is characterized as short term or long term. The goal of recovery efforts is to first establish normalcy, then strive to return the disaster area to what it was before the incident. This may or may not be achievable and depends highly on the nature of the incident.

Laboratory Response Network, CDC

In 1999, the CDC partnered with the Association of Public Health Laboratories and the Federal Bureau of Investigation to form the **Laboratory Response Network**. The goal of this partnership was to bring together a collective body of knowledge and infrastructure needed to facilitate cooperation in the event of an act of terrorism or other public health emergency and to enable rapid identification of a biological agent. The LRN currently has two major components: a well-developed network of public health laboratories dealing with biological agents (Bio-LRN) and a smaller network of public health laboratories dealing with chemical agents. The LRN is a national network of approximately 150 laboratories. The network includes the following types of laboratories:

- **Federal.** These laboratories are at the Centers for Disease Control and Prevention, the U.S. Department of Agriculture, the Food and Drug Administration, the Department of Defense, the Environmental Protection Agency, and other facilities affiliated with federal agencies.
- **State and local public health.** These are laboratories affiliated with state and local departments of health. In addition to being able to test for Category A biological agents, a few LRN public health laboratories are able to measure human exposure to toxic chemicals through tests on clinical specimens.

The LRN is one network that encompasses both bioterrorism and chemical terrorism preparedness and response. LRN bioterrorism preparedness and response activities emphasize local laboratory response by performing the following tasks:

- Helping to increase the number of trained laboratory workers in state and local public health facilities.
- Distributing standardized test methods and reagents to local laboratories and promoting the acquisition of advanced technologies.
- Supporting facility improvements.

The Bio-LRN is a network of about 120 laboratories in all 50 states that include local, state, and federal public health laboratories as well as international, veterinary diagnostic, military, and other specialized laboratories that test environmental samples, animals, and food (see Figure 12-1 for LRN facility locations). Efficient detection and an effective response require the coordination of a network made up of three levels of laboratory that handle progressively more complex testing: sentinel, reference, and national. Figure 12-2 is a graphic depiction of the LRN. Each laboratory's support role and capacity within the LRN structure is detailed as follows.

Sentinel Laboratories

Sentinel laboratories play a key role in the early detection of biological agents. These include environmental, food, veterinary, agriculture, public health, and clinical laboratories. Because of their routine activities, these laboratories have the potential to handle materials that may contain agents that threaten the public's health. Routine assay of human specimens for the presence of microbial agents is an activity that places all clinical

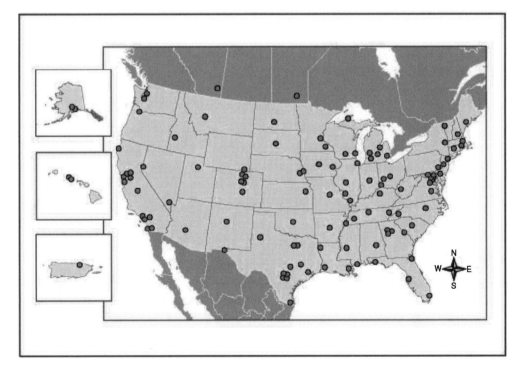

Figure 12-1 The location of LRN facilities in the United States, Canada, and Puerto Rico. (Image courtesy of Centers for Disease Control and Prevention.)

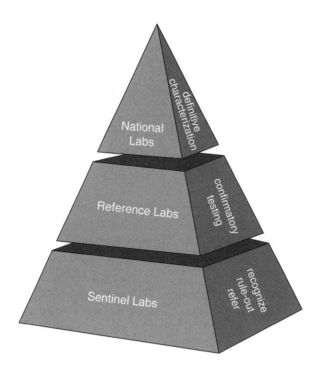

Figure 12-2 The three tiers of the Laboratory Response Network and the functions at each level. Sentinel laboratories, which are the most numerous in the United States, provide communities with the ability to recognize that a biothreat pathogen is present in an environmental or clinical specimen. Their primary role is to "rule out" a positive or refer a positive sample to the next higher level of the LRN. Reference laboratories accept samples and provide "confirmatory testing." There is at least one reference laboratory for each state. At the top of this pyramid are the national laboratories, which provide "definitive" testing and agent characterization. (Image courtesy of Centers for Disease Control and Prevention.)

laboratories in a position to serve in a sentinel capacity within the LRN. By default, these laboratories are on the front line for detecting public health threats caused by agents of bioterrorism or newly emerging infectious disease. Sentinel laboratories

- Are the most numerous in the LRN.
- Made up of private and hospital laboratories that routinely process patient tests.
- May be the laboratories to first test or recognize a suspect organism.
- Conduct tests to "rule out" less harmful organisms.
- Refer samples to a reference laboratory, if they cannot rule out that the sample is a bioterror agent.

Reference Laboratories

Reference laboratories are responsible for investigation or referral of specimens. These include more than 100 state and local public health, military, international, veterinary, agriculture, food, and water testing laboratories. In addition to laboratories located in the United States, facilities located in Australia, Canada, and the United Kingdom serve as reference laboratories abroad. Reference laboratories

- Have specialized equipment and trained personnel.
- Perform tests to detect and confirm the presence of a bioterror agent.

- Are capable of producing conclusive, confirmatory results.
- Include local, state, and federal laboratories.

National Laboratories

The LRN for biological agents includes national laboratories operated by the CDC, U.S. Army Medical Research Institute for Infectious Diseases, and the Naval Medical Research Center. These laboratories are responsible for specialized strain characterizations, bioforensics, select agent activity, and handling highly infectious biological agents. These national laboratories

- Include the CDC, the U.S. Army Medical Research Institute for Infectious Diseases in Maryland, and the Naval Medical Research Center, also in Maryland.
- Perform highly specialized testing to identify specific disease strains and other characteristics of an investigated agent.
- Test certain highly infectious agents that require special handling.

The Bio-LRN has been involved in a number of major testing operations since it was established in 1999. In the 2001 anthrax attacks, Bio-LRN laboratories tested more than 125,000 samples by the time the investigation was completed. Bio-LRN laboratories were involved in developing tests and materials to support the DNA sequencing of the SARS virus, which was identified at the CDC (Centers for Disease Control, 2004). As previously mentioned, Bio-LRN laboratories process all samples from the BioWatch program. Figure 12-3 shows examples of the LRN in action.

Examples of the LRN in Action

Anthrax attacks of 2001—In 2001, just weeks after terrorists attacked the World Trade Center (WTC) in New York City and the Pentagon in Washington, D.C., letters containing spores of anthrax were sent to Florida, New York City, and Washington, D.C. The anthrax spores infected 22 people, killing five. The LRN played a pivotal role in the quick detection of *Bacillus anthracis*, the bacteria that causes anthrax.

On Oct. 4, 2001, CDC confirmed the first case of the 2001 anthrax attacks in a 63-year-old Palm Beach County, FL, man who was exposed to *B. anthracis* at his workplace. The discovery came when clinical specimens taken from the man revealed the organism. The specimens were forwarded to a state public health laboratory, which was an LRN member. The state public health laboratory confirmed the anthrax infection and alerted the CDC.

Investigators collected environmental and clinical samples from the victim's workplace, a local hospital, and from sites in North Carolina where the man had traveled just prior to getting sick. Testing performed by LRN laboratories helped determine that exposure occurred at work after being exposed to anthrax that was mailed to the man's office.

Testing of postal facilities, U.S. Senate office buildings, and newsgathering organizations' offices occurred in the weeks and months that followed. Between October and December of 2001, LRN laboratories successfully and accurately tested more than 125,000 samples, which amounted to more than one million separate bioanalytical tests.

Source: http://www.bt.cdc.gov/lrn/examples.asp

Figure 12-3 Examples of the LRN in action. (Source: Centers for Disease Control and Prevention, LRN web site, www.bt.cdc.gov/lrn.)

The LRN has developed exquisitely sensitive and specific diagnostic protocols to either "rule in" or "rule out" Category A, B, and C biological agents. Each of the LRN laboratory levels has a specified list of diagnostic tests and procedures to identify the biothreat agents. This list is based on the biosafety level classification of each agent and the capacity of each laboratory to meet the biosafety level guidelines specified by the CDC and National Institutes of Health for each organism. Specific biological markers related to virulence or pathogenicity have been incorporated into the agent specific protocols. These protocols and procedures are *sensitive* and not in the public domain; therefore, it is not possible to comment further on these assays.

Important Considerations for Responders

Before submitting a sample to an LRN facility, responders should contact the facility's bioterrorism coordinator to ensure that the sample is taken in accordance with local laboratory procedures. Specific circumstances surrounding the incident should be discussed with the bioterrorism coordinator to ensure that the collection procedures are appropriate. Biosampling techniques can be agent specific and matrix specific (Sanderson et al., 2002). This means that certain biological agents require a specific sampling methodology to best support the testing necessary to identify the analyte or biological marker employed by the definitive assay. In addition, the matrix or environment from which the suspect substance is believed to be (e.g., clean water, waste water, air, soil) may dramatically influence the sampling method employed.

In situations where biological threat agents are suspected, the item(s) should be field safety screened and immediately transported in law enforcement custody to an LRN laboratory. This should be done in coordination with the local FBI WMD coordinator.

Field safety screening should be limited to ruling out explosive devices, radiological materials, corrosive materials, and volatile organic compounds. Currently, *there are no definitive tests for identifying biological agents in the field*. In fact, in 2002, the Department of HHS issued an advisory against first responders employing handheld assays to assist in making conclusive determinations on the scene of a possible biological incident. Additional field testing can mislead response efforts by providing incorrect or incomplete results and destroy limited materials critical for definitive laboratory testing required to facilitate any appropriate public health and law enforcement response.

☐ ☐ ☐ ▬▬▬▬▬▬▬▬▬▬▬▬▬▬▬▬▬▬▬▬▬▬▬▬▬▬▬▬▬▬▬▬▬▬▬▬

The Department of Health and Human Services Advisory

In July 2002, the Department of Health and Human Services issued the following advisory:

The U.S. Department of Health and Human Services at this time recommends against use by first responders of hand-held assays to evaluate and respond to an incident involving unknown powders suspected to be anthrax or other biological agents.

That statement has not been retracted.

▬▬▬▬▬▬▬▬▬▬▬▬▬▬▬▬▬▬▬▬▬▬▬▬▬▬▬▬▬▬▬▬▬▬▬▬ ☐ ☐ ☐

State LRN reference laboratories developed and prepared agent- or test-specific sample collection kits that must be used by responders to collect unknown samples. Samples are not normally accepted by an LRN facility if they were not collected using the specific kit needed to ensure protocols and procedures are consistent with sampling methodology. Working from the statement made in Chapter 2 of this text, do not take bad samples to a good test. Sampling kits normally contain both cotton swabs (for suspected biological samples) and nylon swabs (for suspected chemical samples), tubes, jars, pipettes, labels, wax wrap, marker pens, and a clean metal paint can for overpackaging the samples. All of these items are packaged in a box for storage on hazmat vehicles or in apparatus.

When responders request a sample collection kit, they must meet certain criteria, which include having certified hazardous materials technicians on the team, possessing the appropriate level of personal protective equipment, and having completed state-provided training on sample collection. The recommended level of PPE is Level A (fully encapsulated with self-contained breathing apparatus, or SCBA) for indoor collection and Level B (splash protection with SCBA) for outdoor collection. The LRN stipulates that the FBI's 12-point collection process be used to collect samples. Samples can be (and have been) collected by numerous types of agencies: local hazardous materials response teams, civil support teams, the FBI's Hazardous Materials Response Unit, and local emergency management agencies. All samples must be tested for chemical, explosive, and radiological/nuclear hazards before being transported to the LRN facility. Additionally, all samples must include a chain of custody form and transported to the LRN laboratory under the custody of a law enforcement official. Once the samples have arrived at the LRN facility, they are tested again for radiological hazards before being accepted into the laboratory.

Hazardous Materials Response Unit

The Federal Bureau of Investigation's **Hazardous Materials Response Unit** (HMRU) responds to criminal acts and incidents involving the use of hazardous materials and develops the FBI's technical proficiency and readiness for crime-scene and evidence-related operations in cases involving chemical, biological, and radiological materials and wastes. The FBI HMRU fulfills its mission through an integrated effort involving specialized response teams, a national training program, interagency liaison, technical assistance to FBI field and headquarters divisions, and the development of field response programs. The unit also trains, equips, and certifies FBI field office personnel for hazardous materials operations. The FBI HMRU responds to the scene of a credible act of bioterrorism to ensure that the crime scene is processed in accordance with established protocols for safety and evidence processing. This team has extensive experience from the Amerithrax incident and numerous other events that have taken place over the past few years. Formed in June 1996, the FBI HMRU is an example of a vision made reality in a very short time as the nation was preparing for the 1996 olympics. The unit was envisioned by Dr. Randall Murch, chief of the Scientific Analysis Division of the FBI's Laboratory Division, and Dr. Drew Richardson, the HMRU director. At the time, the unit's philosophy was simple: At the site of a WMD incident, there might be scores of dead people about, but if you could not prove who did it, the likelihood of more victims in future incidents increases. Despite the extreme emotion of the moment, evidence has to be collected (Seiple, 1997).

National Guard WMD Civil Support Teams

The *Defense Against Weapons of Mass Destruction Act of 1996* stipulated that the Department of Defense take on a new role with additional responsibility for supporting the domestic anti-terrorism mission. Specifically, the DOD was mandated by Congress to share its expertise and capabilities for neutralizing, dismantling, and disposing of explosive ordnance, as well as radiological, biological, and chemical materials. In addition, the DOD was asked to work toward the development and deployment of countermeasures against weapons of mass destruction. In May 1998, Presidential Decision Directive (PDD) 62, Protection Against Unconventional Threats to the Homeland and Americans Overseas, directed that the DOD assist other federal agencies train first responders and maintain specially trained military units to assist states with WMD response. Shortly thereafter, the National Guard formed 10 rapid assessment and initial detection units. These teams were designed to provide rapid response to a WMD incident and assist state and local responders. The 10 teams became what is now referred to as **WMD civil support teams** (CST). Since that time, the National Guard has added more teams with the goal of having one for each state. Currently, specific locations for these teams is based on population concentrations and intended to minimize the response times within particular geographic areas. They were also located in order to prevent overlapping team areas of responsibility.

The mission of the WMD-CST is to support local and state authorities at domestic WMD incident sites by identifying agents and substances, assessing current and projected consequences, advising on response measures, and assisting with requests for additional military support. Civil support teams maintain the capability to mitigate the consequences of a WMD event. They are considered to be experts in WMD effects and nuclear, biological, and chemical defense operations. This ambitious mission is accomplished by 22 personnel, highly trained in multiple disciplines covering 14 military occupational specialties. The team is divided into six functional areas or cells: command, operations, logistics/administration, communications, medical, and survey.

Local jurisdictions may request assistance from the CST through their state adjutant general's office for plans, operations, and military support. Direct request for CST assistance is also available through its operation and command sections. First responders are able to directly contact the CST for possible WMD assistance. Interagency training and cross training for the CST and first responding agencies become a valuable tool to develop professional relationships. Furthermore, the CST are able to respond to all counties within the state or region, including distant island communities, by loading and flying vehicles on U.S. Coast Guard or Air National Guard assets. Response time varies due to remoteness of locations; however, all team members are on 24-hour alert at all times (Hurston, Sato, and Ryan, 2006).

□ □ □ ▬▬▬▬▬▬▬▬▬▬▬▬▬▬▬▬▬▬▬▬▬▬▬▬▬▬▬▬▬

Critical Thinking

Imagine that over a 24-hour period 17 patients report to the Emergency Department of a small hospital in a rural community. Clinically, the patients present with fever, malaise, flushing, conjunctivitis, myalgia, abdominal pain, nausea, diarrhea, and a petechial rash. One of the patients is coughing up blood (hemoptysis) and another has seizures in the Emergency Department and falls into a coma. An infectious diseases specialist is called in to determine the cause of this outbreak. The specialist collects blood and urine from most of the patients and orders a battery of tests. Samples are sent on to the hospital laboratory for routine blood and urine tests. A subset of the patient samples is forwarded to a commercial laboratory where more elaborate testing is available. Based on initial findings from the hospital laboratory, the specialist comes up with a differential diagnosis of viral hemorrhagic fever, bacterial sepsis, Rocky Mountain spotted fever or other rickettsial disease, leptospirosis, borreliosis, dengue hemorrhagic fever, septicemic plague, or hemorrhagic smallpox.

The specialist begins to piece together information gathered from the patients and family members. There appears to be one common event shared by all the case patients: All attended a major sporting event, a championship college football game that occurred nearly two weeks previously. The physician has a reasonable suspicion that the cases are all related to an intentional act or at least to some bizarre coincidence.

At this point, isolates from case patients would be forwarded to a regional laboratory in the state's capitol city for further testing. If the isolate is found to test positive for one of the CDC bioterrorism agents (Category A, B, or C), an isolate would be sent to the national laboratory in Atlanta for definitive testing. The state Bureau of Investigation, the Federal Bureau of Investigation, and a local joint terrorism task force would send agents to the community to work with epidemiologists to determine the source of the outbreak. The FBI's Hazardous Materials Response Unit, along with the state's Army National Guard's WMD civil support team might be requested to respond to collect and process evidence within the community. The evidence that these teams collect would be delivered to the laboratory via local, state, or federal law enforcement. Environmental and clinical samples would be gathered from numerous sites. The field collection effort would be enormous and likely to include thousands of samples.

Review the scenario to discuss implications for local emergency managers and response organizations from the jurisdictions that will be included in the response and investigation. Where does the National Incident Management System, Incident Command System, unified command, and the National Response Framework come into play here? What agency will be in charge of the response? What agency will be in charge of the investigation? Consider something like this occuring in your town.

Conclusion

Programs and assets have been assembled internationally, nationally, and regionally to safeguard populations from the threat of biological agents. The programs and assets can be viewed with the framework of comprehensive emergency management, which is made up of mitigation, preparedness, response, and recovery. Nations have come together and taken a stance individually to mitigate the threat. For the most part, these programs produce policy and procedures that support the Biological and Toxin Weapons Convention of 1972. In addition, the best mitigation strategy may be to develop safe and effective vaccines that could prevent disease from some of the most serious biothreat pathogens. Perhaps Project BioShield will one day give us a few of these vaccines.

Nothing is easy about preparing for a biological disaster. The task is further complicated by the added dimension that the disaster you may be preparing for will be due to an intentional, covert act that is strategically employed in the areas where you are weakest. Such is the insidious nature of bioterrorism and biowarfare. Regardless, we may all find ourselves rather "flat-footed" if and when that moment comes, especially if we are unable to recognize early on that the problem exists. This is all the more dangerous if the agent that emerges is highly transmissible from person to person, the incubation period short, and the case fatality rate high. A few examples that come to mind are smallpox, pneumonic plague, and pandemic influenza. Our hope is that BioWatch provides us with early detection, which of course depends on where the sensors are placed and what they monitor. Probably one of the best investments we have made along these lines is the establishment of the Laboratory Response Network. Having the ability to *quickly and definitively identify the problem* is the LRN charter. This extensive and highly capable network stands to *recognize* the threat, which will enable us to focus response efforts and get onto the business of recovery.

Responding to a biological disaster will be frustrating, confusing, and dangerous for first responders, first receivers, and public health officials. Developed countries are far better trained and equipped to deal with the release of a formulated biological agent than they were 10 years ago. However, we have a long way to go before we are truly capable of responding with a standard set of rules and procedures that will enable us to minimize death and restore the community back to its predisaster state. Chapter 13 explores consequence management; that is, what we will do when a biosensor tells us that we have been attacked.

Essential Terminology

- **Australia Group**. An informal forum of countries that, through the harmonization of export controls, seeks to ensure that exports do not contribute to the development of chemical or biological weapons. Coordination of national export control measures assists Australia Group participants to fulfill their obligations under the Chemical Weapons Convention and the Biological and Toxin Weapons Convention to the fullest extent possible.

- **BioSense initiative**. A national program intended to improve the nation's capabilities for conducting near real-time biosurveillance, enabling health situational awareness through access to existing data from health-care organizations across the country.

- **BioShield project**. A comprehensive effort to develop and make available modern, effective drugs and vaccines to protect against attack by biological and chemical weapons or other dangerous pathogens.

- **BioWatch program**. An early warning system that can rapidly detect trace amounts of biological materials in the air, whether they are due to intentional release or minute quantities that may occur naturally in the environment. The system assists public health experts determine the presence and geographic extent of a biological agent release, allowing federal, state, and local officials to more quickly determine emergency response, medical care and consequently management needs.

- **Covert.** Secret or hidden, not openly practiced or engaged in or shown or avowed.

- **Dual-use research of concern.** Research that, based on current understanding, can be reasonably anticipated to provide knowledge, products, or technologies that could be directly misapplied by others to pose a threat to public health and safety, agriculture, plants, animals, the environment, or material.

- **Hazardous Materials Response Unit.** A highly trained unit, belonging to the FBI laboratory services, that responds to criminal acts and incidents involving hazardous materials (hazmat). The unit also develops technical proficiency and readiness for crime-scene and evidence-related operations in cases involving chemical, biological, and radiological materials and wastes and trains U.S. and international law enforcement in these skills. It also provides site safety oversight of FBI personnel operating in other high hazard crime scenes, including collapsed structures and confined spaces.

- **Laboratory Response Network.** A national network of local, state, and federal public health, food testing, veterinary diagnostic, and environmental testing laboratories that provide the laboratory infrastructure and capacity to respond to biological and chemical terrorism, and other public health emergencies. The more than 150 laboratories that make up the LRN are affiliated with federal agencies, military installations, international partners, and state and local public health departments.

- **Mass prophylaxis.** Medical care or measures provided to a large percentage of a population to prevent or protect them from disease. The best example of this is the smallpox eradication campaign that rid the world of one of the worst human diseases in 1980. As a program, mass prophylaxis can be a mitigation measure, a preparedness initiative or a post-event response function.

- **Mitigation.** Measures taken in advance of a disaster aimed at decreasing or eliminating its impact on society and on environment.

- **Overt.** Open and observable, not secret or hidden.

- **Preparedness.** Actions that are undertaken to reduce the negative consequences of events where there is insufficient human control to institute mitigation measures. Commonly, plans, training, exercises, stockpiles, warning systems, and capacity building for response fall into the realm of preparedness.

- **Recovery.** The coordinated process of supporting emergency-affected communities in reconstruction of the physical infrastructure and restoration of emotional, social, economic, and physical well-being. When it comes to bioterrorism and major outbreaks, recovery is often an afterthought.

- **Response.** Activities and programs designed to address the immediate and short-term effects of the onset of an emergency or disaster.

- **Strategic national stockpile.** Large quantities of medicine and medical supplies to protect the American public if there is a public health emergency (e.g., terrorist attack, flu outbreak, earthquake) severe enough to cause local supplies to run out. Once federal and local authorities agree that the SNS is needed, medicines will be delivered to any state in the U.S. within 12 hours in something referred to as a *push pack*. Each state has plans to receive and distribute SNS medicine and medical supplies to local communities as quickly as possible.

- **WMD civil support team.** U.S. National Guard teams made up of 22 highly trained personnel with the mission to deploy rapidly to assist a local incident commander in determining the nature and extent of an attack or incident, provide expert technical advice on WMD response operations, and help identify and support the arrival of follow-on state and federal military response assets. The WMD CST is a joint unit, which can consist of both Army National Guard and Air National Guard personnel.

Discussion Questions

- How does the comprehensive emergency management model relate to countering the threat of biothreat agents?
- Explain the process for getting samples to the LRN.
- What's wrong with performing rapid tests in the field for the detection of biothreat pathogens?
- An act of bioterrorism involving pneumonic plague occurs in your town. Imagine how the situation would unfold: How would it be recognized? What agencies in your local community would respond? What assets at the regional, state, and federal level could you call on to lend assistance? Who would be the incident commander?

Web Sites

Australia Group, available at www.australiagroup.net/en/index.html.

BioSense initiative, available at www.cdc.gov/biosense.

Cities readiness initiative, available at www.bt.cdc.gov/cri.

DHS management of the BioWatch Program (OIG 2007), available at www.dhs.gov/xoig/assets/mgmtrpts/OIG_07-22_Jan07.pdf.

FBI Hazardous Materials Response Unit, available at www.fbi.gov/hq/lab/html/hmru1.htm.

National Science Advisory Board for Biosecurity, available at www.biosecurityboard.gov.

Laboratory Response Network, available at www.bt.cdc.gov/lrn.

Project BioShield home page, available at www.whitehouse.gov/infocus/bioshield.

Weapons of mass destruction civil support teams at GlobalSecurity.org, available at www.globalsecurity.org/military/agency/army/wmd-cst.htm.

Strategic national stockpile, available at www.bt.cdc.gov/stockpile.

References

Bradley, C. A., H. Rolka, D. Walker, and J. Loonsk. 2005. BioSense: Implementation of a national early event detection and situational awareness system [electronic version]. *Morbidity and Mortality Weekly Report* 54 (Supplement):11–19.

Brodsky, B. 2007. *The Next Generation of Sensor Technology for the BioWatch Program*, available at www.nti.org/e_research/e3_92.html.

Caldwell, B. 2006. *Connecting for Biosurveillance: Essential BioSense Implementation Concepts* [electronic version], available at www.amia.org/inside/initiatives/healthdata/biosense_amia_2_presentation4_06.pdf.

Center for Disease Control. 2004. *The Cities Readiness Initiative City-by-City Allocations Formula*, available at http://www.bt.cdc.gov/planning/continuationguidance/pdf/cri-funding-attachl.pdf.

Center for Disease Control. 2006. *The Cities Readiness Initiative Guidance*, available at www.bt. cdc.gov/planning/guidance05/pdf/appendix3.pdf.

Centers for Disease Control. 2007a. *BioSense*, available at www.cdc.gov/biosense.

Center for Disease Control. 2007b. *The Cities Readiness Initiative*, available at www.bt.cdc.gov/cri.

Center for Disease Control. 2007c. *The Cities Readiness Initiative Factsheet*, available at www.bt. cdc.gov/cri/pdf/facts.pdf.

Center for Disease Control. 2007d. *The Cities Readiness Initiative Q&A*, available at www.bt.cdc. gov/planning/guidance05/pdf/qa.pdf.

Cohen, J. M. 2007. United States Department of Homeland Security Science and Technology: Six Years after the Attack: Are We Better Prepared to Respond to Bioterrorism? Hearing before the United States Senate Committee on Homeland Security Government Affairs on October 23.

Crawford, M. 2006. *United States Department of Homeland Security Science and Technology Fact Sheet*, available at www.milnet.com/wh/DoHS/BioWatchFactSheetFINAL.pdf.

Francis, D. 2006. U.S defends tularemia response. Global Security Newswire.

Hupert, N., J. Cuomo, M. A. Callahan, A. I. Mushlin, and S. S. Morse. 2004. *Community-Based Mass Prophylaxis: A Planning Guide for Public Health Preparedness*. Prepared by Weill Medical College of Cornell University, Department of Public Health under Contract No. 290-02-0013-3. AHRQ Pub No. 04-0044. Rockville, MD: Agency for Healthcare Research and Quality.

Hurston, E., A. Sato, and J. Ryan. 2006. National Guard civil support teams: Their organization and role in domestic preparedness. *Journal of Emergency Management* 4, no. 5 (September–October):20–27.

Lindell, M., C. Prater, and R. Perry. 2007. *Introduction to Emergency Management*. Hoboken, NJ: John Wiley and Sons.

Linger, S. 2005. The BioWatch Tool: GIS-Enabled Sensor Siting. URISA 2005 Annual Conference, Geographic Information Systems. In: *Addressing Conference Proceedings, Public Participation GIS Conference Proceedings*.

Loonsk, J. W. 2004. BioSense—A national initiative for early detection and quantification of public health emergencies [electronic version]. *Morbidity and Mortality Weekly Report* 53 (Supplement): 53–55.

Marek, A. 2007. A meager yield from BioShield: A federal effort to protect the public from bio-terrorism isn't off to a strong start. *U.S. News and World Report* (March 18).

Mileti, D. 1999. *Disasters by Design: A Reassessment of Natural Hazards in the United States*. Washington, DC: Joseph Henry Press.

National Association of County and City Health Officials. 2007. *Federal Funding for Public Health Emergency Preparedness: Implications and Ongoing Issues for Local Health Departments*, available at www.naccho.org/documents/SurveyReport_Final.pdf.

Pike, J. 2006. *BioWatch*, available at www.globalsecurity.org/security/systems/biowatch.htm.

Russell, P. 2007. Project BioShield: What it is, why it is needed, and its accomplishments so far. *Clinical Infectious Diseases* 45:S68–S72.

Sanderson, W., M. Hein, L. Taylor, B. Curwin, G. Kinnes, T. Seitz, T. Popovic, H. Holmes, M. Kellum, S. McAllister, D. Whaley, E. Tupin, T. Walker, J. Freed, D. Small, B. Klusaritz, and J. Bridges. 2002. Surface sampling methods for *Bacillus anthracis* spore contamination. *Emerging Infectious Diseases* 8:1145–1151.

Seiple, C. 1997. Consequence management: Domestic response to weapons of mass destruction. *Parameters* (Autumn):119–134.

Shea, D., and S. Lister. 2003. *The BioWatch Program: Detection of Bioterrorism*. Report No. RL 32152; Washington, DC: Congressional Research Service, November 19.

Sokolow, L. Z., N. Grady, H. Rolka, D. Walker, P. McMurray, R. English-Bullard, and J. W. Loonsk. 2004. Practice and experience deciphering data anomalies in BioSense [electronic version]. *Morbidity and Mortality Weekly Report* 54 (Supplement):133–139.

Thoburn, K. K., J. R. Miller, J. I. Tokars, C. Bradley, and D. Zomer. 2006. The New York state BioSense sentinel alert experience [electronic version]. *Advances in Disease Surveillance* 1:68.

Tokars, J. I., G. A. Roselle, L. Brammer, J. Pavlin, R. English-Bullard, S. M. Kralovic, P. Gould, A. Postema, and N. Marsden-Haug. 2006. Monitoring influenza activity using the BioSense system, 2003–2005 [electronic version]. *Advances in Disease Surveillance* 1:70.

U.S. Department of Homeland Security, Office of the Inspector General. 2007. *DHS Management of BioWatch Program*. Publication OIG-07-022. Washington, DC, available at www.dhs.gov/xoig/assets/mgmtrpts/OIG_07-22_Jan07.pdf.

U.S. Government Accountability Office. 2005. *Report to Congressional Requestors: Information Technology—Federal Agencies Face Challenges in Implementing Initiatives to Improve Public Health Infrastructure* [electronic version], available at www.gao.gov/new.items/d05308.pdf.

U.S. Government Accountability Office. 2006. *Report to the Chairman, Committee on Government Reform, House of Representatives, Information Technology: Agencies and OMB Should Strengthen Processes for Identifying and Overseeing High Risk Projects* [electronic version], available at www.gao.gov/new.items/d06647.pdf.

Yates, L. 2007. *CDC BioSense: Capabilities and Capacities for Biosurveillance*. Point Paper. Jacksonville, FL: Jacksonville State University.

13

Consequence Management and a Model Program

Technology is a gift of God. After the gift of life it is perhaps the greatest of God's gifts. It is the mother of civilizations, of arts and of sciences.
—Freeman Dyson

Objectives

The study of this chapter will enable you to

1. Discuss consequence management as it applies to an act of bioterrorism.
2. Define *autonomous detection system* and discuss concerns for employment of such a system.
3. Describe the function and operation of the biohazard detection system, which is deployed throughout the United States Postal Service.
4. Discuss the USPS Continuity of Operations Plan for dealing with a positive biohazard detection system signal.
5. Discuss current initiatives in military biodefense aimed at providing continuous monitoring for biothreat agents.

Key Terms

Consequence management, autonomous detection system, biohazard detection system, concept of operations.

Introduction

In the fall of 2001, letters containing formulated *Bacillus anthracis* spores were mailed to congressional officials and news media personnel. These letters led to the first cases of anthrax related to an intentional release *B. anthracis* in the United States. The cases resulting from this attack were located in five locations: Connecticut; Florida; New Jersey; New York; and of the Washington, D.C. regional area, which includes Maryland and Northern Virginia. The incident, often referred to as Amerithrax, resulted in 22 case patients; 11 of them had cutaneous anthrax and 11 had inhalational anthrax.

Tragically, five of the inhalation anthrax patients died, all from inhalational anthrax. This limited attack, although simple in execution, touched all Americans as they worried about their mail. The actual attack prompted a number of sick individuals to perpetrate hoaxes by enclosing a variety of powdery substances into envelopes and mailing them to a victim. Across the nation, even in unaffected areas, citizens phoned into 911 centers to report suspicious packages, envelopes, and powdery substances. They also brought samples of suspicious powders to officials for testing. Hazardous materials (hazmat) teams and public health laboratories were inundated with an unprecedented amount of work related to these situations and samples.

The response to Amerithrax was complicated by a number of factors. First, the incident occurred when the focus of the nation was centered on response to the terrorist attacks of September 11, 2001. Second, physicians in the United States were not familiar with the clinical presentation, diagnosis, or treatment of anthrax patients. Third, CDC officials, by their own admonition, were not prepared to handle the myriad functions of a large-scale outbreak. In addition, the response was hindered by an enormous crime scene investigation and communication problems between federal agencies that had to coordinate their activities (U.S. General Accounting Office, 2003a).

The attack introduced postal workers to a new and deadly occupational hazard. Nine postal workers were infected and two of them died (Becker, 2004). Amerithrax shocked U.S. Postal Service officials and created great confusion as to how to preserve their business, handle the problem of contamination, and answer all the tough questions that were coming from the American Postal Workers Union (APWU). The USPS closed two postal facilities (Trenton, New Jersey, and Brentwood, Virginia), but other contaminated sites remained open. Here are some important questions that USPS officials needed to answer correctly and expeditiously:

- What should be done to immediately protect the workforce and notify them of the existing threat?
- What was the extent of the contamination (how many facilities)?
- What was the existing threat to postal workers?
- How would the contaminated facilities be cleared and put back into operation?
- What should and could be done if the attacks continued?
- What obligation do USPS officials have to protect their workers from the threat?

How postal officials handled these matters has been the subject of much discussion (Thompson, 2003). Initially, USPS officials were advised by CDC officials that cross-contamination or leakage of *Bacillus anthracis* spores from sealed envelopes would be minimal and unlikely to pose an occupational hazard to postal workers. The discovery of inhalational anthrax in a postal worker in the Washington, D.C., regional area, demonstrated that even individuals who had been exposed only to sealed anthrax letters could contract the inhalational form of the disease. Subsequent inhalational cases in Washington, D.C., New Jersey, New York, and Connecticut underscored that finding (U.S. General Accounting Office, 2003a). In late November 2001, an elderly woman died of inhalation anthrax. Investigators believed that she had received a low level dose of *B. anthracis* spores, but due to her age, she became ill and eventually succumbed to the disease. Investigators focused their attention on the Wallingford, Connecticut, mail processing facility. Even though no postal workers appeared to be ill, the workers were placed on antibiotic therapy as a precaution and the facility was tested for the presence of *B. anthracis* spores. The facility was found to be contaminated with *B. anthracis*; however, USPS officials at the facility informed workers and the union that only "trace" contamination had been found at the facility and decided not to release specific quantitative test results. They believed that the risk to the workers was minimal, none of them was sick and all of them were on prophylactic drugs (U.S. General Accounting Office, 2003b). Although the postal service's communication of anthrax test results appears consistent with its guidelines, its decision not to provide the December 2001 quantified results (i.e., the number of colony-forming units found in the positive samples)—after being requested to do so by an employee union—did not satisfy OSHA disclosure requirements (U.S. General Accounting Office, 2003b). In addition, postal employees called the long-standing distrust of management a communication barrier (Becker, 2004). Subsequently, the APWU applied great pressure for the USPS to institute short- and long-term measures and programs to protect union members from the threat of biological agents.

□ □ □ ▬▬▬▬▬▬▬▬▬▬▬▬▬▬▬▬▬▬▬▬▬▬▬▬

Union Response to USPS Lack of Disclosure

In this time of heightened alert, the employer must provide adequate and timely information that the employee is afforded adequate protection from harm. It is never understandable that an employer can deny or inhibit this opportunity for self protection.
—William Burrus, president, APWU, March 26, 2003

▬▬▬▬▬▬▬▬▬▬▬▬▬▬▬▬▬▬▬▬▬▬▬ □ □ □

General Accounting Office investigators concluded that critical information, which would have alerted public health agencies and USPS to the risks postal employees faced in 2001, was not quickly available. Public health officials initially underestimated the risks posed by the anthrax letters. Both the CDC and the postal service said agency officials would have made different decisions if they had understood earlier that anthrax spores could leak from taped, unopened letters and sicken postal workers (Becker, 2004). Clearly, everyone involved was at a loss for reliable and timely information. These problems, coupled with pressure from the APWU, eventually led government officials to address the lessons learned from Amerithrax. Difficulties encountered from Amerithrax sparked intense interest in bioterrorism preparedness programs and initiatives. One of those initiatives, the biohazard detection system, will be covered in this chapter.

Looking forward, government officials and intelligence analysts predict that terrorists will develop an enhanced capability to use biological agents against us. Accordingly, there appears to be a tremendous potential for large-scale attack with some of the pathogens and toxins that were the subject of Chapters 3, 4, and 5. Further, there is the reality of our day-to-day experience with hoax powders and threats. Dealing with these potentials and realities costs the first responder community millions of dollars annually. In this chapter, we consider the concepts and principles of consequence management as they apply to the release of a formulated biological agent. Following that, we delve into autonomous detection systems and examine in depth a prime example of a device and system that stands to preserve our biosecurity; the USPS biohazard detection system.

Consequence Management

Broadly defined, **consequence management** encompasses measures designed to protect public health and safety, restore essential government services, and provide emergency relief to governments, businesses, and individuals affected by the consequences of disaster. Consequence management is predominately an emergency management function. Relative to terrorism incident operations, consequence management includes measures to protect public health and safety, restore essential government services, and provide emergency relief to governments, businesses, and individuals affected by the consequences of terrorism (Federal Emergency Management Agency, 2001).

Seiple, in a seminal article entitled "Consequence Management: Domestic Response to Weapons of Mass Destruction," stated that consequence management to WMD

> *describes ways and means to alleviate the short- and long-term physical, socio-economic, and psychological effects of a chemical or biological attack. It describes the coordination of international, national, regional, and local assets to deal with the effects of such an attack. The term includes preparatory work in response to a WMD threat—against the Super Bowl, for example—that would include site surveys; assessment of the ability of local hospitals to treat or decontaminate victims; and the size, condition, and locations of local stocks of various antidotes. Preparation could include determining the locations, size, and availability of other national antidote stocks as well as international stocks available to support planning for surge capacity (Seiple, 1997).*

He goes on in this visionary article to make some specific recommendations. First, he proposed that the United States *invest in WMD detection capabilities*, the desired end state being full-spectrum detection. He stated that, "Detection is the first line of defense; it is where tactical consequence management begins." Second, he called for *mandatory consequence management awareness and training*. He suggested that new awareness, education, and training concepts will be the keys to success. This mandatory training would ensure a lowest common denominator of knowledge at the local, regional, and national level. Third, he recommended that we *identify, train, and mentor individuals within organizations*, which would thereby create a new culture determined to deal with the consequences of terrorist use of WMD. He suggested that, if we did not grow such a culture, organizations would not be able to respond effectively and efficiently to either crisis response or consequence management tasks. Last, Seiple recommended that we *develop a tiered continuum of response*. Seiple argued that national assets (e.g., the Hazardous Materials Response Unit and civil support teams) would not be likely to respond to an incident within 6–12 hours. This being true, local responders will have to carry the burden of the immediate response.

It is almost as if Seiple had set the path forward for domestic preparedness and crisis management in the wake of a WMD attack. As has often been emphasized in this text, detection or *Recognition* is the key to the initiation of Avoidance, Isolation, and Notification. Much has been done in the past 10 years to bolster our capability to detect WMD. This coupled with initiatives to advance first responder awareness levels, the formation of the Department of Homeland Security, and the creation of a National Incident Management System, the national response plan, and a national response framework have brought us closer to a state of domestic preparedness.

The key to crisis management is accurate and timely diagnosis of the criticality of the problems and the dynamics of events that ensue. This requires knowledge, skills, courageous leadership full of risk-taking ability, and vigilance. Successful crisis management also requires motivation, a sense of urgency, commitment, and creative thinking with a long-term strategic vision. In managing crises, established organizational norms, culture, rules, and procedures become major obstacles: Administrators and bureaucrats tend to protect themselves by playing a bureaucratic game and hiding behind organizational and legal shelters. A sense of urgency gives way to inertia and organizational sheltering and self-protection by managers and staff alike. Successful crisis management requires sensing the urgency of the matter, thinking creatively and strategically to solving the crisis, taking bold actions and acting courageously and sincerely, breaking away from the self-protective organizational culture by taking risks and actions that may produce optimum solutions in which there would be no significant losers, and maintaining a continuous presence in the rapidly changing situation with unfolding dramatic events (Farazmand, 2001).

The requirements of consequence management and crisis management were combined and addressed in the national response plan. The biological incident annex of the NRP clearly spells out the actions, roles, and responsibilities associated with a response to a biological agent or a disease outbreak requiring federal assistance (Department of Homeland Security, NRP, 2004). However, the NRP applies only to events that are designated as *incidents of national significance*, a term that goes away with the national response framework (2007). This can occur with or without a presidential Stafford Act declaration or a public health emergency declaration by the Health and Human Services secretary.

Autonomous Detection Systems

Release of biothreat agents (BTAs) into public and private organizations is clearly intended by a terrorist to cause widespread panic and catastrophic economic disruption. The ability of authorities to contain and manage an effective response depends on quickly and accurately determining if such a release has genuinely occurred. The ideal detection technology provides both a very rapid and a very accurate test result. Inability to achieve rapid and accurate results would have extraordinary negative outcomes, both in terms of the health and potential mortality to those exposed and the economic costs. False negative results mean that there would be no recognition of the event and no containment of the release. Secondary contamination of work products, workers, or the general public would occur. For anthrax, smallpox, and a few of the other agents, once symptoms occur, the likelihood of death is dramatically increased. For smallpox and many other agents, secondary exposures can occur, with additional people becoming infected. By the time such a situation was finally recognized, decontamination costs would be incredibly high. False positive results, on the other hand, would lead to the unnecessary shutting down of buildings and operations, quarantining people, treating the exposed individuals and subjecting them to potential adverse drug reactions, and generally creating panic.

All current detection technologies, except for the technology described in this chapter, are either too slow or inaccurate (too many false positives or false negatives) or both to enable the rapid and cost-effective management of a potential BTA release. Some of these technologies, such as immunoassay strip tests, are used in the current biothreat environment and may rapidly detect the presence of an agent; however, they are generally insensitive and nonspecific. A definitive confirmation of the results must be made in a special laboratory, such as those of the Laboratory Response Network, using culture methods and molecular methods. Results are not available for 24 hours or more.

The state of the art for accurate detection of *most* BTAs is through genetic analysis. Immunological methods (based on antibody binding) are neither sensitive nor specific enough. Other physical methods, such as mass spectroscopy, are too technologically immature, complicated and expensive, require highly trained operators, and are unwieldy or nonspecific. With genetic assessment tools, such as the polymerase chain reaction, it is possible to detect the presence of the specific genes that actually cause the organism to be virulent, offering the potential to detect engineered organisms (Ryan and McMillan, 2003).

The power of genetic analysis in current systems is offset by the complexity of sample preparation methods and the risk of a contamination of the testing environment by amplified materials. Even in specialized laboratories with highly skilled scientists, false positive rates can exceed 5% because of errors and contamination. As previously mentioned, shortly after Amerithrax, a rash of "white-powder" incidents caused response agencies to deploy their hazmat teams. Commercial diagnostic companies were quick to realize government agencies need to find a rapid and reliable way to discern true threat agents from innocuous materials.

The risk for terrorist events involving the intentional airborne release of infectious agents led to development of new approaches for sampling and testing ambient air both indoors and outdoors (Fitch, Raber, and Imbro, 2003). Handheld assays are essential for making initial determinations from the hot zone. Many biothreat detection products, particularly those involving genetic analysis techniques, are offered today without extensive validation studies or appropriate licenses.

Following Amerithrax, it was clear that sophisticated systems would be needed to protect postal workers and other critical infrastructure (e.g., government offices, military installations, symbolic events, iconic structures). One such approach is the use of an **autonomous detection system** (ADS) that combines automated sampling and on-site testing. An ADS continuously samples the environment (e.g., air or water) and mixes that sample with a special buffer solution. An automated detection assay (e.g., a real-time PCR test or an immunoassay) later analyzes the trapped material at a defined sampling interval. Autonomous detection systems incorporate an alert notification system to trigger a response once a positive signal has been generated. The result is an approximate real-time detection and alerting system (Meehan et al., 2004).

Every agency that deploys an ADS must develop detailed plans for responding to a positive signal (Meehan et al., 2004). In essence, these plans should be formulated into **concept of operation** (CONOPS) documents that embody consequence management principles. Responding to an ADS detection of *B. anthracis* involves coordinating responses with response agencies and other stakeholders. Meehan and colleagues (2004) wrote an extensive report that expresses the government's concerns about ADS deployment and provides guidelines for effective and responsible use of one of these systems. Specifically, the report provides guidelines in the following six areas: response and consequence management planning, including the minimum components of a facility response plan; immediate response and evacuation; decontamination of potentially exposed workers to remove spores from clothing and skin and prevent introduction of the agent into the worker's home and conveyances; laboratory confirmation of an ADS signal; steps for evaluating potentially contaminated environments; and postexposure prophylaxis and follow-up (Meehan et al., 2004). We now explore one such ADS, the biohazard detection system and see how CONOPS has been incorporated into its utilization.

The Biohazard Detection System

Overview

The **biohazard detection system** (BDS) was developed for the United States Postal Service by a consortium of private companies led by Northrop Grumman (Linthicum, Maryland). Subcontractors on the project include Cepheid, Inc. (Sunnyvale, California), Sceptor Industries, Inc. (Kansas City, Missouri), and Smiths Detection (Edgewood, Maryland). The BDS automates and integrates air sampling and subsequent analysis using polymerase chain reaction technology. As letter mail is processed down to a single stream of mail through an automated facer canceller system, it is screened for *Bacillus anthracis* spores using the BDS. Consumables (cartridges and buffer solutions) are replenished daily and weekly with no skilled labor required to operate the system. Deployment of the BDS began in early 2004 and has been completed at 272 sites across the United States. As of 2007, more than 2.6 million tests have been performed during screening of more than 40 billion pieces of mail. There have been no false positives (or true positives) reported. This level of performance has been achieved by the use of two *B. anthracis*-specific target sequences. A sample is called positive only if both sequences are detected. In addition, every test has its own sample processing and internal control to minimize false negative results.

The BDS was designed in response to the anthrax attacks of 2001. The goal was to screen mail for biothreat agents, starting with *B. anthracis* first. The USPS initiated a BDS pilot program in May 2002, followed by a preproduction phase (November 2002–May 2003). Production deployment started in early 2004 and was completed in December 2005. The BDS cabinet holds 10 cartridges and a sufficient supply of water and consumables for a full week of stand-alone operation. Daily maintenance requirements include loading the system with cartridges and other consumables if necessary. Weekly and monthly maintenance activities are performed to ensure that the system performance is optimal at all times (Jarvis and Chegwidden, 2006). At the heart of the BDS lies a biosensor produced by Cepheid, Inc. The biosensor is made up of Cepheid's GeneXpert® instrument and *B. anthracis* detection cartridge, which were developed under design and development protocols according to the best practices detailed in the FDA's quality system requirements. The GeneXpert system was developed as a flexible modular platform suitable for applications in clinical diagnostics, food pathogens, environmental testing, and biothreat testing.

The first test application of the GeneXpert technology in the biothreat arena was initiated in response to the anthrax incident in October 2001. Northrop Grumman selected the GeneXpert module and cartridge system as the key analytical component to its biological detection system because of the attributes just described. Later, in the winter of 2001, the first BDS prototype systems began testing at the Edgewood Aberdeen

Proving Grounds. Over the next eight months, Northrop Grumman sponsored a competition involving a number of candidate technologies to determine which one might possess the ability to detect a small amount of *Bacillus* spores in an envelope. To do this, they used *Bacillus globigii*, a nonpathogenic near neighbor (related species) of *B. anthracis*. The competition demonstrated the GeneXpert to be the only technology capable of detecting *B. globigii* in sealed letters containing as small as 1 milligram (mg) of powdered BG spores (Note: There are 454,000 mg in a pound). No other technology evaluated (12 companies or consortiums competed) demonstrated sufficient sensitivity or selectivity to be considered included in the pilot phase.

Following the successful evaluation of subsequent BDS prototypes, the BDS was selected by the USPS for pilot testing in May 2002. Twelve AFCS sorting machines were fitted with BDS systems, and mail was continuously tested from May 2002 to June 2003. The BDS successfully demonstrated its ability to meet the performance requirements, sensitivity, specificity, and nondeterminate rates and ease of use in the field. Based on the success of the pilot system, a preproduction contract was awarded to the Northrop Grumman Consortium in November 2002, followed by award of a production contract in May 2003. In May 2003, the four-plex assay with fully internally validated quality controls was implemented, and testing continued in more facilities until the USPS was satisfied with the system and a thorough 18-month validation program was completed.

Statement of Required Technical Specifications

To prevent the consequences of slow or inaccurate testing results, key technical specifications were defined that would provide the best solution to the problem outlined previously. The USPS anthrax testing application is an appropriate model. Input was received from experts at the U.S. Army Medical Research Institute for Infectious Diseases, the USPS, the CDC, and leading academic institutions. The USPS intended to safeguard the health of its workforce, minimize cross-contamination of the mail, and strictly avoid false positives or false negatives. System performance parameters specified by the USPS follow:

- *Sensitivity* is a measurement of how few organisms can be present in a sample and still be detected. Based on the specific protocols in the GeneXpert cartridge and knowledge of infectious dose ranges for anthrax, sensitivities were established as
  - Less than 50 *B. anthracis* spores per reaction in a USPS specimen.
  - Less than 30 *B. anthracis* spores per reaction in pure water or buffer.
- *Specificity* is a measure of how often a true negative is called negative by the method. False positive results can cause unnecessary and expensive responses or work stoppages:
  - False positive rate target $\leq 1{:}500{,}000$ (99.9998%).
  - No cross-reactivity with nearest neighbor organisms or those found as normal content of the raw sample.
- *Nondeterminate rate* (due to all test failures, mechanical, software, or reagent) of less than 1%.
- *Speed* of less than 35 minutes to result (after raw sample transfer to cartridge).
- *Algorithm* is a continuous, on-site testing with no human intervention.

Performance Results

The Office of Science and Technology Policy, in the Executive Office of the President, formed an interagency working group (IWG) to critically evaluate the USPS plans and data from BDS pilot studies. In a report from the IWG and the letter from the House of Representatives Committee on Government Reform, dated November 25, 2002, that group concluded that "the BDS and GeneXpert system demonstrated performance consistent with laboratory-based state of the art systems. They found the system fully capable to meet the strict USPS performance requirements" (Office of Science and Technology Policy, 2002).

Overview of the Biosensor

Cepheid developed a system that fully integrates sample preparation, gene amplification, and detection. It consists of an instrument (GeneXpert) and disposable cartridges. The GeneXpert cartridge integrates sample preparation so the user needs no special skills to operate the system. Furthermore, all of the fluids, both sample and processing, are contained within the cartridge, eliminating environment contamination, reagent contamination, and sample-to-sample cross-contamination. False positives due to user mistakes or contamination of the workspace by amplified genetic materials are eliminated. The user simply adds the sample to the cartridge, places the cartridge in the GeneXpert instrument, and 30 minutes later a result is provided. These results are also internally validated so that erroneous but believable results are eliminated.

GeneXpert cartridges (see Figure 13-1) handle large volumes of raw sample, extract and concentrate the target organisms, remove extraneous and inhibiting substances and purify and concentrate the organism's DNA, all automatically. The concentrating of target organisms from large sample volumes enables the GeneXpert to meet the sensitivity requirement.

PCR is a well-established method for the highly sensitive and specific detection of cells at extremely low levels. Gene sequences are amplified from very few copies. Cepheid's technologies enhance the capabilities of this powerful chemistry by employing a unique four-color fluorescent real-time PCR system (see Figure 13-2). Up to four targets or controls can be measured and distinguished simultaneously. For the USPS anthrax test, the assay detects two key virulence genes (pX01 gene [*pag*], and pX02 gene [*capB*]), an internal control designed to emulate those targets, and a separate sample prep control. Detection of the two key virulence genes is the best approach to achieving the specificity requirement. The probability that a test would be simultaneously falsely positive for two separate genes is extremely improbable.

In order to address the issues of false results due to a variety of reagent component failures or micro-fluidic process failures, Cepheid conceived a new approach for quality control of the assay. A *total internal control* method was developed comprising a conventional PCR *internal control*, a separate *sample preparation control*, and a method for evaluating the integrity of the hybridization probes, called a *probe check*. The probe check can actually detect if the hybridization probes have degraded in any way. It can also indicate if reagent reconstitution or reaction tube filling has occurred correctly. These features, in conjunction with manufacturing in a QSR compliant, ISO 13485–certified facility, means no separate external positive and negative controls are required to obtain a valid result. False positive and false negative results are virtually eliminated. Further, the use of the internal controls form key elements of a totally internal control scheme that means *separate positive and negative controls are not required* for routine operation.

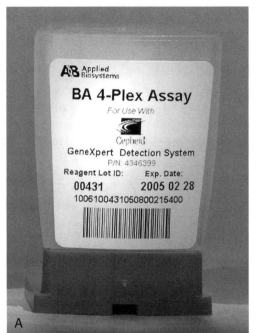
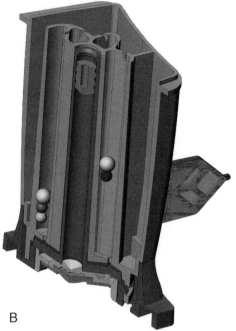

FIGURE 13-1 (a) Actual test cartridge for the biohazard detection system used for sample processing and testing for *Bacillus anthracis* within U.S. Postal Service mail processing facilities. (b) *B. anthracis* cartridge cross-section, artist's rendition, showing inner working parts of the test cartridge. Note macro-fluidic chamber in the center. Flanking that are two chambers that hold the lyophilized reagent beads, which contain all the components needed to perform the real-time PCR. To the extreme right is the wafer-thin test tube that channels the sample and reagent mixture into position with the heating and cooling portion of the GeneXpert biosensor. The entire testing process takes about 30 minutes to perform. (Images courtesy of Cepheid, Inc.)

Cepheid's GeneXpert, shown in Figure 13-3, combines cartridge-based sample preparation with amplification and detection functions performed by processing modules in an integrated automated nucleic acid analysis instrument. These products are designed to purify, concentrate, detect, and identify targeted nucleic acid sequences, taking an unprocessed sample to providing a result in less than 30 minutes. Current techniques for accomplishing this complex series of procedures require extensive manual labor by skilled technicians and can take anywhere from six hours to three days.

□ □ □ ▬▬▬▬▬▬▬▬▬▬▬▬▬▬▬▬▬▬▬▬▬▬▬▬▬▬▬▬▬▬▬▬

USPS Biohazard Detection System

Excerpt from Testimony of Thomas Day, vice president, Engineering, U.S. Postal Service, before the U.S. House of Representatives Committee on Government Reform, Subcommittee on National Security, Emerging Threats, and International Relations, April 5, 2005:

The Postal Service is continuing to improve its processes to protect our employees and our customers from biohazards in the mail. We have installed advanced biohazard detection systems at 107 facilities. Eventually, they will be installed at 282 of our key mail-processing plants.

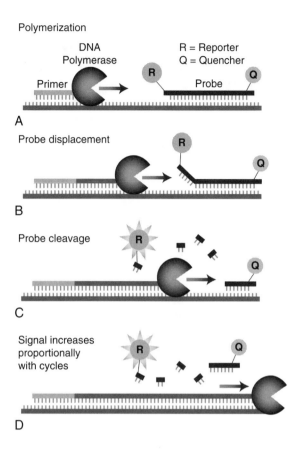

FIGURE 13-2 The BDS uses a real-time PCR assay to detect possible threat agents. The key to the specificity of the BDS anthrax assay is in the use of two targets to identify the presence of *B. anthracis*, pX01 (*pag*) and pX02 (*capB*) sequences. The presence of both targets is required to identify a virulent *B. anthracis* strain. The graphic depiction here shows, in cartoon format, how the process of real-time PCR amplifies and detects specific gene sequences. In A, the probe hybridizes to the gene sequence it was designed for while polymerization is taking place. In B, the probe is displaced by the DNA polymerase and cleaved in C. Finally, in D, the fluorochrome attached to the probe is released into solution and later excited by a specific wavelength of light. This excitation is detected and measured. When that signal exceeds a specific limit, the signal is considered positive. (Image courtesy of Cepheid, Inc.)

To date, the Biohazard Detection System has performed over 550,000 tests involving more than 12 billion pieces of mail. There have been no false positives.

These automated systems, developed with the cooperation of experts from the federal government, the military and the private sector, provide rapid on-site PCR analysis of aerosol samples collected during one of the earliest stages of mail processing. They allow for quick response to a positive test result, triggering the local integrated emergency management plan including cessation of operations and facility shutdown, notification to community first responders, including local public health officials who would make any medical decisions regarding potentially exposed employees and customers.

In addition to the Biohazard Detection System, we are installing a ventilation and filtration system designed to contain the release of biohazards as mail moves through our processing equipment.

In developing and deploying the Biohazard Detection System, we recognized the very real need for standardization of processes to produce reliable, accurate test results in which our stakeholders can have a high level of confidence.

Over the last several years, and as recently as last month, the Postal Service has been the focus of a number of events in which detection systems at other government

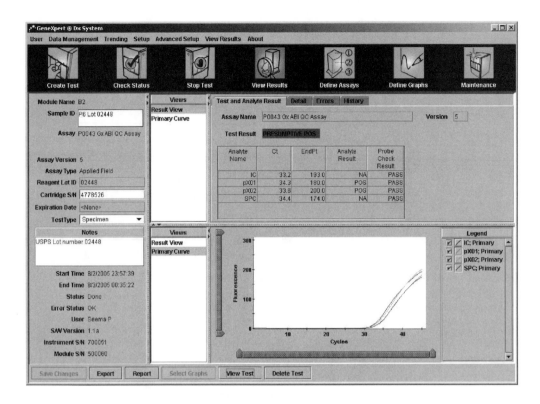

FIGURE 13-3 GeneXpert system showing a presumptive positive test result, which indicates that the sample contained gene sequences for both biological markers for virulent strains of *B. anthracis*. For the test to be positive, both *B. anthracis* markers (*pag* and *cap B*) must be positive and both controls (internal and sample preparation) must also be positive. In addition, the system tests the stability of the reagents with something referred to as a probe check. This sophisticated four-plex assay represents the most exquisitely sensitive and specific rapid commercial test available. Best of all, the technology is incorporated into an autonomous detection system that continuously produces samples, introduces them into the testing apparatus, and alarms postal inspectors when a presumptive positive test result ensues. (Image courtesy of Cepheid, Inc.)

facilities that receive mail have indicated the possible presence of a biohazard. In each of these cases, the Postal Service implemented a response plan that involved sampling and testing, operational adjustments and, where appropriate, preventive medical treatment for our employees.

Ultimately, investigation and further testing determined that the mail was not involved in these incidents and, in fact, that no biohazards were present. The initial positive alerts, however, appear to reflect the varying capabilities of detection equipment as well as sampling and testing protocols relied upon by other agencies.

Source: U.S. General Accounting Office, 2003a.

Development Verification Testing and Field Testing Summary

Sensitivity (limit of detection) was evaluated by the Applied Physics Laboratory of Johns Hopkins, U.S. Army Medical Research Institute for Infectious Diseases, and at CDC LRN, during the pilot phase. In all cases, the measured sensitivity met the requirement, with some tests showing sensitivity as low as 112 spores/ml or about 3.5 spores/reaction (Office of Science and Technology Policy, 2002).

The importance of this low detection limit is that the assay can be very tolerant of variations in sample collection, processing, inhibition, and reagent integrity. At field tests conducted at the Edgewood Chemical and Biological Center in Edgewood, Maryland, all letters containing only 1 milligram of simulant spores were correctly identified.

For specificity, the assay design includes two key genetic markers of virulence for anthrax. U.S. Army Medical Research Institute for Infectious Diseases researchers demonstrated that the assay tests positive for 40 of 40 strains of *B. anthracis* and negative for 54 of 54 nearest neighbor *Bacillus* strains. The ability of the system to meet the demanding false positive rate is based on not only the molecular specificity of the target sequences but on the ability of the system to avoid the pitfalls of cross-contamination as described previously. A positive is obtained when both pX01 and pX02 are positive in the same sample (see Figure 13-3). Based on field test data generated in the validation study made up of over 10,000 tests for pX01 and 500 tests for pX02, with *no false positives*, there was a 99% probability that the system could meet the false positive rate of <1:500,000. It is important to note that this performance exceeds any of the currently approved methods for blood quality screening, which are currently considered the benchmark for clinical performance.

□ □ □ ▬▬▬▬▬▬▬▬▬▬▬▬▬▬▬▬▬▬▬▬▬▬▬▬▬▬▬▬▬▬▬▬

Critical Thinking

In the fall of 2001, we experienced an act of bioterrorism when *Bacillus anthracis* spores were intentionally released through several small envelopes placed in the U.S. mail. The USPS turned to industry and asked for proposals to a solution to this problem. Several small companies teamed up with a major defense contractor, Northrop Grumman, and developed the biohazard detection system. It took two years to fully develop the system and nearly 18 months to validate it. The USPS began deployment of the BDS in late 2004. The system is now fully deployed and actively screening letter mail in 282 mail sorting facilities across the United States. So far, more than 70 billion pieces of mail have been screened and there have been no false positive or true positive results.

Question: Do you believe that having this system in place is the reason why we have not seen another attempt at using the U.S. postal system to disseminate biological agents?

▬▬▬▬▬▬▬▬▬▬▬▬▬▬▬▬▬▬▬▬▬▬▬▬▬▬▬▬▬▬▬▬ □ □ □

New Developments for BDS

The USPS contract with Northrop Grumman called for the eventual development of a three-agent cartridge. In 2007, Cepheid, in collaboration with scientists from the U.S. Army Medical Research Institute for Infectious Diseases, developed a three-agent bio-threat assay for the GeneXpert system. The cartridge is designed for the simultaneous detection of the *Bacillus anthracis*, *Yersinia pestis*, and *Francisella tularensis* in environmental samples.

The three-agent biothreat assay kit consists of a simple two-cartridge system. Either cartridge can be used for screening or to rule out a substance in question. If one of the three targets is detected during a single cartridge test, the second cartridge is used to identify the specific agent in question. The three-agent biothreat assay kit was produced by Cepheid with the same technology employed in the USPS. The GeneXpert system can be run as a stand-alone unit from the USPS. The *Bacillus anthracis* cartridge and the three-agent test may also be purchased by response organizations and used to rule out a suspicious substance or proceeding with appropriate treatment for those exposed to biohazards. At the time of this writing, the USPS has yet to deploy the three-agent cartridge.

□ □ □

BDS Summary

- Has free-standing PCR-based technology.
- Samples air continuously above mail-sorting machines.
- Runs a test every 60 minutes while sorting is under way.
- Takes about 30 minutes to complete the test.
- Tests for a single agent, *Bacillus anthracis*.
- Is automatic: A positive "signal" leads to an alarm, building evacuation, and recall of mail.
- Is exquisitely sensitive and specific.

□ □ □

United States Postal Service CONOPS

The USPS has also installed air ventilation systems above the automated facer canceller systems. In practice, these systems have been designed to minimize the circulation of any aerosolized biological agents. Capturing the release of any materials further mitigates exposure to the workforce.

We now know what makes the BDS function. However, what will occur if a positive alarm sounds from the BDS? In brief, the BDS alarm immediately stops the flow of mail. Contamination is limited to the sorting area inside the postal facility. Postal employees will be required to remove clothing before leaving the site. Public health officials and responders will ensure that employees go through a wet decontamination process before leaving the site. This will greatly reduce the number of spores on exposed skin and hair. Persons living or working in the area around the postal facility are not considered at risk. However, the local health department will conduct surface and air sampling in the area immediately following an alarm.

However, let us look at the concept of operations the USPS will employ. If there is a presumptive positive BDS signal, the BDS will sound a visible and audible alarm, notify on site postal inspectors, and automatically shut down the mail sorting processes for the line where that automated facer canceller system is located (see Figure 13-4).

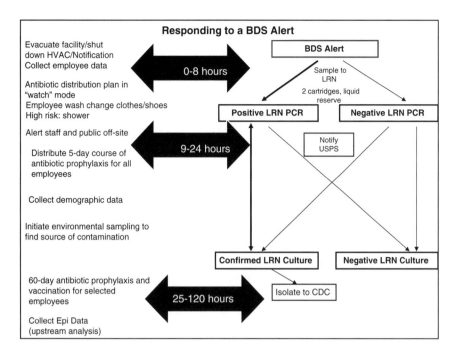

FIGURE 13-4 Some of the essential actions that take place under the BDS CONOPS at different time intervals and depending on the outcome of LRN testing. (Image courtesy of Cepheid, Inc.)

Actions to Protect Personnel and Minimize Exposure

With respect to personnel and actions taken within the first eight hours, the intent is to relocate, enumerate, aggregate, decontaminate, and educate. Immediately on the sounding of the alarm, all personnel evacuate the facility and relocate to a predesignated location. Managers then account for all their employees. All employees aggregate for a briefing and are notified why they have evacuated the building (actual alarm, test, drill, exercise) and what procedures will follow. Workers need to place their outer garments into a plastic bag. They then are directed into a decontamination shelter, where they wash exposed skin with soap and water. They are given a towel to dry off. The towel is placed inside the same plastic bag. They then are given temporary clothing and footwear to don. Postal workers are given a fact sheet on anthrax and issued a supply plan for antibiotic distribution (if needed). They also are directed to shower at home.

The Facility, Notifications, and the Sample

The facility is completely shut down, including the HVAC system, and the building(s) are secured to prevent unauthorized personnel from entry. The BDS alarm should also trigger a number of immediate notifications. The U.S. Postal Inspection Service has a special BDS unit. That unit should be notified immediately. Other stakeholders include local law enforcement, the state health department, hazmat team, and whatever officials and agencies are predesignated by community emergency operations plans. The incident commander must jointly coordinate with USPS, public health, and law enforcement to communicate on facility issues. The governor's office or state public health should communicate with the public at large. The USPS communicates with employees who went home and may not have participated in the post-alarm actions. Following notifications, specially trained postal inspectors prepare to make an entry into the building. The inspectors are in the appropriate protective posture to prevent them from being contaminated by any aerosolized agent. The GeneXpert cartridge containing the presumptive positive sample must be retrieved from the BDS unit. This cartridge is located in a special area within the BDS cabinet that holds archived samples. A chain of custody form is initiated and the cartridge is then placed inside a special biosafety container and handed off to another inspector. Samples are driven or flown to an LRN laboratory by postal inspectors or state police.

Role of the LRN

When the BDS triggers inside a postal facility, postal inspectors need to notify the LRN state reference laboratory that incoming samples are forthcoming. Following transfer of the sample from the USPS to the LRN, the sample buffer remaining inside the spent cartridge must be removed and processed for DNA extraction. This takes about three hours to perform. The sample is then tested using LRN-approved protocols real-time PCR detection of *Bacillus anthracis*. This testing also takes approximately three hours to perform. A portion of the original sample is used to inoculate a culture in an attempt to grow *B. anthracis* colonies. Culturing normally takes more than 24 hours to accomplish. Positive results for PCR and culture have further implications for personnel that were inside the facility at or just before the time when the BDS alarm sounded. Exposed individuals are given three to five days of antibiotics if the LRN test of initial sample via PCR is positive. In this instance, USPS officials contact employees and business visitors to come to a clinic on a staggered schedule to receive antibiotics within 24 hours. The local department of public health will notify potentially exposed public through public service announcements. If cultures are positive, exposed personnel should be directed to return within 60 hours of the alarm to receive enough antibiotics to complete a 30-day regimen. They should also be offered their first dose of anthrax vaccine. The second dose of vaccine should be offered at end of week 2. Exposed personnel should return in 30 days to receive 30 additional days of antibiotics, plus a third dose of vaccine. Note that, if the candidate vaccine for anthrax is under investigational new drug restrictions, these mass prophylaxis procedures are complicated by a consenting process, as required by the FDA. This adds considerable complexity and time to the process.

Coordination Is the Key to a Functional CONOPS

To ensure the functionality of the BDS CONOPS, it is essential for USPS officials to conduct periodic "service talks" with their employees. The talks are designed to inform the employees on the capabilities of the BDS and the postalarm activities. Local public health departments collocated with BDS-serviced postal facilities should develop a good working relationship with USPS plant management and integrate themselves into the CONOPS to facilitate future interactions. Periodically, all parties should conduct simulated evacuation drills aimed at dealing with personnel accountability issues and decontamination procedures, and to conduct some public education about anthrax as a disease and the antibiotics and vaccine that may be used to counter the threat.

Conclusion

The Amerithrax incident was a wake-up call for government officials and the American public. It demonstrated to us how vulnerable we all are to the threat of terrorism. This threat applies to the average citizen and is extended to the employees of the U.S. Postal Service. Amerithrax nearly brought the postal system to its knees. Clearly, a solution was needed to protect workers and ensure the safety and integrity of the U.S. mail. The commercial sector worked quickly and efficiently to build the solution that the USPS needed. Autonomous detection systems are built from impressive and intricate technologies. These systems enable us to monitor the environment for a potential attack from a bioterrorist. The biohazard hazard detection system is a perfect example of a model system. It is intended to take advantage of exposure surveillance compared to disease surveillance, which reduces the time for detecting a bioterrorist attack, thereby reducing the risk of disease through postexposure prophylaxis. Consequence management and CONOPS are important, well-thought-out programs aimed at taking advantage of these systems to the fullest extent possible. Other organizations are looking to take advantage of ADS technologies. However, the cost is high and the question will always be, When you get a positive, what are you going to do about it?

Essential Terminology

- **Consequence management.** The embodiment of measures designed to protect public health and safety, restore essential government services, and provide emergency relief to governments, businesses, and individuals affected by the consequences of disaster.

- **Autonomous detection system (ADS).** A comprehensive effort to combine numerous state-of-the-art technologies to achieve automated method for environmental sampling and on-site testing. The system involves no human intervention for routine functioning and alerts the user when a positive signal is generated.

- **Biohazard detection system (BDS).** A state-of-the-art system that automatically samples the air above lines that process mail inside USPS facilities. The system incorporates an air collection device, which mixes the air sample with a buffer solution. The buffer solution is automatically injected into a cartridge that is fed into a biosensor unit. The biosensor then performs real-time PCR on the sample and renders a result in about 30 minutes. If the sample tests positive for *Bacillus anthracis*, the system sounds an alarm and automatically shuts down the mail processing line. The BDS is a product of Northrop Grumman.

- **Concept of operations (CONOPS).** A plan for taking action in the midst of a crisis situation. The plan, as it applies to a positive BDS signal, involves actions designed to protect the workforce and the public. Furthermore, it establishes procedures aimed at retrieving the sample from the BDS and speeding it to an LRN facility for definitive testing. The BDS CONOPS establishes follow-up procedures that are triggered by LRN test results.

Discussion Questions

- How do the CONOP measures for the BDS compare to the recommendations of Meehan and colleagues (2004), previously outlined in the section on autonomous detection systems?
- How do the actions outlined in the CONOPS section of this chapter fall into line with RAIN?
- What are the benefits and features of having an ADS installed? What are the liabilities?

Web Site

USPS Biohazard Detection System Site, available at www.nalc.org/depart/safety/USPSBDS.html.

References

Becker, A. 2004. Postal service urged to hone plans for coping with anthrax. [University of Minnesota]. *Center for Infectious Disease Research and Policy News* (September 15).

Department of Homeland Security, NRP. 2004. *Biological Incident Annex.*

Farazmand, Ali, ed. 2001. *Handbook of Crisis and Emerency Management.* New York and Basel: Marcel Dekker.

Federal Emergency Management Agency. 2001. *The Disaster Dictionary—Common Terms and Definitions Used in Disaster Operations.* No. 9071.1-JA Job Aid. Washington, DC: FEMA, May.

Fitch, J. P., E. Raber, and D. R. Imbro. 2003. Technology challenges in responding to biological or chemical attacks in the civilian sector. *Science* 302:1350–1354.

Jarvis, K., and K. Chegwidden. 2006. Experience to date with biohazard detection system (BDS) at USPS. American Society for Microbiology annual conference, Poster 292.

Meehan, P., N. Rosenstein, M. Gillen, R. Meyer, M. Kiefer, S. Deitchman, R. Besser, R. Ehrenberg, K. Edwards, and K. Martinez. 2004. Responding to detection of aerosolized *Bacillus anthracis* by autonomous detection systems in the workplace. *Morbidity and Mortality Weekly Report* 53:1–11.

Office of Science and Technology Policy. 2002. *Review of the United States Postal Service's (USPS) Biohazard Detection Systems (BDS) Pilot Project.* Report of the Intra-Agency Working Group, November 25.

Ryan, J., and W. McMillan. 2003. *Biothreat.* Sunnyvale, CA: Cepheid, Inc.

Seiple, C. 1997. Consequence management: Domestic response to weapons of mass destruction. *Parameters* (Autumn) 119–134.

Thompson, M. 2003. *Killer Strain: Anthrax and a Government Exposed.* Collingdale, PA: DIANE Pub Co.

U.S. General Accounting Office. 2003a. *U.S. Postal Service: Better Guidance Is Needed to Improve Communication Should Anthrax Contamination Occur in the Future.* No. GAO-03-31. Washington, DC: General Accounting Office.

U.S. General Accounting Office. 2003b. *Bioterrorism: Public Health Response to Anthrax Incidents of 2001.* No. GAO-04-152. Washington, DC: General Accounting Office.

14

Future Directions for Biosecurity

Nothing in life is to be feared. It is only to be understood.
—Marie Curie

Objectives

The study of this chapter will enable you to

1. Discuss how the future of biosecurity relates to advancements in biotechnology.
2. List and describe scientific methods that may lead to the advancement of more deadly bioweapons.
3. Discuss new strategies for prevention, preparedness, and containment.

Key Terms

Binary bioweapons, designer genes, gene therapy, stealth viruses, host-swapping diseases, designer diseases.

Introduction

Biosecurity has become an essential element of national security for many developed countries. Sophisticated biodefense programs have grown beyond protecting deployed military forces and have become part of homeland defense. The importance of agriculture and the threat of emerging diseases have given rise to the emergence of biosecurity systems and containment strategies that serve to protect crops, livestock, and human populations from the threat of foreign disease agents. These systems and containment strategies have taken years to develop and are likely to become more comprehensive and prominent as the future unfolds.

When looking back on the topic of biosecurity, we appreciate that many of the concerns we had came from the possibility that harmful biological agents had fallen into the wrong hands. Indeed, the technological advances in biowarfare from the Cold War era have already been used against us (Miller et al., 2002). The recent experience with anthrax-laced letters is indicative of this, but what does that portend? Might there be a more spectacular event in our near future? We, the authors, believe that the future of biosecurity will be dictated by advances in dual-use research and limited outbreaks due to emerging and reemerging disease threats.

Looking toward the future, it is clear that, as the power of biological science and technology continues to grow, it will become increasingly possible that we may face an attack with a pathogen that has been deliberately engineered for increased virulence. This enhanced virulence could take the form of resistance to antibiotic drugs, increased infectiousness (pathogenicity), or a new virulent pathogen made by combining genes from more than one organism. Threats arising from deliberate human action are not the only dangers we confront, because naturally occurring infectious diseases emerge or reemerge on a regular basis (Garrett, 1995). A current example of this is the emergence of *bird flu* due to H5N1 avian influenza virus (see Figure 14-1). The pathogen emerged in 1997 and, in a 10-year period, was responsible for the culling of nearly 300 million birds and more than 200 associated human deaths. The disease emerged in Hong Kong but, in the course of 10 years, spread across Asia, into Africa and Europe. Most human deaths reported have come from Cambodia, Indonesia, Thailand, and Vietnam. There have been two likely small clusters of human-to-human transmission of the H5N1 virus, and it is possible that other such transmissions have occurred. It is also possible that the H5N1 virus, through genetic mutation or recombination with a human-adapted influenza virus, could become easily transmissible among people. Given the poor condition of public health systems in

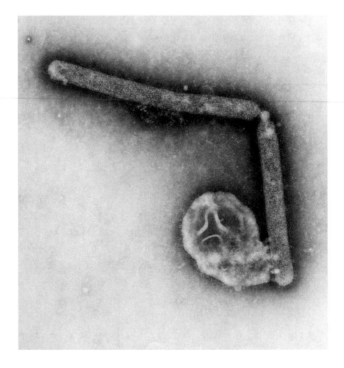

FIGURE 14-1 This transmission electron micrograph, taken at a magnification of 108,000 times, reveals the structural details of two avian influenza A (H5N1) virions, a type of bird flu virus, which is a subtype of avian influenza A. At this magnification, one may note the stippled appearance of the roughened surface of the proteinaceous coat encasing each virion. Although this virus does not typically infect humans, in 1997, the first instance of direct bird-to-human spread of influenza A (H5N1) virus was documented during an outbreak of avian influenza among poultry in Hong Kong. The virus caused severe respiratory illness in 18 people, of whom, 6 died. Since that time, there have been outbreaks in numerous countries, which have resulted in the culling of nearly 300 million birds and more than 200 associated human deaths. Public health officials fear that a mutation in this virus may lead to one that is transmissible from human to human, potentially sparking the next influenza pandemic. (Image courtesy of the Centers for Disease Control; Cynthia Goldsmith and Jackie Katz.)

many underdeveloped regions and the speed of modern air travel, the consequences of such an event would be severe. However, biosecurity programs sponsored by the World Health Organization and its partners, including the Centers for Disease Control and Prevention, have managed to bring sufficient attention and resources to the problem that a pandemic may have been averted. When public health strategies and biosecurity programs are successful, it is hard to know just how far the problem may have gone without intervention. Certainly, the world did not benefit from such programs, modern day technologies, containment strategies, and surveillance infrastructure when the 1918 Spanish flu circled the globe, leaving an estimated 40 million people dead in its wake.

With respect to dual-use research, genetic engineering is becoming routine and commonplace. Molecular genetics, genomic sequencing, and gene splicing therapies have dual-use potential. Paradoxically, the same biotechnology for developing a new drug or new vaccine may be used to develop more virulent biological weapons. As such, science that can be used to save lives may also be used to take lives (Ainscough, 2002). An outbreak of a biologically engineered pathogen might have greater disease potential than recently discovered naturally emerging diseases. A terrorist attack with a biologically engineered agent may unfold unlike any previous event. The pathogen may be released covertly, so there will be a delay between exposure and onset of symptoms. Days to weeks later, when people do develop symptoms, they could immediately start spreading contagious diseases. By that time, many people will likely be hundreds of miles away from where they were originally exposed, possibly at multiple international sites. Acutely ill victims may present themselves in large numbers to emergency rooms and other medical treatment facilities (Ainscough, 2002).

□ □ □ ▬▬▬▬▬▬▬▬▬▬▬▬▬▬▬▬▬▬▬▬▬▬▬

Michael Ainscough on Future Wars

The 20th century was dominated by physics, but recent breakthroughs indicate that the next 100 years likely will be "the Biological Century." There are those who say: "the First World War was chemical; the Second World War was nuclear; and that the Third World War—God forbid—will be biological.
—Michael J. Ainscough

▬▬▬▬▬▬▬▬▬▬▬▬▬▬▬▬▬▬▬▬▬▬▬ □ □ □

In 1960, the U.S. government formed a secret group of academic scientists, the Jason Group, to advise senior officials and help them find solutions to particularly difficult technical problems, mostly having to do with defense (Finkbeiner, 2006). In 1997, this group addressed the problem of next-generation bioweapons threats (Block, 1999). The report they produced explored a wide range of possibilities open to genetically engineered pathogens, including some that could be achieved with current state-of-the-art techniques and others that would be realized in the near future. The prospects for future bioweaponry advanced by technology are quite sobering (Block, 1999). In fact, technology over the past 20 years enabled scientists to engineer pathogens to be qualitatively different from conventional bioweapon agents. In terms of bioweaponry, this includes the ability to give these "classic" pathogens attributes that might make them safer to handle, more virulent, more transmissible, harder to detect, and easier to disseminate (Block, 1999).

In their 1997 report, several broad classes of unconventional pathogens were identified by the Jason Group (Block, 1999). These include **binary bioweapons**, which are two-component systems, relatively safe to handle but becoming deadly when the two components come together on deployment. The same technology has been employed with chemical weapon systems. The Jason Group also postulated the existence of **designer genes**, whereby specific unnatural gene sequences are built into viruses or other life forms to incorporate into the genome of the unsuspecting host, which later becomes the victim. On a similar note, they suggested that, once **gene therapy** becomes a medical reality, the technology that should one day allow medicine to repair or replace defective genes in a diseased individual might be subverted to introduce pathogenic sequences into healthy individuals. In addition, **stealth viruses** could be fashioned by a researcher to infect the host but remain silent, until activated by some physiological or environmental trigger. New zoonotic agents, referred to by Jason as **host-swapping diseases**, might be developed specifically for bioweapon purposes by modifying existing pathogens to seek human hosts. Finally, detailed knowledge of biochemical signaling pathways could conceivably be used to create **designer diseases.**

Soviet Superbugs

These possibilities, for the most part, were actually stark realities of what some bioweapons experts refer to as the Soviet Superbug program. As discussed in Chapter 1, while the United States and her allies were dismantling their bioweapons programs in the 1970s, the Soviets, under *Biopreparat*, were assembling a huge bioweapons production capacity, comprising dozens of production facilities and as many as 60,000 personnel. This massive program aimed to build offensive capabilities by mass producing many of the Categories A and B agents. More important, the Soviet bioweapons program also created research institutions with top secret goals and objectives to employ biotechnology toward creating pathogens and toxins with superior capability. As we know now, the Soviets were producing *Bacillus anthracis* spores by the ton. We know that Soviet strains of *B. anthracis* were engineered to carry a form of antibiotic resistance; however, we did not know whether the NATO conventional anthrax vaccine was effective against all Soviet variants. Ken Alibek, a former high-ranking official in the Soviet bioweapons program, testified in 1998 before the United States Congress (Alibek, 1998). Here is a chilling excerpt of what he had to say:

> It is important to note that, in the Soviet's view, the best biological agents were those for which there was no prevention and no cure. For those agents for which vaccines or treatment existed—such as plague, which can be treated with antibiotics—antibiotic-resistant or immunosuppressive variants were to be developed.

Another famed Soviet bioweapons expert and researcher, Dr. Sergei Popov, was interviewed by a journalist from the public television show NOVA. (An excerpt from the interview, entitled "Creating 'Superbugs'" can be accessed on the Internet; see NOVA, 2001.) In the interview, Popov admitted that the Soviets were producing synthetic genes to give microbes properties that they did not possess in nature. When Popov was asked by the interviewer, "What would be the point of that?" he replied, "Imagine a new weapon which is difficult to diagnose initially and then which is impossible to treat with conventional antibiotics." Popov explained that "the idea was that a new weapon has to have new and unusual properties, difficult to recognize, difficult to treat." By his own admonition, the goal of his research program was to create a more deadly biological weapon. He briefly described the goal of Project Bonfire, which dealt with the creation and potential exploitation of antibiotic-resistant strains of bacteria. Under Project Bonfire, the Soviets were able to produce a strain of *Yersinia pestis* that was shown to be resistant to almost 10 antibiotics. And a recombinant strain of anthrax had resistance to 10 antibiotics. In the Hunter Program, Popov explained that whole genomes of different viruses were being combined together to produce completely new hybrid viruses. They wanted to combine two microorganisms in one, say, a combination of encephalomyelitis virus and smallpox. Purportedly, this completely artificial agent would manifest as illness with new symptoms, probably with no known way to treat it. And, what would be the purpose and danger of this, one might ask. In Popov's own words,

> *Essentially, the major feature would be a kind of surprise effect. Nobody would recognize it. Nobody would know how to deal with it. But nobody could predict the result of that kind of genetic manipulation.*

As for the term *Superbug*, how does this exactly work? The concept sounds reminiscent of the legend of the Trojan horse. Popov explained the idea was to create a bacterial agent that harbored a virus. The virus would remain silent until the bacterial infection is treated. So, if the bacterial disease was recognized and treated with an antibiotic, there would be a release of virus. After the initial bacterial disease was completely cured, there would be an outbreak of a viral disease on top of this. According to Popov, a good example of this Superbug model would be plague bacteria, which is relatively easy to treat with antibiotics, and viral encephalomyelitis inside. So, in case of biological attack, people would be treated against plague, and after that, the weakened host would manifest with a highly fatal infection affecting the brain and central nervous system. Remember that the encephalitides are normally transmitted by arthropod vectors, making them unlikely candidates and impractical for biowarfare. In the Superbug model, the need for a vector is eliminated. Regardless, imagine the insidious nature of this scenario and the resultant fear, panic, social disruption, medical management issues, and implications for public health.

□ □ □ ▬▬▬▬▬▬▬▬▬▬▬▬▬▬▬▬▬▬▬▬▬▬▬▬▬▬

Critical Thinking

Biotechnology today is capable of most of the possibilities about which the Jason Group warned us. Some genetically engineered agents may have already been produced and stockpiled by bioweapons experts in the former Soviet Union. Consider these scenarios or possibilities:

- What if an agent could be developed that specifically targeted one or another population group? Or, what if some group could be protected against infection in advance?

- What if one could engineer a viral disease with the lethality of a hemorrhagic fever virus but the communicability of influenza?

- What if a highly lethal disease like smallpox was hard to diagnose because it did not form pustules?
- What if a pathogen was designed to give a false negative result on a gold standard diagnostic assay?
- What if a highly lethal pathogen with a short incubation period had never even been encountered before? How long would it take public health officials to develop a new diagnostic test and write a case definition?
- What if some pathogen could produce a localized outbreak then render itself harmless? Conversely, what if a pathogen could continually alter itself in such a way as to evade treatment?

The Dark Specter of Terrorism

It is perfectly clear to us now just how massive the Soviet bioweapons program was. Following the leadership of Gorbachev and Yeltsin, bioweapons war stocks of the former Soviet Union were destroyed; much of it at one of the most remote spots on earth, an arid island in the Aral Sea, which was formerly known to be the world's largest biological-warfare testing ground, Vozrozhdeniye Island. So, what remains of the former Soviet arsenal and where are all the seed stocks from the bioengineering efforts of Project Bonfire and the Hunter Program? Have deadly Superbugs been sequestered for dark days ahead? Further, what other countries have had and remain actively engaged in bioweapons production and research? The Office of the Secretary of Defense identified countries that maintain various levels of offensive biological warfare capabilities or research facilities. China, Iran, Israel, Libya, North Korea, Syria, and Taiwan are believed to have produced operational quantities of biological weapons (U.S. Congress, Office of Technology Assessment, 1993). The Henry L. Stimson Center also identified Egypt, Israel, and Taiwan as countries of proliferation concern (Block, 1999). The al Qaeda network is reported to have sought to purchase biological agents, and some on-site reports suggest that their rudimentary laboratory facility at Tarnak Farm, Afghanistan, was being set up for biological and chemical agent production.

The technology required to mass produce biological agents (e.g., yeast, bacteria, and viruses) is relatively inexpensive. Beer, cosmetics, pharmaceuticals, and vaccine production facilities alike use much of the same equipment, making it relatively easy to acquire. If there is any doubt about this, explore the possibility of setting up your own laboratory by shopping online with one of the Internet auctioneers to see how readily available and inexpensive laboratory equipment and fermentation chambers are. Most microbial agents needed for biological weapons may be naturally sourced. "It is difficult to gauge the extent of biological weapons development in other nations since production facilities require little space and are not easy to identify. The acquisition and dissemination of even the most highly restricted organism, *Variola major*, is not an implausible scenario" (Inglesby, O'Toole, and Henderson, 2000).

In the age of terrorism, our adversaries no longer wear uniforms and fight us on a battlefield with clearly defined boundaries and objectives. The threat is now asymmetric, and as such, biological weapons will always be an option. Belligerents, allured by the potentially deadly power of weapons of mass destruction, strive to acquire them (Ainscough, 2002). Yet, when biological weapons have been employed in battle, they have proven relatively ineffective. They have been undependable and uncontrollable (Zilinskas, 2000). Because they have been difficult to deploy reliably, their military value has been marginal. Stabilizing biological agents and deploying them, either overtly with sophisticated weaponry or covertly without endangering the perpetrator or friendly forces, requires expertise not widely held (Ainscough, 2002). Possibly, with the capabilities of biological engineering and a new generation of weapons, this may change.

Critical Thinking: Possible Future Bioweapons Scenarios

Dr. Jim Davis (2002) stated that the three most likely bioweapons scenarios that the United States and its allies might face in the future are the following:

- An agroterrorist event against the United States.
- A bioweapons attack on U.S. and allied troops in the Middle East.
- A bioterrorist attack against a large population center in the United States or an allied state.

Based on what you know now and the current world situation, are these three possibilities still valid? What has changed since 2002 to make these three scenarios more or less likely?

Well-developed militaries are trained and equipped to operate in chemical and biological environments. Vulnerable civilian populations have neither the protective equipment or defensive training and are therefore totally unprepared for a biological attack. Naturally, these civilian populations are the most likely "soft" target for a bioterrorist objective. According to Sprinzak (2001), the "megalomaniacal hyperterrorists" of the modern era are innovative and resourceful. They are always looking for ways to surprise and devastate the enemy. They think big, seeking to go beyond "conventional" terrorism, and unlike most terrorists, could be willing to use weapons of mass destruction. If the intent of terrorists is to inflict mass casualties, then biological agents are likely to be used (Ainscough, 2002).

Biological Warfare

Nuclear warfare threat has been one of the main driving forces for cultural, political, economical and social changes in the late twentieth century. Biological warfare threat is about to take over. However, while nuclear warfare was a concrete possibility, biological warfare is just an elusive risk.
—Emilio Mordini, 2005

Bioweapons counterproliferation expert Dr. Jim Davis stated there are at least six reasons why senior officials and skeptics believe a significant bioweapons attack will not occur (Davis, 2002). These reasons, which he characterizes as myths and false assumptions, are as follows:

Myth 1. There never really has been a significant bioweapons attack. Counter: From our readings in Chapter 1, we know this is not true.

Myth 2. The United States has never been attacked by a bioweapons agent. Counter: Consider Amerithrax and the Rajneeshee incident as significant bioweapons attacks on U.S. soil.

Myth 3. You have to be extremely intelligent, highly educated, and well funded to grow, weaponize, and deploy a bioweapons agent. Counter: If you can source the agent and know something about fermentation processes, you can make a crude but effective agent concoction. Terrorist groups with relatively few resources and a lot of "want to" could manage to pull together a bioweapons attack. In addition, a small group with connections may be able to procure a small amount of formulated material, which may be enough to introduce a disease with a high degree of person-to-person transmissibility.

Myth 4. Biological warfare must be too difficult because, when it has been tried, it has failed. Counter: Certainly, there are those that would argue Aum Shinrikyo's blunder with anthrax is an indication that well-funded terrorism is no guarantee for success. On many fronts, evil doing is not easy. However, that is no guarantee that subsequent attempts would not be successful. It only takes one successful attempt to make the point that it is easier to prepare for bioterrorism than to explain the lack of preparation after an attack.

Myth 5. There are moral restraints that have and will keep bioweapons agents from being used. Counter: If a terrorist can fly a jumbo jet into a high-rise office building filled with thousands of innocent people, there really are no moral boundaries when it comes to terrorism.

Myth 6. The long incubation period required for bioweapons agents before onset of symptoms makes bioweapons useless to users. Counter: Do not make the mistake of questioning the motives or means of a terrorist. A long incubation period may work to someone's advantage, especially if the act is covert and the perpetrator is looking to disseminate the agent along a broad front or from numerous points of release to make containment more difficult.

New Strategies for Prevention, Preparedness, and Containment

Hospitals will bear the brunt of caring for the sick and dying should a biological weapon be used. Yet few hospitals are prepared to cope with even a handful of cases of a highly contagious, life-threatening disease; and few hospitals are prepared to manage even a modest surge in the numbers of seriously ill patients. Hospital leaders should examine current policies in relation to this threat and develop new policies as appropriate. Infection control practices are but one critical component of such planning efforts (Inglesby et al., 2000). As previously discussed in Chapters 6 and 11, response organizations and community officials have increased their awareness to this threat, but it remains one of the least understood. Much more effort along these lines to heighten awareness and bolster surveillance is needed. We cannot allow this relative period of quiescence following Amerithrax to lull us into a state of ill preparedness.

Homeland Security Presidential Directive 18, released in early 2007, outlines strategies for medical countermeasure research, development, and acquisition, and frames the spectrum of biological threats in four distinct categories:

- **Traditional agents.** Naturally occurring microorganisms or toxin products with the potential to be disseminated to cause mass casualties. Examples include *Bacillus anthracis* (anthrax) and *Yersinia pestis* (plague).

- **Enhanced agents.** Traditional agents that have been modified or selected to enhance their ability to harm human populations or circumvent available countermeasures. An example is drug-resistant pathogens such as extensively drug-resistant TB (see Figure 14-2) or multidrug-resistant plague.

- **Emerging agents.** Previously unrecognized pathogens that might be naturally occurring and present a serious risk to human populations. Tools to detect and treat these agents might not exist or be widely available. An example is severe acute respiratory syndrome (SARS) or "bird flu" (avian influenza).

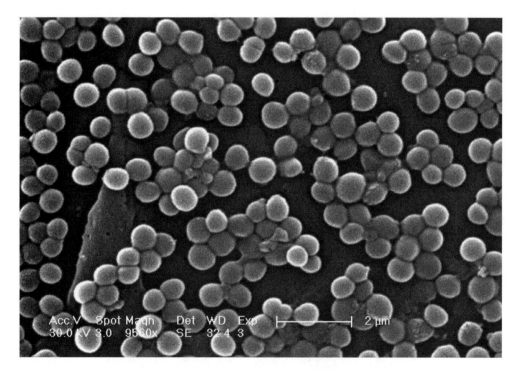

FIGURE 14-2 This scanning electron micrograph depicts numerous clumps of methicillin-resistant *Staphylococcus aureus* bacteria, commonly referred to as MRSA, magnified 9,560 times. Recently recognized outbreaks, or clusters, of MRSA in community settings have been associated with strains that have some unique microbiologic and genetic properties, compared with the traditional hospital-based MRSA strains, which suggests some biologic properties, such as virulence factors like toxins, may allow the community strains to spread more easily or cause more skin disease. Antibiotic-resistant bacteria, such as MRSA, and drug resistant strains of *Mycobacterium tuberculosis* (the etiologic agent of TB), will become increasingly important in public health and infection control settings. There is also the potential that they may be exploited due to the difficulty of control. (Image courtesy of the Centers for Disease Control Public Health Image Library. Photomicrograph by Janice Haney Carr and Jeff Hageman.)

- **Advanced agents.** Novel pathogens or other biological materials that have been artificially engineered in the laboratory to bypass traditional countermeasures or produce a more severe or otherwise enhanced spectrum of disease. An example is multidrug-resistant anthrax.

These designations expand on the traditional classifications of Category A, B, and C agents, because they address the fact that future threats are likely to be unanticipated and ill defined. While appropriate and effective for the highest priority traditional threats, such as smallpox and anthrax, developing medical countermeasures using a conventional "one bug–one drug" approach will rapidly prove unsustainable as the list of threats increases to include enhanced, emerging, and advanced agents. Responding to traditional and new types of threats requires the capability to rapidly identify unknown or poorly defined agents, quickly evaluate the efficacy of available interventions, and develop and deploy novel treatments to prevent or mitigate medical consequences and the subsequent impact on society. Certainly, the importance of the LRN and the establishment of regional centers of excellence for biodefense and emerging infectious diseases have been realized (see Figure 14-3). Maintaining this vital capability to guide recognition of the threat is costly but essential.

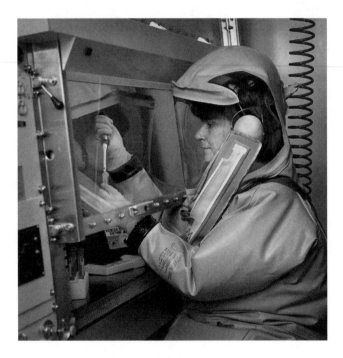

FIGURE 14-3 A scientist in the process of transferring specimens in one of the CDC biosafety level-4 laboratories, located in Atlanta, Georgia. The scientist wears a protective airtight suit equipped with a helmet and face mask. She is seated at a negatively pressurized laminar flow hood that allows no air flow to escape back into the lab environment. Using this negatively pressurized, hooded environment, any airborne pathogens or toxic vapors are drawn back into the hooded container and up into a filtered ventilation system, thereby, avoiding the spread of contaminants through the laboratory. Although these facilities are very costly to staff and maintain, they are vital and give us the ability to investigate unknown threats and emerging diseases. Regional centers of excellence have given the United States biosafety level-4 capacity. (Image courtesy of the CDC, Public Health Image Library.)

The Future of Biodefense Research

Scientific research will be needed to identify new diagnoses, prevention, or treatment for infectious disease. Commensurate with this, the infectious diseases community might elect to encourage and reward basic science research efforts that seek to produce novel diagnostic technologies, preventive, or therapeutic interventions for the diseases caused by biological weapons. That agenda was outlined by Dr. Anthony Fauci, director of the National Institutes of Health (Fauci, 2005).

Developing medical countermeasures against a finite number of known or antici-pated agents is a sound approach for mitigating the most catastrophic biological threats. Responding to enhanced, emerging, and advanced agents, however, demands new para-digms, which allow for more rapid and cost-effective development of countermeasures. The National Institutes of Health, in collaboration with other agencies, established a solid framework of research and product development resources for biodefense. The pro-gram outlined in 2007 calls for new approaches to provide the flexibility required to meet the challenges of nontraditional threats. The National Institute for Allergy (2007) and Infectious Diseases identified three "broad-spectrum" strategies to create a more responsive biodefense capability (see Figure 14-4). These strategies are described next.

Broad-Spectrum Activity

Broad-spectrum activity is a characteristic that enables a particular product to mitigate biological threats across a wide range or class of agents. Multiplex diagnostics possessing broad-spectrum activity rapidly differentiate a variety of common and lesser-known pathogens in a single clinical sample, identify drug sensitivities, and determine how a sample pathogen is related to known pathogens. Consider the lab-on-a-chip concept, whereby a clinical specimen is placed on a microchip-like device, which has a complex microarray of DNA- or RNA-based diagnostics. The chip allows the processing unit to test for dozens of possibilities simultaneously based on DNA- or RNA-hybridization modalities. Some exciting new developments along these lines have occurred already.

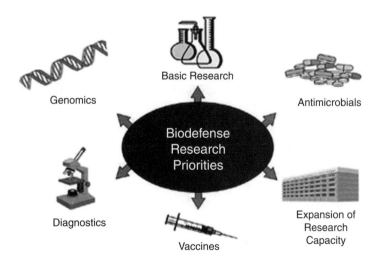

FIGURE 14-4 Priorities for biodefense research, as established by the National Institutes of Health director, Dr. Anthony S. Fauci.

Vaccines demonstrating broad-spectrum activity include cross-protective and multiple-component vaccines. Cross-protective vaccines induce an immune response against constant components of a microbe and, therefore, are effective against pathogens that evolve or "drift" naturally or deliberately. A universal influenza vaccine is an example of a cross-protective vaccine. Multiple-component vaccines include, within a single vaccine, elements that protect against viruses or microbes that are different but usually closely related. An example of a multiple-component vaccine is a hemorrhagic fever vaccine that contains elements of Ebola, Marburg, and Lassa viruses.

For a number of traditional threats, safe and effective treatments are either nonexistent, of limited usefulness, or susceptible to emerging antimicrobial resistance and genetically engineered threats. A limited number of antiinfectives with broad-spectrum activity directed at common, invariable, and essential components of different classes of microbes could be effective against both traditional and nontraditional threats. This approach would allow a small number of drugs to replace dozens of pathogen-specific drugs. Additionally, the strategies to overcome antibacterial resistance could extend the clinical utility of existing broad-spectrum antiinfectives and have immediate benefits. Treatments that target host immune responses have the potential to be effective against multiple diseases. These immune modulators reduce morbidity and mortality by controlling responses that contribute to disease (e.g., cytokine storms) or nonspecifically activating the host's natural immune defenses to induce a faster, more potent protective response.

Broad-Spectrum Technology

Broad-spectrum technology refers to capabilities, such as temperature stabilization or delivery method, that can be engineered into a wide array of existing and candidate products. Developing countermeasures that will be useful in responding to future threats represents a major challenge, given the capabilities that these products must possess. They should be safe and effective against multiple pathogens in people of any age and health status. To be appropriate for storing in the strategic national stockpile, the products should be suitable for long-term storage at room temperature, have simple compact packaging, be easily delivered in a mass casualty setting, confer protection with limited dosing, and have single dose delivery devices that can be self-administered. Added to these factors is the potential need to produce additional quantities with little notice, requiring manufacturers to take the costly step of keeping production facilities on standby. A recent example of this is the relatively rapid creation and production of a vaccine for H5N1 "bird flu," which is already FDA approved with 5 million doses placed in the strategic national stockpile.

Broad-Spectrum Platforms

Broad-spectrum platforms are standardized methods that can be used to significantly reduce the time and cost required to bring medical countermeasures to market. For example, a proven monoclonal antibody fermentation and purification method can be applied to rapidly develop any therapeutic monoclonal antibody, avoiding lengthy development work. Other examples of platform technologies include screening systems, in-vitro safety testing, expression modules, manufacturing technologies, and chemical synthesis designs. The potential to rapidly apply such platform methods to developing new countermeasures will considerably shorten and streamline the process.

Bioweapons and Scientists

The community of biologists in the United States has maintained a kind of hand-wringing silence on the ethics of creating bioweapons—a reluctance to talk about it with the public, even a disbelief that it's happening. Biological weapons are a disgrace to biology. The time has come for top biologists to assert their leadership and speak out, to take responsibility on behalf of their profession for the existence of these weapons and the means of protecting the population against them, just as leading physicists did a generation ago when nuclear weapons came along. Moral pressure costs nothing and can help; silence is unacceptable now.
—Richard Preston (1998)

Conclusion

It is clear that security and defense against biological threats, whether natural or the result of deliberate human action will continue to be a high priority for the foreseeable future. Biological warfare and bioterrorism are multifaceted problems requiring multifaceted solutions (Block, 1999). We need our best critical thinkers and biological researchers to solve this constantly evolving problem. Fortunately, the same advances in genomic biotechnologies that can be used to create bioweapons can also be used to set up countermeasures against them. The probability of a terrorist use of a genetically engineered biological agent on a given city is very low, but the consequence of such an event would obviously be very high. With maximum casualties the likely goals, metropolitan areas are most at risk for an attack. However, the indiscriminate nature of biological warfare and bioterrorism puts all communities at risk. This dilemma is the challenge of local communities, which are sensitive to the need for preparedness but have finite resources. Community officials must have a plan and sufficient medical and public health resources accessible to sustain a response for up to 24 hours. Robust federal assistance would be made available promptly, but it would not be immediate. At present, all military and civilian populations throughout the world are vulnerable to a bioweapons attack. We remain grossly ill-prepared to respond to an epidemic caused by a novel genetically engineered biological agent.

President Nixon said it best when he stated, "Mankind already carries in its own hands too many of the seeds of its own destruction." We know that he was forewarning us that further advances in biowarfare and the production of bioweapons could ultimately end in our own demise. Acting responsibly, he put an end to our biological weapons arsenal and focused our assets on biodefense rather than biooffense. Currently, we have in place sophisticated and well-developed biosecurity and biodefense programs. These programs are essential to countering the asymmetric warfare threat, but they are costly and perishable. Future directions in biosecurity and biodefense may very well be determined by the "next event." However, it is our opinion that the most likely events are those that naturally and accidentally threaten human and animal health through the emergence of novel pathogens and the reemergence of others in light of new environmental or societal factors.

Essential Terminology

- **Binary bioweapons.** A two-component system consisting of innocuous parts that are mixed immediately prior to use to form the pathogen. This process occurs frequently in nature. Many pathogenic bacteria contain multiple plasmids (small circular extrachromosomal DNA fragments) that code for virulence or other special functions. Virulent plasmids can be transferred among different kinds of bacteria and often across species barriers (Block, 1999).

- **Designer diseases.** The possibility that science one day might allow a researcher to propose the symptoms of a hypothetical disease and then design or create the pathogen to produce the desired disease complex. Designer diseases may work by turning off the immune system, by inducing specific cells to multiply and divide rapidly (like cancer), or possibly by causing the opposite effect, such as initiating programmed cell death (apoptosis). This futuristic biotechnology would clearly indicate an order of magnitude of advancement in offensive biological warfare or terrorism capability (Block, 1999).

- **Designer genes.** The entire genomes of numerous organisms have been published in unclassified journals and on the Internet. Now that the codes are known, it seems only a matter of time until microbiologists develop synthetic genes, synthetic viruses, or even complete new organisms. Some of these could be specifically produced for biological warfare or terrorism purposes (Block, 1999).

- **Gene therapy as a weapon.** Gene therapy will revolutionize the treatment of human genetic diseases. The goal is to effect a permanent change in the genetic composition of a person by repairing or replacing a faulty gene. The same technology could be subverted to insert pathogenic genes in a targeted host of population (Block, 1999).

- **Stealth viruses.** The concept of a stealth virus is a cryptic viral infection that covertly enters human cells (genomes) then remains dormant for an extended time. However, a signal by an external stimulus could later trigger the virus to activate and cause disease. This mechanism, in fact, occurs fairly commonly in nature. For example, many humans carry herpes virus, which can activate to cause oral or genital lesions. Similarly, varicella virus sometimes reactivates in the form of herpes zoster (shingles) in some people who had chicken pox earlier in life. However, the vast majority of viruses do not cause disease (Block, 1999).

- **Host-swapping diseases.** Viruses that "jump species" may occasionally cause significant disease. Manageable infectious agents can be transformed naturally into organisms with markedly increased virulence (Block, 1999).

Discussion Questions

- What is the most likely reason for biosecurity programs to increase in scope and complexity?
- Is a major act of bioterrorism likely in the next five years? If not, what will that do to existing research programs and surveillance systems like BioWatch?
- Imagine that bioweapons programs come back into prominence and there is a renewed interest in creating "Superbugs" in sophisticated state-sponsored programs. How could technology today give a military advantage to a country?

• What would be the likely outcome if an adversary overtly used a biological weapon against its enemy? What sort of a response would the international community pursue? Might it provoke the use of a nuclear weapon?

Web Sites

Regional centers of excellence for biodefense and emerging infectious diseases (10 centers, located nationwide, provide resources and communication systems that can be rapidly mobilized and coordinated with regional and local systems in response to an urgent public health event), available at www.niaid.nih.gov/research/resources/rce.

National biocontainment laboratories (NBLs) and regional biocontainment laboratories (RBLs) (2 NBLs and 13 RBLs are available or under construction for research requiring high levels of containment and are prepared to assist national, state, and local public health efforts in the event of a bioterrorism or infectious disease emergency), available at www.niaid.nih.gov/topics/BiodefenseRelated/Biodefense/research/resources/NBL_RBL.

The Biodefense and Emerging Infections Research Resources Repository (offers reagents and information essential for studying emerging infectious diseases and biological threats), available at www.beiresources.org.

References

Ainscough, M. 2002. Next generation bioweapons: Genetic and BW. In: *The Gathering Biological Warfare Storm*, ed. J. Davis and B. Schneider, Chapter 9. Mongomery, AL: USAF Counterproliferation Center, Air War College, Air University, Maxwell Air Force Base.

Alibek, K. 1998. Terrorist and intelligence operations: Potential impact on the US economy. Statement before the Joint Economic Committee, U.S. Congress (May 20), available at www.house.gov/jec/hearings/intell/alibek.htm.

Block, S. 1999. Living nightmares: Biological threats enabled by molecular biology. In: *The New Terror: Facing the Threat of Biological and Chemical Weapons*, ed. S. Drell, A. Sofaer, and G. Wilson, p. 60. Stanford, CA: Hoover Institution Press.

Davis, J. 2002. A biological warfare wake-up call: Prevalent myths and likely scenarios. In: *The Gathering Biological Warfare Storm*, eds. J. Davis and B. Schneider, Chapter 10. Mongomery, AL: USAF Counterproliferation Center. Air War College, Air University, Maxwell Air Force Base.

Fauci, A. 2005. Testimony before the Committee on Homeland Security, Subcommittee on the Prevention of Nuclear and Biological Attack United States House of Representatives by the Director of the National Institute of Allergy and Infectious Diseases, National Institutes of Health, U.S. Department of Health and Human Services (July 28).

Finkbeiner, A. 2006. *The Jasons: The Secret History of Science's Postwar Elite*. New York: Viking Books.

Garrett, L. 1995. *The Coming Plague: Newly Emerging Diseases in a World Out of Balance*. New York: Farrar, Straus and Giroux.

Inglesby, T., T. O'Toole, and D. A. Henderson. 2000. Preventing the use of biological weapons: Improving response should prevention fail. *Clinical Infectious Diseases* 30:926–929.

Miller, J., S. Engelberg, and W. Broad. 2002. *Germs: Biological Weapons and America's Secret War*. New York: Simon and Schuster.

Mordini, E. 2005. Biowarfare as a biopolitical icon. *Poiesis and Praxis: International Journal of Technology Assessment and Ethics of Science* 3:242–255.

National Institute of Allergy and Infectious Diseases. 2007. *Strategic Plan for Biodefense Research, 2007 Update.* Washington, DC: U.S. Department of Health and Human Services, National Institutes of Health.

NOVA. 2001. Soviet "Superbugs," interview between NOVA and Sergei Popov, available at www.pbs.org/wgbh/nova/bioterror/biow_popov.html.

Preston, R. "Taming the Biological Beast." Op-Ed, New York Times, Apr. 21, 1998.

Sprinzak, E. 2001. The lone gunman. *Foreign Policy* (November–December):72–73.

U.S. Congress, Office of Technology Assessment. 1993. *Technologies Underlying Weapons of Mass Destruction.* OTA-BP-ISC-115. Washington, DC: Government Printing Office.

Zilinskas, R. 2000. *Biological Warfare: Modern Offense and Defense.* Boulder, CO: Lynne Rienner Publishers.

Index

Note: Page numbers followed by 'f' indicate figures 't' indicate tables.